Total Body PET Imaging

Editors

RAMSEY D. BADAWI
JOEL S. KARP
LORENZO NARDO
AUSTIN R. PANTEL

PET CLINICS

www.pet.theclinics.com

Consulting Editor
ABASS ALAVI

January 2021 • Volume 16 • Number 1

ELSEVIER

1600 John F. Kennedy Boulevard ● Suite 1800 ● Philadelphia, Pennsylvania, 19103-2899

http://www.pet.theclinics.com

PET CLINICS Volume 16, Number 1
January 2021 ISSN 1556-8598, ISBN-13: 978-0-323-76146-8

Editor: John Vassallo (j.vassallo@elsevier.com)
Developmental Editor: Casey Potter

PET Clinics (ISSN 1556-8598) is published quarterly by Elsevier Inc., 360 Park Avenue South, New York, NY 10010-1710. Months of issue are January, April, July, and October. Periodicals postage paid at New York, NY, and additional mailing offices. Subscription prices per year are $254.00 (US individuals), $501.00 (US institutions), $100.00 (US students), $282.00 (Canadian individuals), $514.00 (Canadian institutions), $100.00 (Canadian students), $275.00 (foreign individuals), $514.00 (foreign institutions), and $140.00 (foreign students). To receive student and resident rate, orders must be accompanied by name of affiliated institution, date of term, and the signature of program/residency coordinator on institution letterhead. Orders will be billed at individual rate until proof of status is received. Foreign air speed delivery is included in all Clinics subscription prices. All prices are subject to change without notice. POSTMASTER: Send address changes to PET Clinics, Elsevier Health Sciences Division, Subscription Customer Service, 3251 Riverport Lane, Maryland Heights, MO 63043. **Customer Service: 1-800-654-2452 (U.S. and Canada); 314-447-8871 (outside U.S. and Canada). Fax: 314-447-8029. E-mail: journalscustomerservice-usa@elsevier.com (for print support); journalsonlinesupport-usa@elsevier.com (for online support).**

Reprints. For copies of 100 or more of articles in this publication, please contact the Commercial Reprints Department, Elsevier Inc., 360 Park Avenue South, New York, NY 10010-1710. Tel.: 212-633-3874; Fax: 212-633-3820; E-mail: reprints@elsevier.com.

PET Clinics is covered in MEDLINE/PubMed (Index Medicus).

Contributors

CONSULTING EDITOR

ABASS ALAVI, MD, MD (Hon), PhD (Hon), DSc (Hon)
Professor of Radiology and Neurology
Director of Research Education
Department of Radiology
Perelman School of Medicine
University of Pennsylvania
Philadelphia, Pennsylvania, USA

EDITORS

AUSTIN R. PANTEL, MD, MSTR
Assistant Professor of Radiology, Department
of Radiology, University of Pennsylvania,
Hospital of the University of Pennsylvania,
Philadelphia, Pennsylvania, USA

JOEL S. KARP, PhD
Professor of Radiologic Physics, Department
of Radiology, University of Pennsylvania,
Philadelphia, Pennsylvania, USA

LORENZO NARDO, MD, PhD
Assistant Professor, Department of Radiology,
University of California Davis, Sacramento,
California, USA

RAMSEY D. BADAWI, PhD
Professor, Departments of Radiology and
Biomedical Engineering, University of
California Davis, Davis, Sacramento, California,
USA

AUTHORS

YASSER G. ABDELHAFEZ, MD,
EXPLORER Molecular Imaging Center, UC
Davis Health, Sacramento, California, USA

ABASS ALAVI, MD, MD (Hon), PhD (Hon), DSc (Hon)
Professor of Radiology and Neurology
Director of Research Education
Department of Radiology
Perelman School of Medicine
University of Pennsylvania
Philadelphia, Pennsylvania, USA

RAMSEY D. BADAWI, PhD
Professor, Departments of Radiology and
Biomedical Engineering, University of
California Davis, Davis, Sacramento, California,
USA

DENIS BECKFORD-VERA, PhD
Department of Radiology and Biomedical
Imaging, University of California, San
Francisco, San Francisco, California, USA

PACO E. BRAVO, MD
Division of Nuclear Medicine and Clinical
Molecular Imaging and Division of
Cardiothoracic Imaging, Department of
Radiology; Division of Cardiovascular
Medicine, Department of Medicine,
Perelman School of Medicine, University of
Pennsylvania, Philadelphia, Pennsylvania,
USA

ABHIJIT J. CHAUDHARI, PhD
Department of Radiology, University of
California, Davis, Sacramento, California,
USA

SHUGUANG CHEN, BSc
Department of Nuclear Medicine, Zhongshan Hospital, Fudan University, Institute of Nuclear Medicine, Fudan University, Shanghai Institute of Medical Imaging, Shanghai, China.

SIMON R. CHERRY, PhD
Professor, Departments of Biomedical Engineering and Radiology, University of California, Davis, California, USA

AUSTIN L. CHIEN, BA
Rutgers Robert Wood Johnson Medical School, Piscataway, New Jersey, USA

RHEA CHITALIA, BS
Graduate Student, Department of Radiology, University of Pennsylvania, Philadelphia, Pennsylvania, USA

MARIA CHONDRONIKOLA, PhD, RDN
Assistant Professor, Department of Nutrition, University of California, Davis, Davis, California, USA

MARGARET E. DAUBE-WITHERSPOON, PhD
Senior Research Investigator, Department of Radiology, University of Pennsylvania, Philadelphia, Pennsylvania, USA

JACOB G. DUBROFF, MD, PhD
Assistant Professor of Radiology, Division of Nuclear Medicine and Clinical Molecular Imaging, Perelman School of Medicine at the University of Pennsylvania, Philadelphia, Pennsylvania, USA

LARS EDENBRANDT, MD, DMSc
Professor/Chief Physician, Department of Clinical Physiology, Region Västra Götaland, Sahlgrenska University Hospital, Gothenburg, Sweden; Professor/Chief Physician, Department of Molecular and Clinical Medicine, Institute of Medicine, SU Sahlgrenska, Göteborg, Sweden

OKE GERKE, MSc, PhD
Chief Consultant, Biostatistician, Department of Nuclear Medicine, Odense University Hospital, Department of Clinical Research, University of Southern Denmark, Odense C, Denmark

ALI GHOLAMREZANEZHAD, MD
Keck School of Medicine, University of Southern California, Los Angeles, California, USA

POUL FLEMMING HØILUND-CARLSEN, MD, DMSc, Prof (Hon)
Professor of Clinical Physiology, Head Research, Department of Nuclear Medicine, Odense University Hospital, Department of Clinical Research, University of Southern Denmark, Odense C, Denmark

TIMOTHY J. HENRICH, MD
Division of Experimental Medicine, University of California, San Francisco, San Francisco, California, USA

PENGCHENG HU, MD, PhD
Department of Nuclear Medicine, Zhongshan Hospital, Fudan University, Institute of Nuclear Medicine, Fudan University, Shanghai Institute of Medical Imaging, Shanghai, China

TERRY JONES, DSc
Department of Radiology, University of California Davis Medical Center, Sacramento, California, USA

JOEL S. KARP, PhD
Professor of Radiologic Physics, Department of Radiology, University of Pennsylvania, Philadelphia, Pennsylvania, USA

GUOBING LIU, MD, PhD
Department of Nuclear Medicine, Zhongshan Hospital, Fudan University, Institute of Nuclear Medicine, Fudan University, Shanghai Institute of Medical Imaging, Shanghai, China

DAVID A. MANKOFF, MD
Gerd Muehllehner Professor, Vice-Chair for Research, Department of Radiology, Associate Director of Education and Training, Abramson Cancer Center, Department of Radiology, University of Pennsylvania, Hospital of the University of Pennsylvania, Philadelphia, Pennsylvania, USA

SAMUEL MATEJ, PhD
Department of Radiology, University of Pennsylvania, Philadelphia, Pennsylvania, USA

LORENZO NARDO, MD, PhD
Associate Professor, Department of Radiology,
University of California Davis, Sacramento,
California, USA

AUSTIN R. PANTEL, MD, MSTR
Assistant Professor of Radiology, Department
of Radiology, University of Pennsylvania,
Hospital of the University of Pennsylvania,
Philadelphia, Pennsylvania, USA

REZA PIRI, MD
Department of Nuclear Medicine, Odense
University Hospital, Department of Clinical
Research, University of Southern Denmark,
Odense C, Denmark

PATRICIA M. PRICE, MD
Department of Surgery and Cancer, Imperial
College, London, United Kingdom

JINYI QI, PhD
Department of Biomedical Engineering,
University of California, Davis, Davis,
California, USA

CHAMITH S. RAJAPAKSE, PhD
Department of Radiology, University of
Pennsylvania, Philadelphia, Pennsylvania,
USA

WILLIAM Y. RAYNOR, BS
Department of Radiology, University of
Pennsylvania, Drexel University College of
Medicine, Philadelphia, Pennsylvania, USA

JOSE A. RODRIGUEZ, MD
Division of Nuclear Medicine and Clinical
Molecular Imaging, Department of Radiology,
Perelman School of Medicine, University of
Pennsylvania, Philadelphia, Pennsylvania, USA

SOUVIK SARKAR, MD, PhD
Assistant Professor, Division of
Gastroenterology and Hepatology, University
of California, Davis, Davis, California, USA

SENTHIL SELVARAJ, MD, MA
Division of Cardiovascular Medicine,
Department of Medicine, Perelman School of
Medicine, University of Pennsylvania,
Philadelphia, Pennsylvania, USA

HONGCHENG SHI, MD, PhD
Department of Nuclear Medicine, Zhongshan
Hospital, Fudan University, Institute of Nuclear
Medicine, Fudan University, Shanghai Institute
of Medical Imaging, Shanghai, China

BENJAMIN A. SPENCER, PhD
EXPLORER Molecular Imaging Center, UC
Davis Health, Sacramento, California, USA

XIULI SUI, MD
Department of Nuclear Medicine, Zhongshan
Hospital, Fudan University, Institute of Nuclear
Medicine, Fudan University, Shanghai Institute
of Medical Imaging, Shanghai, China

ASHESH A. THAKER, MD
Assistant Professor of Radiology, Division of
Neuroradiology, University of Colorado School
of Medicine, Aurora, Colorado, USA

HENRY F. VANBROCKLIN, PhD
Department of Radiology and Biomedical
Imaging, University of California San Francisco,
San Francisco, California, USA

VARSHA VISWANATH, PhD
Postdoctoral Researcher, Department of
Radiology, University of Pennsylvania,
Philadelphia, Pennsylvania, USA

GUOBAO WANG, PhD
Department of Radiology, University of
California Davis Medical Center, Sacramento,
California, USA

THOMAS J. WERNER, MSE
Department of Radiology, University of
Pennsylvania, Philadelphia, Pennsylvania, USA

YING WANG, PhD
United Imaging Healthcare, Shanghai, China

HAOJUN YU, BSc
Department of Nuclear Medicine, Zhongshan
Hospital, Fudan University, Institute of Nuclear
Medicine, Fudan University, Shanghai Institute
of Medical Imaging, Shanghai, China

XUEZHU ZHANG, PhD
Department of Biomedical Engineering,
University of California, Davis, Davis,
California, USA

Contents

Total-body PET imaging using long axial FOV scanners brings new imaging opportunities and allows novel and improved modeling and ways of processing the data. One unique aspect of total-body imaging is simultaneous coverage of the entire human body, which makes it convenient to perform total-body dynamic PET scans. Therefore, four-dimensional dynamic PET reconstruction and parametric imaging are of great interest in total-body imaging. This article covers some basics of PET image reconstruction and then focuses on three and four-dimensional PET reconstruction for total-body imaging. Challenges and opportunities in total-body PET image reconstruction are also discussed.

The high sensitivity and total-body coverage of total-body PET scanners will be valuable for a number of clinical and research applications outlined in this article.

New protocols for imaging cancer have been developed to take advantage of the improved imaging capabilities of long axial field-of-view PET scanners. Both research and clinical applications have been pursued with encouraging early results. Clinical studies have demonstrated improved image quality and the ability to image with less injected activity or for shorter duration. With the increased sensitivity inherent in total-body PET scanners and new imaging paradigms, new challenges in image interpretation have emerged. New research applications have also emerged, including dosimetry, cell tracking, and dual-tracer applications.

Obesity and associated metabolic syndrome are a global public health issue. Understanding the pathophysiology of this systemic disease is of critical importance for the development of future therapeutic interventions to improve clinical outcomes. The multiorgan nature of the pathophysiology of obesity presents a unique challenge. Total-body PET imaging, either static or dynamic, provides a vital set of tools to study organ crosstalk. The visualization and quantification of tissue metabolic kinetics with total-body PET in health and disease provides essential information to better understand disease physiology and potentially develop diagnostic and therapeutic modalities.

Total-body PET enables high-sensitivity imaging with dramatically improved signal-to-noise ratio. These enhanced performance characteristics allow for decreased PET scanning times acquiring data "total-body wide" and can be leveraged to decrease the amount of radiotracer required, thereby permitting more frequent imaging or longer imaging periods during radiotracer decay. Novel approaches to PET imaging of infectious diseases are emerging, including those that directly visualize pathogens in vivo and characterize concomitant immune responses and inflammation. Efforts to develop these imaging approaches are hampered by challenges of traditional imaging platforms, which may be overcome by novel total-body PET strategies.

contributions to basic science and clinical medicine, PET has not been used to explore nervous system physiology and disease throughout the remainder of the body. Our understanding of neurologic disorders has also changed during this period, and we are beginning to realize that many neuropsychiatric diseases manifest throughout the entire body. Thus, whole-body PET imaging with the Explorer instrument represents an exciting tool to address important questions in pathophysiology and develop novel pharmacologic strategies.

PET CLINICS

PET CLINICS

PROGRAM OBJECTIVE
The goal of the PET Clinics is to keep practicing radiologists and radiology residents up to date with current clinical practice in positron emission tomography by providing timely articles reviewing the state of the art in patient care.

TARGET AUDIENCE
Practicing radiologists, radiology residents, and other health care professionals who provide patient care utilizing radiologic findings.

LEARNING OBJECTIVES
Upon completion of this activity, participants will be able to:
1. Review initial experiensces of Total-body (TB) PET/CT implementation in various clinical settings.
2. Discuss aspects of scanner design of long axial field of view (AFOV) systems and how these choices affect system performance.
3. Recognize potential applications of TB PET imaging in oncology and metabolic disease, atherosclerosis, musculoskeletal disease, infection, cardiac disease, and neurological disease.

ACCREDITATION
The Elsevier Office of Continuing Medical Education (EOCME) is accredited by the Accreditation Council for Continuing Medical Education (ACCME) to provide continuing medical education for physicians.

The EOCME designates this journal-based CME activity for a maximum of 13 *AMA PRA Category 1 Credit*(s)™. Physicians should claim only the credit commensurate with the extent of their participation in the activity.

All other health care professionals requesting continuing education credit for this enduring material will be issued a certificate of participation.

DISCLOSURE OF CONFLICTS OF INTEREST
The EOCME assesses conflict of interest with its instructors, faculty, planners, and other individuals who are in a position to control the content of CME activities. All relevant conflicts of interest that are identified are thoroughly vetted by EOCME for fair balance, scientific objectivity, and patient care recommendations. EOCME is committed to providing its learners with CME activities that promote improvements or quality in healthcare and not a specific proprietary business or a commercial interest.

The planning committee, staff, authors, and editors listed below have identified no financial relationships or relationships to products or devices they or their spouse/life partner have with commercial interest related to the content of this CME activity:
Yasser G. Abdelhafez, MD; Abass Alavi, MD, MD (Hon), PhD (Hon), DSc (Hon); Denis Beckford-Vera, PhD; Paco E. Bravo, MD; Abhijit J. Chaudhari, PhD; Regina Chavous-Gibson, MSN, RN; Shuguang Chen, BSc; Austin L. Chien, BA; Rhea Chitalia, BS; Maria Chondronikola, PhD, RDN; Jacob G. Dubroff, MD, PhD; Lars Edenbrandt, MD, DMSc; Oke Gerke, MSc, PhD; Ali Gholamrezanezhad, MD; Poul Flemming Høilund-Carlsen, MD, DMSc, Prof (Hon); Pengcheng Hu, MD, PhD; Terry Jones, DSc; Joel S. Karp, PhD; Guobing Liu, MD, PhD; David A. Mankoff, MD; Austin R. Pantel, MD, MSTR; Reza Piri, MD; Patricia M. Price, MD; Chamith S. Rajapakse, PhD; William Y. Raynor, BS; Jose A. Rodriguez, MD; Souvik Sarkar, MD, PhD; Senthil Selvaraj, MD, MA; Hongcheng Shi, MD, PhD; Benjamin A. Spencer, PhD; Xiuli Sui, MD; Ashesh A. Thaker, MD; Henry F. VanBrocklin, PhD; John Vassallo; Vignesh Viswanathan; Varsha Viswanath, PhD; Guobao Wang, PhD; Thomas J. Werner, MSE; Ying Wang, PhD; Haojun Yu, BSc; Xuezhu Zhang, PhD

The planning committee, staff, authors, and editors listed below have identified financial relationships or relationships to products or devices they or their spouse/life partner have with commercial interest related to the content of this CME activity:
Ramsey D. Badawi, PhD: receives research support from United Imaging Healthcare Co., Ltd.

Simon R. Cherry, PhD: receives research support from Canon Medical Research USA, Inc. and United Imaging Healthcare Co., Ltd.

Margaret E. Daube-Witherspoon, PhD: receives research support from Koninklijke Philips N.V. and Siemens Medical Solutions USA, Inc.

Timothy J. Henrich, MD: receives research support from Bristol-Myers Squibb Company, Gilead Sciences, Inc., and Merck Sharp & Dohme Corp., a subsidairy of Merck & Co., Inc.

Samuel Matej, PhD: is a consutlant/advisor for Siemens Medical Solutions USA, Inc.

Lorenzo Nardo, MD, PhD: is a consultant/advisor and receives research support from United Imaging Healthcare Co., Ltd.

Jinyi Qi, PhD: receives research support from Canon Medical Research USA, Inc.

UNAPPROVED/OFF-LABEL USE DISCLOSURE
The EOCME requires CME faculty to disclose to the participants:

1. When products or procedures being discussed are off-label, unlabelled, experimental, and/or investigational (not US Food and Drug Administration [FDA] approved); and
2. Any limitations on the information presented, such as data that are preliminary or that represent ongoing research, interim analyses, and/or unsupported opinions. Faculty may discuss information about pharmaceutical agents that is outside of FDA-approved labelling. This information is intended solely for CME and is not intended to promote off-label use of these medications. If you have any questions, contact the medical affairs department of the manufacturer for the most recent pre-scribing information.

TO ENROLL

To enroll in the PET Clinics Continuing Medical Education program, call customer service at 1-800-654-2452 or sign up online at http://www.theclinics.com/home/cme. The CME program is available to subscribers for an additional annual fee of USD 254.00

METHOD OF PARTICIPATION

In order to claim credit, participants must complete the following:
1. Complete enrolment as indicated above.
2. Read the activity.
3. Complete the CME Test and Evaluation. Participants must achieve a score of 70% on the test. All CME Tests and Evaluations must be completed online.

CME INQUIRIES/SPECIAL NEEDS

For all CME inquiries or special needs, please contact elsevierCME@elsevier.com

Errata

The article "Reinventing Molecular Imaging with Total-Body PET, Part II: Clinical Applications" by Drs. Babak Saboury, Michael A. Morris, Moozhan Nikpanah, Thomas J. Werner, Elizabeth C. Jones, and Abass Alavi (October 2020, Volume 15, issue 4, pp463-475) should contain the following acknowledgment: The authors would like to acknowledge contributions from William Raynor, who provided original images for this article.

Also in the October 2020 issue (Volume 15, number 4), in the article, "Recent Advances in Computed Tomography and MR Imaging" (pp. 381-402), one author's name was misspelled. The correct spelling is Jina Pakpoor.

PET Clin 16 (2021) xv
https://doi.org/10.1016/j.cpet.2020.10.001

Preface
Total Body PET: Exploring New Horizons

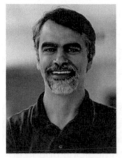

Ramsey D. Badawi, PhD

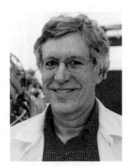

Joel S. Karp, PhD

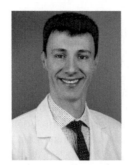

Lorenzo Nardo, MD, PhD

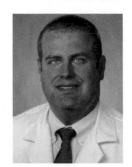

Austin R. Pantel, MD, MSTR

Editors

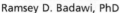

In this special issue of *PET Clinics*, we provide the readers with a complete update of where total body (TB) PET stands at the present time, together with some views on future applications for this transformative technology. TB PET is a 30-year-old idea finally brought to fruition in 2018, by the EXPLORER Consortium, with the beginning of human imaging with TB PET/CT scanners in the United States and in China. The EXPLORER Consortium has developed 2 different scanner designs with axial fields-of-view (AFOV) significantly beyond that of existing systems: the uEXPLORER, manufactured by United Imaging Healthcare, and the PennPET Explorer, manufactured at the University of Pennsylvania. At the time of this writing, TB PET has been in clinical operation for a little over a year at the University of California at Davis, at Zhongshan Hospital, and at several other sites in China with the uEXPLORER scanner, and for research investigations at the University of Pennsylvania with the PennPET Explorer scanner. The clinical and research potentials are just beginning to be explored.

TB PET is characterized by exceptional signal collection efficiency resulting from close-to-maximal geometric coverage, and by the ability to simultaneously collect signal from multiple organs and potentially the entire body. These features allow the clinician, or research investigator, to select a variety of protocols not available before,

including ultrafast or ultralow dose scanning, scanning with unprecedented image quality, scanning at much later time points after radiotracer injection, and, for the first time with any imaging modality, the ability to simultaneously capture radiotracer kinetics across the entire body. All these capabilities have now been demonstrated in the early use of these instruments, and examples of such studies are presented in this issue. Many of the potential applications of TB PET imaging are discussed in the following articles, including oncology and metabolic disease, atherosclerosis, musculoskeletal disease, infection, cardiac disease, and neurologic disease. Perhaps even more transformative, these capabilities may enable wider application of PET scanning in the management and understanding of human health; some of these possibilities are discussed herein.

We expect that the enthusiasm for TB PET imaging will lead to the introduction of other systems that offer similar, or possibly superior performance compared with the 2 EXPLORER designs. In particular, it is already becoming clear that we will see a range of AFOV for new instruments since it is not yet known what the optimal axial coverage should be for a TB PET instrument, or if indeed there is a single such optimum. Ultimately, the primary use of the scanner should dictate its configuration, which may also be constrained by cost. The many applications discussed in the following

PET Clin 16 (2021) xvii–xviii
https://doi.org/10.1016/j.cpet.2020.09.005
1556-8598/21/© 2020 Published by Elsevier Inc.

articles provide guidance and inspiration for future designs.

TB PET is in its infancy and yet has already shown quite astonishing results. This issue of *PET Clinics* sets the stage for the next phase of exploration.

Ramsey D. Badawi, PhD
Department of Radiology
University of California Davis
4860 Y Street, Suite 3100
Sacramento, CA 95817, USA

Joel S. Karp, PhD
Department of Radiology
University of Pennsylvania
3620 Hamilton Walk
John Morgan Building - Room #154
Philadelphia, PA 19104-6112, USA

Lorenzo Nardo, MD, PhD
Department of Radiology
University of California Davis
4860 Y Street, Suite 3100
Sacramento, CA 95817, USA

Austin R. Pantel, MD, MSTR
Department of Radiology
University of Pennsylvania
3400 Spruce Street
1 Silverstein, Suite 130
Philadelphia, PA 19104, USA

E-mail addresses:
rdbadawi@ucdavis.edu (R.D. Badawi)
joelkarp@pennmedicine.upenn.edu (J.S. Karp)
lnardo@ucdavis.edu (L. Nardo)
austin.pantel@pennmedicine.upenn.edu
(A.R. Pantel)

Clinical Implementation of Total-Body PET/CT at University of California, Davis

Lorenzo Nardo, MD, PhD[a], Yasser G. Abdelhafez, MD[b],
Benjamin A. Spencer, PhD[b], Ramsey D. Badawi, PhD[a,c],*

KEYWORDS

- Positron emission tomography • Total-body PET • Human imaging

KEY POINTS

- Human imaging on the total-body positron emission tomography (PET)/computed tomography (CT) at U.C. Davis has demonstrated superb image quality using both [18]F- and ^{68}Ga-based radiotracers.
- The increased sensitivity and spatial resolution of total-body PET/CT creates new challenges in imaging interpretation that must be overcome for optimal integration into the clinical workflow.
- The large gain in sensitivity and total-body coverage enables a range of different acquisition protocols; work on understanding how best to use these for maximal clinical benefit is ongoing.

INTRODUCTION

Following initial tests in humans at the United Imaging Healthcare (UIH) factory in Shanghai and receipt of Food and Drug Administration (FDA) 510(k) clearance, a UIH uEXPLORER total-body (TB) positron emission tomography (PET)/computed tomography (CT) scanner was installed at the EXPLORER Molecular Imaging Center (EMIC), UC Davis, in May 2019. EMIC is a satellite imaging and research clinic located approximately 1.5 miles from the UC Davis Medical Center (UCDMC). UCDMC contains a National Cancer Institute–designated Comprehensive Cancer Center, 2 medical cyclotrons and a commercial radiopharmaceutical production facility (PETNET), a specialized not-for-profit radiopharmaceutical production facility (Optimal Tracers), and a well-equipped radiochemistry research laboratory (the Sutcliffe laboratory). In the Spring of 2019, the existing clinical PET operation at UCDMC consisted of 2 standard PET/CT scanners providing oncologic, cardiac, and neurologic PET imaging services, with a volume of approximately 20 cases per day (of which approximately 8 were cardiac studies). The UCDMC patient enrollment area is large and extends from the Central Valley to the greater Northern California region outside the San Francisco Bay Area.

EMIC was created with the objective to provide both clinical and research imaging services to UC Davis and to the community, with the intention of allocating equal scanner time to the clinical and research missions. This article focuses on the clinical implementation of TB PET/CT at EMIC (Fig. 1).

Results from the initial tests in humans had demonstrated that this scanner was capable of delivering exceptional image quality with ^{18}F-fluorodeoxyglucose (^{18}F-FDG), with high resolution and low noise.[1] Our clinical implementation philosophy evolved through extensive discussions, but we converged on a view that because EMIC had a rare opportunity to implement protocols that could deliver unprecedented image quality for clinical purposes, that we should do so. This

Funding: NIH R01 CA249422; NIH R01 CA206187.
[a] Department of Radiology, U.C. Davis, Sacramento, CA, USA; [b] EXPLORER Molecular Imaging Center, UC Davis Health, 3195 Folsom Blvd., Suite 120, Sacramento, CA 95816, USA; [c] Department of Biomedical Engineering, U.C. Davis, Davis, CA, USA
* Corresponding author. Department of Radiology, 4860 Y Street, Suite 3100, Sacramento, CA 9581, USA
E-mail address: rdbadawi@ucdavis.edu

PET Clin 16 (2021) 1–7
https://doi.org/10.1016/j.cpet.2020.09.006
1556-8598/21/© 2020 Elsevier Inc. All rights reserved.

pet.theclinics.com

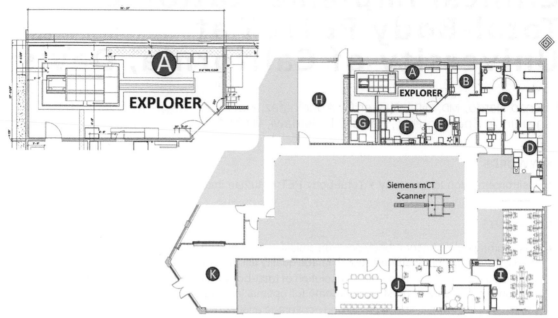

Fig. 1. EMIC site layout. (*A*) EXPLORER scanner room. (*B*) Scanner control room. (*C*) Uptake rooms and restroom. (*D*) Radiopharmaceutical (Hot) laboratory. (*E*) Nurse and technologist workstation. (*F*) Metabolite laboratory. (*G*) Computing hardware room. (*H*) Future cyclotron room. (*I*) Research laboratory and image viewing workstations (*J*) Conference room and office space. (*K*) Patient reception and waiting room. The gray area outlines the affiliated imaging center (Northern California PET Imaging Center) housing a Siemens mCT PET/CT scanner.

presented both an opportunity and a risk for clinical implementation, because our radiologists could not have had prior experience in reading such high-fidelity PET images before. This is of course a persistent issue in the field of radiology due to the constant development of more sophisticated tools, for example, the case of small pulmonary embolism detected with high-resolution CT.[2] In many ways, our challenge echoed that of the early pioneers of clinical PET in the late 1980s and early 1990s, although, of course, the basics of FDG-PET imaging were far better understood in 2019 than they were 30 years before that. Similar to what Maisey[3] did when implementing clinical PET for the first time in the United Kingdom, we used a team approach, involving nuclear medicine physicians, radiologists, physicists, technologists, and oncologists to develop the protocols and to understand the results.[3]

18F-FDG: STUDIES IN HEALTHY SUBJECTS

Our first human imaging studies were performed on healthy subjects who had given informed consent under an institutional review board–approved protocol. This protocol had multiple arms and was aimed at providing preliminary data to guide future research studies, but the arm of most interest to the development of our

clinical protocols involved injecting 370 MBq (10 mCi) of ^{18}F-FDG, performing an initial dynamic scan for 60 minutes, and following it with 20-minute scans at 1.5, 3, 6, 9, and 12 hours postinjection (**Fig. 2**). The data acquired from the first subjects enrolled enabled us to develop our initial image reconstruction protocols, as well as allowing us to gain initial understanding of issues relating to minimization of patient motion[4] and how to perform bolus injections given the constraints of the long gantry.[5] In particular, we learned that although the count density in the data supported image reconstructions with isotropic voxels of size of approximately 1 mm, handling these very large PET datasets, with their corresponding CT datasets, was a significant challenge to our data bandwidth capabilities and our Picture Archiving and Communication System workstations. We also found that the expected significant reduction in blood pool activity at 3 hours postinjection resulted in markedly clear images with high contrast, and without a major noise penalty. Correlation of results from human subjects data with additional experiments performed on large cylindrical phantoms[6] suggested that injecting a somewhat smaller amount of activity might achieve a better trade-off between effective dose and data quality at 1 hour postinjection.

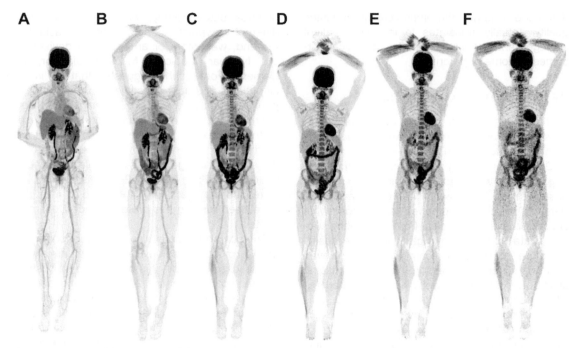

Fig. 2. A 51-year-old woman, healthy volunteer. Dynamic scan was acquired for 60 minutes after injection of 348 MBq of ^{18}F-FDG. (*A*) Reconstruction of the last 20 minutes of dynamic acquisition; (*B–F*) 20-minute duration scans obtained at 90 minutes, and 3, 6, 9, and 12 hours postinjection. Patient was fed with high-protein snack after the 3-hour scan.

INTERACTIONS WITH ONCOLOGISTS

We used a gradual approach to the clinical implementation of TB PET/CT. The first step involved educating the clinical oncologists in the advantages and possible risks of performing TB PET/CT with our high-performance protocols. Our understanding of the risks primarily involved the possibility of false positive results due to the increased potential for detection of smaller or milder FDG uptake foci that might not be seen on conventional PET/CT, the significance of which might be open to misinterpretation. We then worked with a select team of providers who were allowed to order TB PET/CT scans, but only after a discussion between the radiologist and patient. In addition, all the initial cases were presented and further discussed at interdisciplinary conferences where the images were closely scrutinized.

At this point, the referring physicians appeared to divide into 2 groups: those who were enthusiastic about the image quality, and those who were concerned about decreased confidence in interpretation due to the high level of detail that the images provided. Again, this is a common problem encountered as radiological instrumentation and methods improve, and we heard similar stories from colleagues who had been involved in the early adoption of the prior generation of high-performance PET scanners. Both positions have merit and we forged an approach that was a synthesis of optimism tempered by caution and humility. As a matter of caution, we stress the possibility of encountering the risk of false positives during discussions with the referring physicians, in particular when selecting patients to be scanned with TB PET/CT. The direct and continuous collaboration between the radiologists and the oncologists mitigates this risk to acceptable levels for both parties. On the positive side, we note that we are much less prone to error because of the significant reduction in image noise that improves confidence in regions such as the liver. Furthermore, we find ourselves able to more confidently characterize small lesions with CT correlates as benign or malignant.

After approximately 100 clinical cases, we felt comfortable enough to expand the pool of referring physicians, but we still insist on a direct conversation between the referring physician and a radiologist before accepting a new referral.

Moving forward, we have begun a National Cancer Institute–funded clinical study to directly compare TB PET/CT with conventional PET/CT in the initial staging of patients with a range of different cancers. In our early results, we find, as expected, that the difference in image quality is astonishing, but the aim of the study is to determine whether the improvement in image quality actually translates to improved patient management. We will learn more as clinical outcomes become apparent.

^{18}F-FDG: PROTOCOL SELECTION

On the strength of our analysis of the human images and of our phantom studies, we began by injecting 185 MBq (5 mCi) of ^{18}F-FDG, and imaging for 20 minutes starting at 90 minutes postinjection (Fig. 3). However, although imaging at 90 minutes postinjection has plenty of precedent (e.g. Refs.[7,8]), we found ourselves feeling somewhat uncomfortable. It was clear from our healthy subjects data that additional gains in image quality could be obtained by scanning later; however, with only 4 uptake rooms in the center, imaging at 3 hours postinjection would have generated significant logistical challenges. Furthermore, it is also the case that some guidelines for patient management with FDG-PET, specifically, Deauville criteria for lymphoma,[9] are based on imaging at 1 hour postinjection. We felt strongly that imaging at 1 hour postinjection was a decision based on legacy protocols that would result in significant wasted performance for a scanner such as this, and would be a disservice both to our patients and to the future of the field. To resolve this dilemma, we turned to a number of internationally eminent experts in clinical PET for advice, and,

perhaps unsurprisingly, we obtained as many different viewpoints as people who we asked. In the end, we opted for an approach devised by our Nuclear Medicine Medical Director, Dr. Cameron Foster, who suggested that we image all patients at 2 hours postinjection, but that lymphoma patients should also be imaged at 1 hour postinjection. The early scan could then be used in the context of the Deauville criteria without modification, while still providing the patient with the excellent image quality available from the 2-hour scan (Fig. 4). For 2-hour scanning, we increased the injection to 296 MBq (8 mCi). We have been running this protocol since December 2019.

The scan duration is also a protocol parameter that warrants discussion. Because data are always acquired in list mode, it is possible to reconstruct shorter scans from the 20-minute-long acquisitions. Using data from our healthy subjects and from our first patients, we reconstructed a number of 5-minute and 10-minute scans and reviewed the resulting image quality. Although the shorter scans were of diagnostic quality, it was felt that the 20-minute scans remained noticeably better. Following our philosophy of aiming for the best possible image quality, we have continued with the 20-minute acquisition protocol, reserving shorter scans only for those patients who experience excessive discomfort or who have difficulty in remaining still. On the topic of motion, we

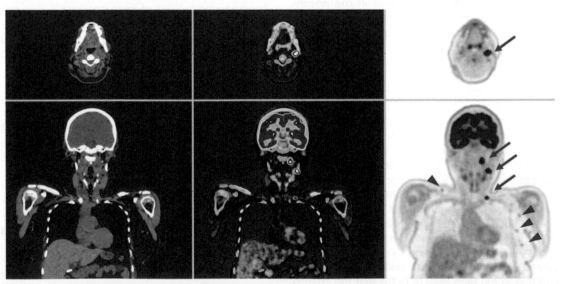

Fig. 3. Patient with diffuse large B-cell lymphoma. The scanning protocol consisted of intravenous injection of 193 MBq of [18]FDG, 90-minute uptake time, and 20-minute scan. Axial (top row) and coronal (bottom row) CT images (left), fused PET/CT images (center), and PET images (right) are shown. The 3 lesions in the left cervical and supraclavicular regions are highlighted by the red arrows representing lymphoma. Several other lymph nodes with lower FDG avidity are noted in the left axilla and right supraclavicular region (arrowhead). These findings were interpreted as benign lymph nodes.

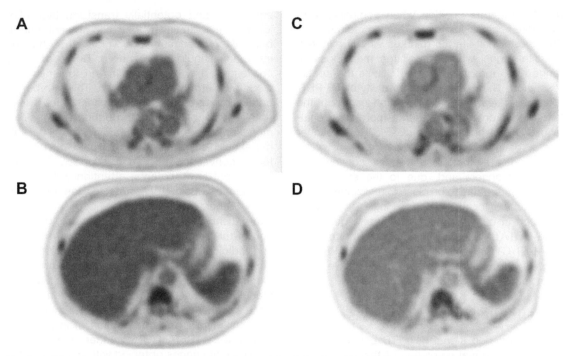

Fig. 4. A 60-year-old man suffering from lymphoma. After injection of 296 MBq of ^{18}F-FDG, 20-minute scans were obtained at 60 (*A, B*) and 120 minutes (*C, D*). Images are displayed using the same window level. Comparing the mediastinal (*top row*) and upper abdominal region (*bottom row*) between 60-minute and 120-minute scans, both blood pool activity within the aorta and the liver uptake significantly decrease. Both mediastinal blood pool and liver uptake are used to normalize lesions and assess Deauville score.

have noticed that because the entire patient remains in the field of view for the entire scan, motion is a larger issue for a 20-minute TB PET/CT scan than it would be for a 20-minute conventional PET/CT scan. Motion correction is now an active area of research within our group.

INITIAL EXPERIENCE WITH ^{18}F-FLUCICLOVINE AND ^{68}GA-DOTATATE

With ^{18}F-Fluciclovine, we acquire 25 minutes of data starting at the time of injection. Data are reconstructed for clinical interpretation starting at 4 minutes postinjection. Our preference would be to inject no more than 185 MBq (5 mCi); however, the label requires a prescription of 370 MBq (10 mCi). Regulations permit a 20% deviation from this value and we aim for the lower end of this range (296 MBq, 8 mCi). There are substantial differences between a ^{18}F-Fluciclovine scan obtained on a TB PET/CT scanner and on a conventional PET/CT scanner. First, the images can be acquired in the entire body at the same time; this allows for early time point scans, especially in the upper part of the body where the radiotracer distribution in the muscles in a conventional PET/ CT scanner often interferes with the evaluation.

Second, it delivers better image quality in the pelvic area, which is the site where disease recurrence rate is higher in patients scanned for biochemical recurrence of prostate cancer. The high sensitivity of the scanner permits reconstruction of short-duration frames while keeping the noise manageable. In routine clinical examination, we use the analysis of a series of short-duration frames (e.g. 2 minutes) to determine when the bladder starts filling and avoid misinterpreting urinary activity as recurrent disease, especially when motion artifacts are present; this is particularly helpful in individuals with very prompt radiotracer excretion. Together, these advantages are highly significant.

In prior studies, the use of ^{18}F-Fluciclovine has been found to be less sensitive than prostate-specific membrane antigen (PSMA)-PET for distant metastases.[10] We do not know if TB PET/ CT will offer equally significant benefits for PSMA-PET, but our initial experience with ^{18}F-Fluciclovine does suggest that the head-to-head comparison between ^{18}F-Fluciclovine and PSMA should be revisited in this context.

The other FDA-approved radiotracer that we have been using clinically is ^{68}Ga-DOTATATE. The ^{68}Ga-based radiotracers are in a disadvantageous position when compared with the more imaging-friendly ^{18}F-based radiotracers. The shorter half-life (68 minutes vs 109 minutes) limits the signal, whereas the larger mean positron range (3.66 mm vs 0.66 mm)[11] limits the spatial resolution. The exceptional sensitivity of TB PET/CT ameliorates the signal limitation issue, but the larger positron range presents more of a challenge. This is because the uEXPLORER scanner has a spatial resolution of close to 3 mm, which is considerably better than most conventional PET/CT scanners and, due to the exceptional sensitivity, appears to be close to realizable in clinical practice for ^{18}F-FDG imaging. As a result, although in our experience the image quality of ^{68}Ga-DOTATATE remains noticeably better with TB PET/CT than with conventional PET/CT (**Fig. 5**), the gains are not as stark as we have seen with ^{18}F-based radiotracers.

PRESENT AND FUTURE CHALLENGES

The unpreceded signal gain, TB coverage, and exceptional spatial resolution of the TB PET/CT scanner provide the physical explanation of its enhanced, and potentially transformative, clinical potential; however, they also present a number of challenges for which the hosting institution should be prepared. Some of these challenges may be found in the logistics and workflows around the scanner. The number of uptake rooms is a critical consideration. If long uptake time or if high throughput is desired, more uptake rooms (potentially, considerably more), will be required than would be needed for a conventional PET/CT scanner. In high-throughput environments, attention will need to be paid to dosimetry issues for the technologists. Other challenges arise from integration into patient care. During the initial years of adoption of this technology, it will not be possible to find radiologists and oncologists with prior experience of the modality, and oncologists and radiologists will need to engage in a mutual learning/teaching process, much as we have done. Even once experience has been gained, a major clinical challenge is the comparison of images obtained with TB PET/CT scanner and prior or subsequent images obtained with a conventional PET/CT scanner (see **Fig. 5**). Radiologists are

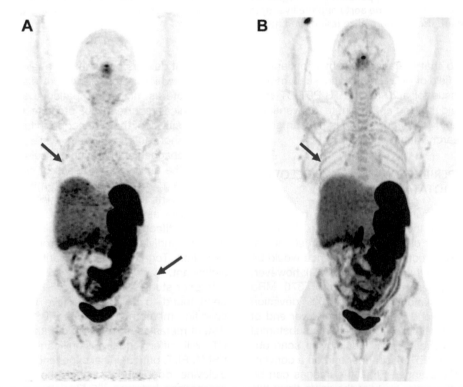

Fig. 5. Patient with Cushing syndrome post bilateral adrenalectomy. A dose of 167 MBq of ^{68}Ga DOTATATE was injected and a 20-minute scan was performed starting at 60 minutes after injection. (*A*) Baseline scan obtained using a conventional PET/CT scanner. (*B*) A 6-month follow-up scan obtained on TB scanner. A lower background noise and higher signal is noted, allowing for clearer visualization of the liver. In addition, the increased signal level on the TB scanner results in new or better visualization of bone marrow details (*arrows*).

already familiar with the difficulties of comparing scans obtained on different devices; however, when a TB PET/CT scan is compared with others, this issue becomes more critical because of the substantial different image quality and potentially (and certainly for ^{18}F-FDG in our hands) different protocols that lead to different radiotracer biodistribution.

SUMMARY/FUTURE DIRECTIONS

We have successfully integrated TB PET/CT into our clinical practice. At our center, the smooth transition was made possible because of the strong research environment, the diverse imaging team, and the productive collaboration between imaging physicians and oncologists who all worked together to improve patient care. Our next step is to rethink ways to image with TB PET/CT, improving old clinical protocols, implementing the use of different radiotracers, and establishing a new clinical routine in which both research and clinical work can further thrive.

ACKNOWLEDGMENTS

The authors thank the EXPLORER team at UC Davis for their hard work and strong support. In particular we thank the technologists: Denise Caudle, Heather Hunt, Kristin McBride, Mike Nguyen, Michael Rusnak; the radiologists: Marwah Helmy, Elizabeth Moore, Fatma Sen, Cameron Foster, Rosalie Hagge, Thomas Loehfelm, Matthew Bobinski, Nancy Pham; the physics team: Benjamin Spencer, Eric Berg, Edwin K. Leung, Negar Omidvari, Emilie Roncali, Anthony Siebert, Linda Kroger; the supporting and supervisory staff: Stephen Wetzel, Dana Little, Ellie Nash, Lynda Painting, Ofilio Vigil, Elizabeth Lincoln, Michelle Verdier-Fontes, Kathy Cruz Rodriguez, Jeanee Cooper, Carla Andalis; the ethics experts in the institutional review board team: John Tupin, Amanda Carioggia, Royce Yokoi; WeiPing Liu and Jeffrey Schmall and United Imaging Engineer team; the oncologist experts: Ken Yoneda, Merin Stephen, Tianhong Li, Primo Lara, Karen Kelly, Aaron Rosenberg, May Cho, Joseph Tuscano, Mamta Parikh, Edward Kim, Amanda Kirane, Marcio Malogolowkin, David Cooke, Lisa Brown, and Johnathan Riess.

DISCLOSURE

R.D. Badawi has research support from United Imaging Healthcare. L. Nardo has is principal investigator of a service agreement with United Imaging Healthcare; UC Davis has a revenue-sharing agreement with United Imaging Healthcare that is based on uEXPLORER sales.

REFERENCES

1. Badawi RD, Shi H, Hu P, et al. First human imaging studies with the EXPLORER total-body PET scanner. J Nucl Med 2019;60(3):299–303.

2. Desai SR. Unsuspected pulmonary embolism on CT scanning: yet another headache for clinicians? Thorax 2007;62(6):470–2.

3. Maisey M. The introduction and development of clinical PET in the United Kingdom. In: McCready R, Gnanasegaran G, Bomanji JB, editors. A history of radionuclide studies in the UK: 50th anniversary of the British Nuclear Medicine Society. Cham (Switzerland): 2016. p. 103–10. https://doi.org/10.1007/978-3-319-28624-2.

4. Rusnak M, McBride K. Total-body PET patient positioning for optimal diagnostic and research scans. J Nucl Med 2020;61(supplement 1):3122.

5. McBride K, Hunt H, Rusnak M, et al. Bolus injection technique for uEXPLORER 18F-FDG PET/CT dynamic scans. J Nucl Med 2020;61(supplement 1):3084.

6. Leung E, Zhang X, Berg E, et al. Relationships between noise-equivalent count rates for extended NEMA NU 2-like scatter phantoms and a human subject scanned using the EXPLORER total-body PET scanner. J Nucl Med 2019;60(supplement 1):1385.

7. Nahmias C, Wahl LM. Reproducibility of standardized uptake value measurements determined by 18F-FDG PET in malignant tumors. J Nucl Med 2008;49(11):1804–8.

8. Davies A, Tan C, Paschalides C, et al. FDG-PET maximum standardised uptake value is associated with variation in survival: analysis of 498 lung cancer patients. Lung Cancer 2007;55(1):75–8.

9. Meignan M, Gallamini A, Meignan M, et al. Report on the first international workshop on interim-PET scan in lymphoma. Leuk Lymphoma 2009;50(8):1257–60.

10. Calais J, Fendler WP, Herrmann K, et al. Comparison of (68)Ga-PSMA-11 and (18)F-fluciclovine PET/CT in a case series of 10 patients with prostate cancer recurrence. J Nucl Med 2018;59(5):789–94.

11. Jødal L, Le Loirec C, Champion C. Positron range in PET imaging: an alternative approach for assessing and correcting the blurring. Phys Med Biol 2012;57(12):3931–43.

Total-Body PET/Computed Tomography Highlights in Clinical Practice
Experiences from Zhongshan Hospital, Fudan University

Xiuli Sui, MD[a,b,c,1], Guobing Liu, MD, PhD[a,b,c,1], Pengcheng Hu, MD, PhD[a,b,c], Shuguang Chen, BSc[a,b,c], Haojun Yu, BSc[a,b,c], Ying Wang, PhD[d], Hongcheng Shi, MD, PhD[a,b,c,*]

KEYWORDS

- Lesion detectability • Short acquisition time • Total-body PET/CT • Dynamic acquisition

KEY POINTS

- Total-body PET/CT imaging provides more comprehensive disease assessment.
- Total-body PET/CT provides a wider choice of protocols, such as low or extra low dose scanning, fast scanning, and high-quality imaging scanning.
- Late time-point postinjection scanning can provide imaging with high lesion-to-background ratio.
- Total-body PET/CT dynamic scanning can be used for radiotracer kinetics studies and for radiotracer angiography.

INTRODUCTION

The Department of Nuclear Medicine, Zhongshan Hospital, Fudan University, was established in 1958, and it is one of the cradles of clinical nuclear medicine in China. It is the National Key Clinical Specialty, the National Demonstration Base of Standardized Training for Residents and the National Base of Clinical Drug Trials.

The department covers an area of approximately 5600 square meters, and consists of 4 centers: the PET Molecular Imaging Center, the Single Photon Functional Imaging Center, the Radionuclide Targeting Therapy Center, and the Molecular Probe Research and Development Center. The 2 imaging centers have 11 scanners in total with 4 clinical whole-body PET/computed tomography (CT) scanners (including the world's first total-body PET/CT scanner), one clinical whole-body PET/MR scanner, 3 single-photon emission CT (SPECT)/CT scanners with diagnostic CT capability, and other imaging modalities, including a dedicated cardiac gamma

Funding: This research was supported in part by the National Key Research and Development Program of China (2016YFC10103908), the National Natural Science Foundation of China (81471706, and 81671735), Shanghai Science and Technology Project (17511104201), Shanghai Municipal Key Clinical Specialty(shslczdzk03401) and the Shanghai "Rising Stars of Medical Talent" Youth Development Program (Receiver: Dr. Liu).

[a] Department of Nuclear Medicine, Zhongshan Hospital, Fudan University, Shanghai, China; [b] Institute of Nuclear Medicine, Fudan University, Shanghai, China; [c] Shanghai Institute of Medical Imaging, Shanghai, China; [d] United Imaging Healthcare, Shanghai, China

[1] The authors contributed equally to this study.

* Corresponding author. Department of Nuclear Medicine, Zhongshan Hospital, 180 Fenglin Road, Shanghai, China.

E-mail address: Shi.hongcheng@zs-hospital.sh.cn

PET Clin 16 (2021) 9–14
https://doi.org/10.1016/j.cpet.2020.09.007

camera (D-SPECT) and a dedicated breast gamma camera.

The first PET/CT scanner in Zhongshan Hospital, Fudan University, was a Discovery VCT from GE Healthcare (Chicago, IL), installed in 2009. The second and third ones were from United Imaging Healthcare (Shanghai, China), installed in 2015 and in 2018, respectively. Since 2017, more than 16,000 PET/CT examinations have been performed each year in our department.

The total-body PET/CT scanner (uExplorer) was installed in April 2019. Site preparation, installation, and equipment adjustment were completed in 4 weeks. A clinical trial, consisting of fludeoxyglucose F 18 (^{18}F-FDG) total-body PET scans performed on 84 volunteers, was completed in the subsequent 30 days. The resulting information was used to meet the request of product registration in China. Finally, uExplorer was approved by the China Food and Drug Administration in December 2019.

The advantages of total-body PET/CT compared with conventional PET/CT, such as high-sensitivity total-body dynamic scanning, and its potential clinical applications, such as short-duration scanning, low-dose imaging, and radiotracer kinetic studies throughout the entire body have been previously introduced.[1,2] How then to maximize its advantages in the clinical space? There are currently no guidelines or clinical application experiences available for reference. We have explored how to use the total-body PET/CT scanner best in clinical practice based on our knowledge and experience. We share our initial experience and some typical cases as follows.

TOTAL-BODY PET/COMPUTED TOMOGRAPHY IMAGING

A conventional PET/CT scan usually covers a scan range from the vertex to the mid-thigh with 4 to 6 bed positions, depending on the height of the patient and the axial length of the scanner. A longer scan range of the entire body should be used as necessary according to the patient's medical history or physical examination.[3] The uEXPLORER PET/CT scanner with an axial field of view (AFOV) of 194 cm can cover the entire body (from vertex to toe) in one bed position for most patients. Total-body PET/CT imaging can then provide more information to improve the diagnostic accuracy and evaluate the patient's status more objectively. Compared with conventional PET/CT scanners, total-body PET/CT imaging can provide complementary information, such as detection of unsuspected lesions

(**Fig. 1**), and incidental findings not directly related to the disease for which the patient was scanned (**Fig. 2**).

HIGH-QUALITY PET IMAGING

PET examination primarily provides functional imaging. Along with offering an aligned anatomic image for correlation, the CT component can supply information for PET attenuation correction. Many factors affect PET image quality. For example, conventional PET scanners only have an AFOV of 15 to 30 cm, which restricts the detection efficiency for coincidence events emitted from the patient. This results in noisy PET images, which must be smoothed, leading to poorer resolution. Although conventional PET imaging can meet the clinical need in most cases, there is no doubt that the low level of coincidence detection efficiency limits its ability to detect small lesions or lesions with low avidity for the radiotracer. Total-body PET, with its extra-high sensitivity can acquire enough coincidence events to reconstruct sufficiently high-quality images to detect such small or low-avidity lesions, and provide both more functional and anatomic information than conventional PET in reasonable acquisition times (**Fig. 3**). We have found that this higher image quality provides more accurate information for diagnosis or evaluation (**Fig. 4**); however it should be noted that in the areas of the lower lung and upper abdomen, image quality remains compromised by respiratory motion.

LOWER DOSE INJECTION OR SHORTER ACQUISITION TIME

It has been reported that the total-body PET imaging geometry with time-of-flight effects included could provide gains of up to 40-fold in effective count rate for total-body applications compared with a conventional 22-cm axial FOV scanner.[4,5] The high sensitivity of total-body PET scanners provides more choices for nuclear medicine physicians, such as use of low injected activity or short scan duration. Lower administered activity requires longer scan times, and conversely, a shorter scan time requires a larger administered activity.[6] In our department, we use 3 protocols for uEXPLORER, a regular dose (3.7 Mbq/kg) with 0.5 to 2 minutes of scan duration, a low-dose (1.85 Mbq/kg) with 3 to 5 minutes of scan duration, and an extra low dose (0.37 Mbq/kg) with 7 to 15 minutes of scan duration. The protocol and acquisition time are selected according to the patient's health condition, the nature of the disease, and the purpose of the examination. In

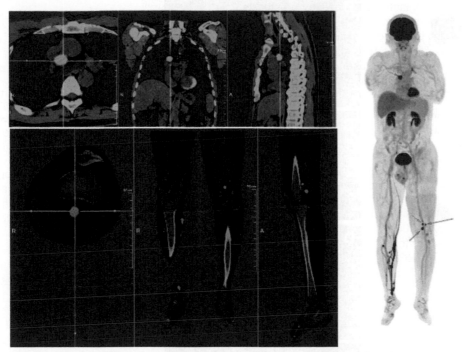

Fig. 1. Left feet melanoma with lymph nodal metastases in left popliteal fossa and mediastinum. A 60-year-old man with history of melanoma. Status post left thumb and second toe resection, popliteal fossa lymph node dissection performed 8 months ago. PET/CT imaging (dose 3.7 Mbq/kg, acquisition time 5 minutes) demonstrated an FDG avid lymph node in mediastinum and a group of FDG avid lymph nodes in left popliteal fossa. Ultrasound-guided bronchoscopy biopsy of the mediastinal lymph showed metastatic melanoma.

most cases, the image quality is good enough for clinical application using our regular protocols. Although the low-dose protocol (1.85 Mbq/kg and 10-minute scans) is the first choice in our department, as the image quality is very good with reasonable scan time (see **Figs. 3** and **4**), in some cases it is preferred to lengthen the acquisition time to get more reliable information for evaluation of the disease, especially for the liver (see **Fig. 4**). The image quality of extra low dose (0.37 Mbq/kg) with 7 to 15 minutes of scan time is sufficient for diagnosis. However, more cases are required to verify the sensitivity and accuracy of this approach in the clinical practice.

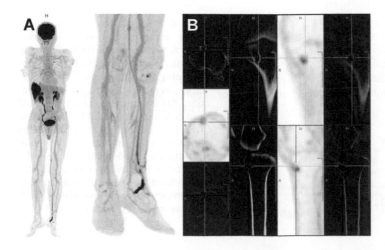

Fig. 2. A patient with cholangiocarcinoma and a benign tumor in right tibia plateau. A 63-year-old man with a liver mass found on CT. Total-body 18F-FDG PET/CT (dose 3.7 Mbq/kg, acquisition time 5 minutes) was performed for further evaluation. Multiple liver lesions were found and pathologic diagnosis on the hepatic segmentectomy specimens demonstrated high-grade intrahepatic cholangiocarcinoma. At the time of the staging PET/CT scan, incidentally, a small FDG avid focus was found located in right tibial plateau (A). Combining with diagnostic CT images (B) the lesion was diagnosed as a benign lesion.

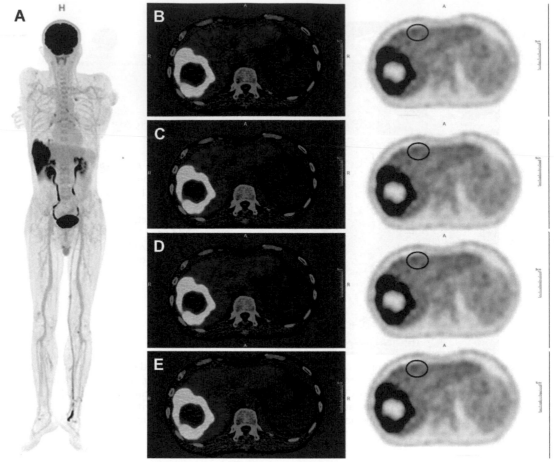

Fig. 3. Liver noise decreases by increasing acquisition time. The same patient as in **Fig. 2**. Acquisition times were 1 (*A* and *B*), 3 (*C*), 5 (*D*), and 10 (*E*) minutes, from top to bottom, respectively. There are a number of foci in the liver parenchyma apparent in the short-duration images (eg, within the oval) that resolve on the longer duration images, indicating that they are caused by noise.

EXTENDED UPTAKE TIME IMAGING

It has been recommended that ^{18}F-FDG-PET scanning should be performed after 50 to 60 minutes of uptake time.[6] However, the contrast between lesion and the background of the PET images acquired at this time point may not be optimal because the background activity is still high. Usually, the FDG accumulated in the lesion

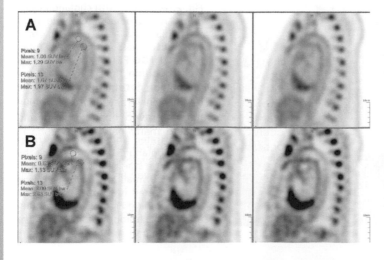

Fig. 4. Delayed imaging provides more accurate diagnostic information. A 19-year-old girl with Takayasu Arteritis underwent FDG PET/CT (dose 3.7 Mbq/kg, acquisition time 15 minutes) to evaluate status of inflammation. PET images acquired 2 hours (*A*) and 5 hours (*B*) after FDG injection. The blood pool activity decreases (standardized uptake value mean [SUVmean] 1.06–0.63) while the aortic wall FDG avidity increases (SUVmean from 1.61 to 2.00). The ratio between aortic wall and blood pool activity increases from 1.57 to 3.17.

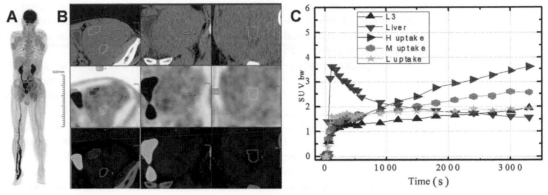

Fig. 5. Differences in FDG avidity within the tumor mass reflects tumor heterogeneity. A 63-year-old man with mantle cell lymphoma underwent 60-minute dynamic total-body PET/CT scan for evaluation of disease status (*A* and *B*). The TACs extracted from regions of interest in different areas in the tumor mass demonstrate the tumor heterogeneity. From the TACs (*C*), it can be seen that the radiotracer delivery was likely the same across the mass but the FDG uptake rate in different areas was different.

increases while distribution in the background (blood pool or normal tissue) decreases with increasing uptake duration. Therefore, delaying the start of PET imaging may allow for greater contrast between the organs or lesions of interest and surrounding structures,[7] and thus improved lesion detectability. However, the total count rate from the patient body decreases with time, which acts to increase noise and thus to decrease lesion detectability. Due to the limited sensitivity of the conventional PET scanners, delayed imaging should be performed within 2 hours after the injection, whereas the ultra-high sensitivity of the uEXPLORER can provide the possibility to acquire images with a 5-hour uptake time to generate images with both high tissue-to-background ratio and manageable noise levels (**Fig. 5**).

TOTAL-BODY DYNAMIC STUDY

It is well known that the dynamic study could provide information for accurate tracer kinetic analysis in studies of physiology, biochemistry, and pharmacology.[1,8] We performed 15 minutes to 75 minutes total-body dynamic acquisition in complex cases according to the clinical information. In clinical practice, time activity curves (TACs) were

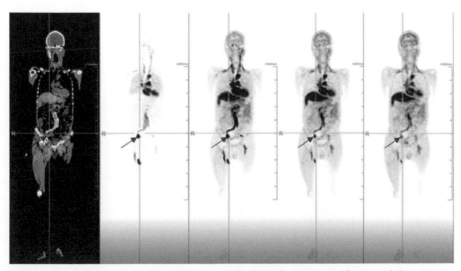

Fig. 6. Radiotracer angiography. A 71-year-old man with clipped aneurysm of internal iliac artery underwent total-body PET/CT scan. The dynamic imaging demonstrated that blood flow existed in the aneurysm at the arterial phase.

calculated by drawing regions of interest in different lesions or different areas of the same lesion to get the information of tumor biological characteristics (**Fig. 6**). Dynamic imaging can also be used as radiotracer angiography to recognize the blood vessel disease.

Perspectives

We have found that the total-body PET/CT scanner (uEXPLORER) with its distinguished physical performance meets multiple current clinical needs; and it provides many potential future application areas. Its clinical application right now is in its infancy and the best clinical performance of total-body PET/CT remains to be determined by means of close cooperation between nuclear medicine physicians and physicists.

DISCLOSURES

Dr. Ying Wang is an employee of United Imaging Research. The other authors working with Zhongshan Hospital have full control of the data and declare that they have no conflict of interest.

REFERENCES

1. Badawi RD, Shi H, Hu P, et al. First human imaging studies with the EXPLORER total-body PET scanner. J Nucl Med 2019;60(3):299–303.

2. Zhang X, Cherry SR, Xie Z, et al. Subsecond total-body imaging using ultrasensitive positron emission tomography. Proc Natl Acad Sci U S A 2020;117(5): 2265–7.

3. Osman MM, Chaar BT, Muzaffar R, et al. 18F-FDG PET/CT of patients with cancer: comparison of whole-body and limited whole-body technique. AJR Am J Roentgenol 2010;195(6):1397–403.

4. Poon JK, Dahlbom ML, Moses WW, et al. Optimal whole-body PET scanner configurations for different volumes of LSO scintillator: a simulation study. Phys Med Biol 2012;57:4077–94.

5. Badawi RD, Poon JK, Surti S, et al. EXPLORER, an ultrasensitive total-body PET scanner: application feasibility simulations. Paper presented at: the World Molecular Imaging Congress, Savannah,Georgia, USA, September 18–21, 2013.

6. Boellaard R, Delgado-Bolton R, Oyen WJ, et al. FDG PET/CT: EANM procedure guidelines for tumour imaging: version 2.0. Eur J Nucl Med Mol Imaging 2015;42(2):328–54.

7. Chan WL, Ramsay SC, Szeto ER, et al. Dual-time-point (18)F-FDG-PET/CT imaging in the assessment of suspected malignancy. J Med Imaging Radiat Oncol 2011;55:379–90.

8. Rahmim A, Lodge MA, Karakatsanis NA, et al. Dynamic whole-body PET imaging: principles, potentials and applications. Eur J Nucl Med Mol Imaging 2019; 46(2):501–18.

Update on the PennPET Explorer
A Whole-body Imager with Scalable Axial Field-of-View

Austin R. Pantel, MD, MSTR, Varsha Viswanath, PhD, Joel S. Karp, PhD*

KEYWORDS

- Positron emission tomography • Whole-body imager • EXPLORER • Human imaging
- Instrumentation

KEY POINTS

- Performance testing of the prototype PennPET Explorer, with a 64-cm axial field of view, validated many of the theoretic benefits of a long axial field-of-view scanner.
- The prototype PennPET Explorer produced images of higher quality than a commercial positron emission tomography scanner with standard axial FOV. The ability to image with less injected activity and with shorter scan duration also was realized.
- The PennPET Explorer recently has been expanded to an axial field-of-view of 1.12 m, with excellent results in preliminary performance testing and a human study.
- Future studies with the PennPET Explorer will focus on optimizing the performance of the scanner for total-body imaging and investigating translational applications.

INTRODUCTION

Advances in positron emission tomography (PET) instrumentation have revolutionized clinical PET imaging. Modern PET scanners can image the entire body over multiple bed positions, typically in 10 minutes to 15 minutes, enabling efficient molecular characterization of disease. Ultimately, however, the limited axial field of view (AFOV) of commercial scanners limits overall sensitivity and the ability to image disparate organ simultaneously.[1]

Motivated by the theoretic benefits of an increased AFOV, the National Institutes of Health–funded EXPLORER Consortium led to the development of 2 total-body (TB) scanners[2]: the PennPET Explorer, based at the University of Pennsylvania, and the uEXPLORER, based at University of California, Davis. Herein, the PennPET Explorer is discussed; the uEXPLORER is

discussed in detail separately in this issue of *PET Clinics*. Both scanners are based on technology from commercial PET scanners with collaboration from industry partners: United Imaging Healthcare (Shanghai, China) for the uEXPLORER and Philips Healthcare (Cleveland, Ohio) for the PennPET Explorer. Although the 2-m AFOV of the uEXPLORER makes it truly a total-body imager and is greater than that of the AFOV of the PennPET Explorer, both instruments image all major organs in the body with high sensitivity in a single bed position.[3-6]

The PennPET Explorer, the long AFOV PET scanner housed at the University of Pennsylvania, has completed initial preliminary testing of a prototype configuration. Many of the underlying benefits of such an extended AFOV instrument have been realized, both with physical measurements and early human studies.[5,6] Impelled by such results, the PennPET Explorer

Funding: NIH R01-CA206187, R01-CA113941, R01-CA225874, and KL2TR001879.
University of Pennsylvania, 3620 Hamilton Walk, 154 John Morgan Building, Philadelphia, PA 19104, USA
* Corresponding author.
E-mail address: joelkarp@pennmedicine.upenn.edu

1556-8598/21/© 2020 Elsevier Inc. All rights reserved.

currently is being expanded from 3 rings to 6 rings for an AFOV of 1.4 m. Recently, evaluation of both phantom and human imaging, with 5 rings and an AFOV of 1.12 m, has been performed.

In this article, the development of the PennPET Explorer is summarized. Initial designs considerations, including the choice of AFOV, is examined. Performance evaluation and human imaging of the system to its current AFOV are described.

DESIGN CONSIDERATIONS

Based on a scalable design, the PennPET Explorer is composed of individual ring segments, enabling interim testing of the system with any number of rings, up to its final configuration of 6 rings. Each ring measures 76.4 cm in diameter and 22.9 cm axially, with 16.4 cm of active detectors. Gaps between the rings enable an overall AFOV greater than the sum of its component ring segments (eg, the prototype 3 ring system had gaps of 7.6 cm between each ring, noting a sensitivity cost, described later).[5]

The PennPET Explorer utilizes a detector tile of 64 lutetium-yttrium oxyorthosilicate scintillation crystals, the same detector tile as the commercial Philips Vereos PET-CT scanner. An 8 × 8 array of crystals is coupled to a digital silicon photomultiplier composed of 16 dies of 4 pixels so that 1:1 crystal-sensor coupling is realized. Improved timing performance with the PennPET Explorer is achieved though cooling the detector modules to 5°C, lower than the 18°C of the commercial Philips Vereos. Sensor calibration can be performed for each ring simultaneously in approximately an hour and does not need to be recalibrated routinely.[5]

Philips Vereos electronic components are utilized similarly. With each ring performing independently, data are collected first on independent solid-state drives on each ring with minimal dead time and then combined into a time-sorted coincidence list data set. Image reconstruction is performed with time-of-flight list-mode ordered subset expectation maximization into 2-mm³ voxels for whole-body imaging. Smaller voxels, for example 1 mm³, may be utilized for studies that emphasize detailed structures, such as those in the brain.[5]

PERFORMANCE CHARACTERIZATION OF PennPET EXPLORER PROTOTYPE

A prototype 3-ring scanner was first tested to study the capabilities of an extended AFOV system, noting the scalable design enables incremental expansion. With an active 64-cm AFOV, an acceptance angle of ±40° was achieved in the center of the AFOV; gaps between rings, however, decrease the overall sensitivity by a factor of 2. Despite this limitation, a total sensitivity of 54 kilocounts per second (kcps)/MBq was achieved with a 70-cm line source at a radius of 0 cm and 57 kcps/MBq at a radius of 10 cm, far surpassing the sensitivity of commercially available scanners.[5]

Additional performance measures validated the system design. The trues count rate increased linearly over a range up to 40 kBq/mL, far greater than a dose that would be administered for a clinical study, with a stable scatter fraction of 32%. The noise-equivalent count rate increased consistently over the entire range, measuring greater than 1000 kcps, with activities greater than 30 kBq/mL. The full system timing resolution 256 ps was measured, with only a modest loss (10–15 ps) when compared with the intrinsic timing resolution of individual ring segments. A spatial resolution of 4.0 mm was achieved in the center of the field of view. Lesion torso phantom experiments demonstrated the ability of the PennPET Explorer to accurately quantify lesional uptake with scans shorter than 1 minute and with acceptable noise.[5] Satisfactory physical performance provided the impetus to move forward with early human testing of the device. It was fortuitous that the standard National Electrical Manufacturers Association (NEMA) phantoms could be used for these measurements, because the prescribed sensitivity line and scatter/count-rate phantom are both 70 cm long. For total-body PET scanners with AFOV greater than 70 cm, specifically, the uEXPLORER and the current configuration of the PennPET Explorer, these NEMA measurements need to be reconsidered. The authors are in agreement with some of the proposals put forth in Spencer and colleagues[3] that these phantoms should be extended to the length of an average adult (170–175 cm) in order to provide a more realistic characterization of the performance benefits of TB-PET scanners.

CHOICE OF AXIAL FIELD OF VIEW

In designing long AFOV systems, the choice of axial FOV becomes paramount. The benefit of imaging the entire body simultaneously must be tempered against clinical/research needs, incremental physical performance gains, and cost.

Clearly, a 2-m AFOV, such as that with the uEXPLORER, enables imaging of the entire body of the vast majority of patients, given an average height of approximately 160 cm to 175 cm.[7] Most malignancies, however, do not routinely affect the distal extremities, and the entire brain often is not included in the AFOV in fluorodeoxyglucose (FDG)-PET oncologic imaging due to reduced sensitivity secondary to physiologic uptake. The majority of FDG-PET scans are performed from the skull base to thigh.[8] A whole-body scan is performed for certain malignancies—including cutaneous lymphomas and melanomas—but these represent a minority of total PET scans performed. A whole-body imager capable of scanning the skull base to thighs in a single bed position should suffice for most oncology indications. For neurologic imaging, the entire brain is contained within the AFOV of a single bed position, so benefits of a long AFOV scanner mostly are secondary to performance gains and possibly for kinetic applications. Axial coverage must be considered in the context of performance gains, described later.

The sensitivity of extended FOV scanners varies with axial position in the scanner and should be matched to clinical/research indication. As discussed in the article by Daube-Witherspoon and Cherry, "Scanner design considerations for long axial field-of-view PET systems," in this issue, and also by Surti and colleagues,[1] the axial sensitivity is peaked at the center of the scanner but is relatively flat due to attenuation of oblique lines of response through the body. Thus, the sensitivity gains at the center of the scanner do not markedly improve beyond a 70-cm AFOV, noting this AFOV was approximately the coverage provided by the prototype PennPET Explorer, discussed previously. Expanding a scanner beyond 70 cm, however, does increase the axial extent where high sensitivity is maintained. For example, a 140-cm AFOV scanner, the planned final AFOV of the PennPET Explorer, maintains high sensitivity across the central 80 cm of the AFOV, enabling high-sensitivity imaging of the majority of organs in the field-of-view.[1] Scanning with a limited number of bed positions (eg, 2–3) with a long AFOV scanner of modest axial length, for example, less than 1 m, can mitigate sensitivity losses at the periphery of the AFOV, although at the expense of increased scan time.

Scanner cost has an impact on scanner design, and, ultimately, adoption of this technology as a clinical or research tool. Increased sensitivity with resultant decreased scan time can improve clinical throughput, justifying such an investment. As a research tool, initial costs may limit such scanners to large academic institutions. Modifications of long AFOV scanners—such as sparse arrangement of crystals, using less detectors, or utilizing alternative materials, for example,

Bismuth germanate (BGO) or plastic scintillators—may decrease costs further and drive a broader dissemination of TB-PET and a wider adoption of this technology.[1]

HUMAN STUDIES ON THE PROTOTYPE PennPET EXPLORER

Following the physical performance studies, described previously, human subjects were imaged on the PennPET Explorer (detailed by Pantel and colleagues[6]). Specific imaging protocols were tailored to investigate potential applications of this long AFOV scanner. Healthy patients were imaged first, followed by patients with disease and subjects imaged with research radiotracers.

To facilitate direct comparison with state-of-the-art PET, subjects were imaged on the PennPET Explorer after standard-of-care PET imaging. The example in **Fig. 1**, a 16-minute scan on the PennPET Explorer, was considered to have superior imaging quality compared with the clinical PET scan with similar scan duration and matched reconstruction parameters. PennPET images demonstrate structural detail not easily seen on standard-of-care (SOC) scans; for instance, vessels walls, delineation of muscles, and vertebral body detail are appreciated on the PennPET Explorer. Images of the brain with the PennPET Explorer demonstrate qualitatively better definition of the basal ganglia compared with SOC imaging. Such detailed PET images may enable better delineation of disease. In a subject with metastatic colon cancer, FDG-PET imaging with the PennPET revealed an epiphrenic lymph node that was not appreciated on SOC imaging.[6] Increased sensitivity for detection of disease may be of particular importance in identifying sites of disease in biochemically recurrent prostate cancer with ^{18}F-fluciclovine or prostate-specific membrane antigen agents.

Such a scanner can be used to produce qualitatively superior images due to the increased count statistics, or, alternatively, the high sensitivity of the PennPET Explorer can be leveraged to image with shorter scan durations or with lesser injected activity. The PennPET Explorer scan subsampled to emulate a 2-minute scan demonstrated comparable, if not superior, image quality than the full SOC PET. To demonstrate this difference in sensitivity, subsampling the SOC PET to the same 2-minute scan resulted in marked image degradation. On the PennPET, transverse imaging through the liver demonstrated preserved image quality in scans as short as 37 seconds. If injected activity is maintained, shorter scans may be obtained, increasing clinical throughput. A clinical subject

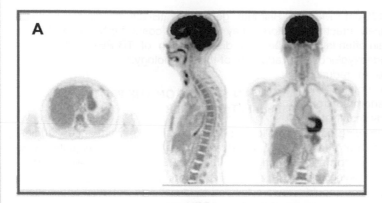

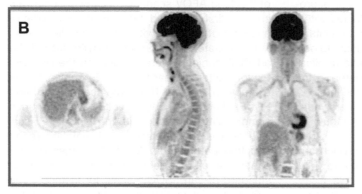

Fig. 1. (*A*) FDG scans of normal subject acquired on the prototype Penn-PET Explorer with 3 rings and 64-cm AFOV. The scan was acquired for 16 minutes after a 15-mCi dose at 1.5 hours postinjection. (*B*) The list data were filtered to extract one-eighth the counts to emulate a 2-minute scan.

with metastatic neuroendocrine tumor demonstrated similar, if not superior, image quality with ^{68}Ga-DOTATATE–PET imaged at 3.5 hours postinjection compared with 65 minutes postinjection on the commercial scanner, although only one-fifth of the activity was present at the time of scanning on the PennPET Explorer compared with the SOC scan.[6] Given relatively stable kinetics of ^{68}Ga-DOTATATE over this time interval,[9] preserved image quality on the delayed PennPET is secondary to differences in scanner performance and not radiotracer distribution. Delayed imaging with FDG, as described in the clinical patient, discussed previously, leverages both inherent advantages of the scanner and a favorable kinetic profile with trapping of FDG in malignancy.[6]

In particular, these studies demonstrate that with an AFOV of 64 cm, the head and abdomen can be imaged in a single bed position with high sensitivity or, alternatively, neck to pelvis, as is typical for routine SOC imaging. The high count-rate capability of the PennPET Explorer and extended AFOV both benefit dynamic image analysis as well as static imaging. The large AFOV ensures the inclusion of large vascular structure in the AFOV for an image-derived input function. With fine temporal sampling afforded by increased count statistics, relatively noise-free input curves

can be constructed, as shown in the article by Viswanath and colleagues, "Analysis of 4D data for total-body PET imaging," in this issue. The blood input function curves demonstrate the expected transit of the radiotracer through the vasculature. As the radiotracer bolus moves distally, partial-volume effects and dispersion become apparent. The selection of different arterial input function ultimately may affect kinetic parameter estimation for dynamic studies, necessitating correction if only a small vasculature structure is contained within the AFOV, as may be the case with conventional scanners. The ability of the PennPET Explorer to capture an arterial input function as well as time activity curves for all lesions in 1 AFOV represents a significant increase in the ability to analyze the whole-body kinetics of radiotracers.[6]

Two experimental research radiotracers were imaged on the PennPET Explorer after imaging on the standard-of-care PET scanner. Imaging of ^{18}F-NOS on the PennPET demonstrated unexpected ocular uptake of the radiotracer. The head was excluded from the AFOV of the research scan, which studied uptake of this radiotracer in the lungs. This finding underscores the potential advantage of including the entire body in early studies with a new radiotracer. Lastly, a subject was imaged with ^{18}F-fluortriopride. Prior dosimetry studies demonstrated that the gallbladder wall received the highest radiation dose, and stimulation of gallbladder contraction with a fatty meal can decrease the absorbed dose.[10] Dynamic imaging performed after the subject drank Ensure (Abbott Laboratories; Abbott Park, IL, USA) demonstrated gallbladder emptying, as expected. These research studies support the utility of the PennPET Explorer in imaging research tracers with increased sensitivity and demonstrate the potential of a scanner with axial coverage of 64 cm or greater for dynamic imaging of multiple organs.

RECENT PROGRESS: EXPANSION OF THE PennPET EXPLORER FROM THE PROTOTYPE CONFIGURATION

The initial imaging studies on the prototype PennPET Explorer validated many of the theoretic benefits of a long AFOV scanner. Image quality of the PennPET Explorer exceeded that of a commercial PET scanner and could be leveraged for several clinical and research indications.[6] These initial experiments provided the impetus to expand the PennPET Explorer from the prototype configuration in the laboratory to its final form in a dedicated imaging suite.

The prototype PennPET Explorer was constructed in the laboratory of the Physics and Instrumentation Group in the Department of Radiology at the University of Pennsylvania, facilitating physical performance testing and development as well as enabling the early human studies. After the successful initial testing, described previously, the instrument was disassembled and rebuilt in a new

imaging suite in the University of Pennsylvania School of Medicine, close to the Cyclotron Facility, to facilitate delivery of radiotracers. Two additional rings and a dedicated computed tomography (CT) scanner since have been added to the prototype. A recent picture of the PennPET Explorer is shown in **Fig. 2** before the covers are added.

Note that the initial imaging studies, described previously, necessitated a separate CT performed in the clinic and registered to the PET image to provide for attenuation correction. With approximately 950 ft^2 of space, the dedicated imaging suite contains a hot laboratory and uptake room, obviating measuring the dose in the clinic prior to injection. An uptake room and bathroom further established the new space as independent of the clinic. The relatively close distance to the clinic, however, enhances the ability to scan subjects after imaging on SOC PET. A 1.4-m PET with integrated CT can fits in a typical PET scan room, facilitating integration of such a machine into existing infrastructure; this scanner room is 400 ft^2, 27 ft × 15 ft. In contrast, a 2-m AFOV scanner may necessitate a room larger than currently is used for SOC commercial PET scanners.

With a total of 5 rings, the AFOV of the PennPET Explorer has been expanded to 1.12 m. Performance evaluation of this updated configuration is ongoing to demonstrate the enhanced capability afforded by higher sensitivity and larger axial coverage. Shown in **Fig. 3** are representative phantom studies performed to validate the upgrade data processing software with the expanded axial length and unrestricted acceptance angle (±56°). These initial studies also are used to validate the quantitative accuracy of the

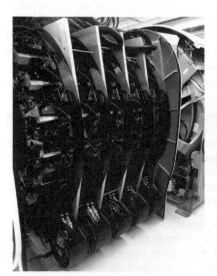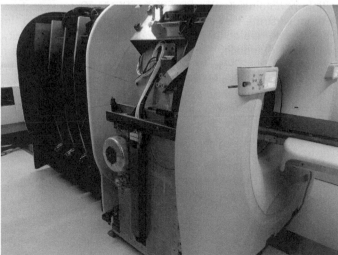

Fig. 2. PennPET Explorer in current configuration (without cosmetic covers) with 5 rings for an AFOV of 1.12 m, together with in-line CT scanner.

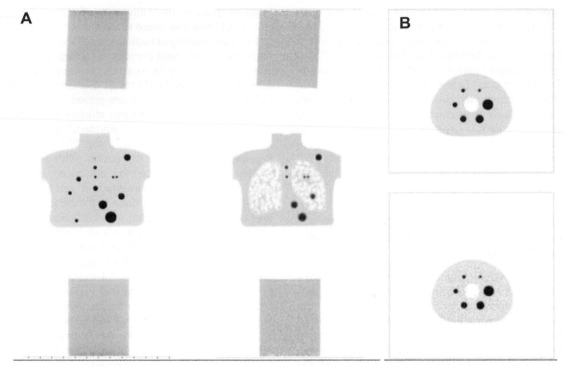

Fig. 3. (*A*) Maximum intensity projection (MIP) (*left*) and representative 2-mm thick coronal image (*right*) of the CTN torso phantom, with lesions ranging from 7 mm to 37 mm. Because the axial length of the CTN phantom is only 29 cm, 2 additional 20-cm× 30-cm phantoms are included to fill the 1.12 m AFOV of PennPET Explorer. (*B*) NEMA Image Quality (IQ) phantom with lesions ranging from 10 mm to 37 mm (*top*). Transverse image (2-mm thick) of 30-minute scan and (*bottom*) 3-minute scan. The NEMA specification dictates a 30-minute scan to cover 1 m.

images and SUV calibration and help to design the dose and scan protocols for human imaging studies. The axial image of the Clinical Trials Network (CTN) torso phantom underscores the fact that currently there are not phantoms to routinely measure performance over a large AFOV, and these tests must be constructed with multiple phantoms. The images of the NEMA IQ phantom illustrate that excellent quality and low noise behavior are achieved in 3 minutes (NEMA background variability ranges from 9.0% to 3.3% for 10-cm–37-cm spheres), whereas the prescribed scan duration by NEMA of 30 minutes (to cover 100 cm) leads to unprecedented low noise behavior (background variability ranges from 4.0% to 2.4%). The corresponding CRC values are 40% to 72% for the mean values and 80% to 113% for the maximum values for 10-mm to 37-mm spheres, using the list-mode time-of-flight ordered subset expectation maximization algorithm with reconstruction parameters optimized for human imaging.

Human imaging on this expanded PennPET Explorer recently has begun; the capability with an FDG scan is illustrated in **Fig. 4**. Following the administration of 10 mCi of FDG for the SOC clinical scan, imaging on the PennPET was performed for 10 minutes, with postinjection time of 1 hour and 45 minutes. As seen in **Fig. 4**, the expanded AFOV imaged from the skull vertex to the mid-thighs in this subject of average height (155 cm), capturing all internal organs in the chest, abdomen, and pelvis. Similar to studies on the prototype, excellent anatomic detail was achieved—vessel walls and small brain structures are appreciated. Images of the liver exhibit low noise and uniformity, as expected in normal tissue. These features may enable increased detection of disease in the liver or other organs.

FUTURE STUDIES ON THE PennPET EXPLORER

Future human studies on the PennPET Explorer will further validate the system and test its capabilities. An institutional review board–approved protocol currently enables imaging the following scenarios on the PennPET Explorer:

1. Patients undergoing clinical PET imaging also may be scanned on the PennPET Explorer (ie, imaging the same injected dose). This has been done previously with the prototype device, allowing comparison of the 2 instruments, as described. Imaging on the PennPET

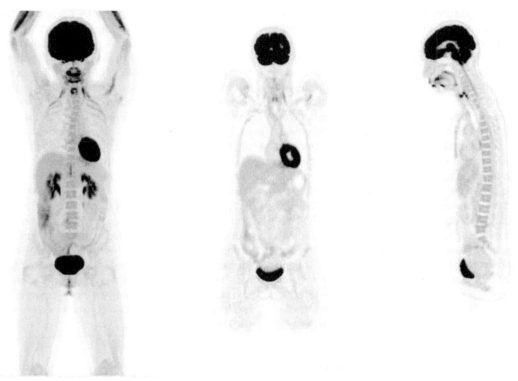

Fig. 4. Representative images of FDG study on PennPET Explorer with 5 rings and 1.12-m AFOV, MIP (*left*), coronal (*middle*), and sagittal (*right*), both 2-mm thick. Scan was acquired after an SOC scan, with 10-mCi dose for 10 minutes at 1 hour and 45 minutes postinjection.

Explorer may take place before or after the SOC clinical scan, or both. A Food and Drug Administration (FDA)–approved radiotracer would be imaged in this application.

2. Subjects enrolled in another research study may be scanned on the PennPET Explorer. This application may image an experimental radiotracer or an FDA-approved radiotracer used for research purposes.

3. Subjects may be imaged with an FDG-approved radiotracer on the PennPET Explorer as a research study. In this scenario, no concomitant imaging would be performed. These studies would be tailored to assess specific features of the PennPET Explorer.

Planned human studies on the PennPET Explorer are described elsewhere in this issue of *PET Clinics*. These studies can be divided into 2 broad groups: (1) studies testing and optimizing the performance of the system for clinical applications and (2) studies investigating research applications of the PennPET Explorer. Through continued feedback between physical performance testing/simulations and human studies, applications of the PennPET Explorer—and long AFOV scanners, in general— should continue to evolve.

As detailed previously, the ability of the PennPET Explorer to image with shorter scan duration/less injected activity and to obtain delayed images previously has been demonstrated. The new PennPET Explorer facility will further facilitate additional studies in these domains. By imaging clinical patients after SOC imaging, the limits of detectability and quantification on the PennPET Explorer can be studied. Breath-hold imaging of 20 seconds to 30 seconds also will be studied on clinical patients with indeterminate lung nodules. Delayed imaging protocols will study the intrinsic ability of the scanner to leverage favorable delayed radiotracer kinetics of FDG to increase lesional contrast and detectability. These studies represent the translation of prior phantom and human studies on the prototype PennPET Explorer that demonstrated clinically acceptable performance for detecting lesions in 1 minute or less in the lung and liver.[11] Patients with varying body habitus will be studied, noting larger patients benefit more from time-of-flight gains.[12] Lastly, incorporation of a joint reconstruction algorithms will be studied,[13] possibly obviating CT and, in combination with low-dose imaging, dramatically reducing radiation exposure. Such a combination could facilitate pediatric imaging and more frequent follow-up in certain clinical settings.

The PennPET Explorer is intended to be used principally as a research tool to facilitate the development of new radiotracers and investigations of underlying causes of disease. The increased sensitivity of the instrument permits more delayed imaging of novel radiotracers, enabling better estimates of radiotracer dosimetry and cell tracking studies. Imaging out to 24 hours after injection of FDG in humans on the PennPET Explorer[6] and to 30 days after injection of ^{89}Zr-antibody, as demonstrated in rhesus monkeys on the mini-EXPLORER PET scanner,[14] support the utility of long AFOV devices for this application. Improved cell tracking studies may have particular use in predicting and monitoring response to immunotherapy, noting increased utilization of these therapies in modern oncology.[15] Furthermore, biodistribution studies of novel radiotracers will benefit from the whole-body coverage of the PennPET Explorer as well as novel studies exploring the interaction of radiotracer between organs.

As a tool to study in vivo biology, the increased sensitivity of the PennPET Explorer may allow for sequential dynamic imaging with 2 PET radiotracers. Phantom and lesion embedding studies with ^{18}F-fluorothymidine on the PennPET Explorer have shown the ability to accurately estimate kinetic parameters, with doses as low as 0.5 mCi to 2 mCi.[16] These studies provide guidance for imaging with a low dose of the first tracer and then injecting a typical dose of a second radiotracer (eg, 10–15 mCi of FDG), to enable imaging sequentially with 2 radiotracers labeled with the same isotope (eg, ^{18}F) so that multiple facets of biology can be measured sequentially. On current state-of-the-art commercial scanners, such studies must be obtained on separate days to allow for decay of the first radiotracer prior to injection of the second. In a research protocol, the authors currently are imaging ^{18}F-fluoroglutamine followed by FDG on a separate day at the University of Pennsylvania but plan to image these radiotracers sequentially in a single session on the PennPET Explorer so that glucose and glutamine metabolism can be assessed simultaneously. Kinetic analysis of dynamic images can further maximize the data yield of the single imaging session.[17]

SUMMARY

Extensive physical performance testing and a small cohort of human studies with the PennPET Explorer demonstrated many of the expected benefits of such a long AFOV PET scanner. These encouraging results include early testing with 3 rings and an AFOV of 64 cm and more recent testing following the expansion of the system to 5 rings with a current AFOV of 1.12 m. The scanner was designed to be scalable, thereby enabling expansion to any number of rings, but the early studies acquired with 3 rings illustrate the power of TB-PET imaging with even a modest AFOV— albeit 2 times to 3 times that of standard clinical PET-CT instruments. Planned studies at the University of Pennsylvania are being designed to leverage the capabilities of the expanded AFOV (1.12 m to 1.4 m) and both clinical and research applications will be explored. These translational studies should further drive instrumentation development, which, in turn, will inform future human studies. Over the next few years, the clinical and research benefits of these powerful scanners should become clear and will help determine the most useful AFOV or optimal range of axial length for TB-PET instruments.

DISCLOSURE

Support for development of the PennPET was received from Philips Healthcare and from the Department of Radiology at the University of Pennsylvania.

REFERENCES

1. Surti S, Pantel AR, Karp JS. Total body pet: why, how, what for? IEEE Trans Radiat Plasma Med Sci 2020;4(3):283–92.
2. Cherry SR, Badawi RD, Karp JS, et al. Total-body imaging: transforming the role of positron emission tomography. Sci Transl Med 2017;9(381):eaaf6169.
3. Spencer BA, Schmall JP, Berg E, et al. Performance evaluation of the EXPLORER Total-body PET/CT scanner based on NEMA NU-2 2018 standard with additional tests for extended geometry. Manchester (United Kingdom): Conference Record of the IEEE NSS/MIC; 2019.
4. Badawi RD, Shi H, Hu P, et al. First human imaging studies with the EXPLORER total-body PET scanner. J Nucl Med 2019;60(3):299–303.
5. Karp JS, Viswanath V, Geagan MJ, et al. PennPET Explorer: design and preliminary performance of a whole-body imager. J Nucl Med 2020;61(1):136–43.
6. Pantel AR, Viswanath V, Daube-Witherspoon ME, et al. PennPET Explorer: human imaging on a whole-body imager. J Nucl Med 2020;61(1):144–51.
7. Fryar CD, Gu Q, Ogden CL, et al. Anthropometric reference data for children and adults: United States, 2011-2014. Vital Health Stat 3 2016;(39):1–46.

8. Boellaard R, Delgado-Bolton R, Oyen WJ, et al. FDG PET/CT: EANM procedure guidelines for tumour imaging: version 2.0. Eur J Nucl Med Mol Imaging 2015;42(2):328–54.

9. Velikyan I, Sundin A, Sörensen J, et al. Quantitative and qualitative intrapatient comparison of 68Ga-DOTATOC and 68Ga-DOTATATE: net uptake rate for accurate quantification. J Nucl Med 2014;55(2): 204–10.

10. Doot RK, Dubroff JG, Scheuermann JS, et al. Validation of gallbladder absorbed radiation dose reduction simulation: human dosimetry of [(18)F] fluortriopride. EJNMMI Phys 2018;5(1):21.

11. Viswanath V, Daube Witherspoon ME, Karp JS, et al. Numerical observer study of lesion detectability for a long axial field-of-view whole-body PET imager using the PennPET Explorer. Phys Med Biol 2020; 65(3):035002.

12. Karp JS, Surti S, Daube-Witherspoon ME, et al. Benefit of time-of-flight in PET: experimental and clinical results. J Nucl Med 2008;49(3):462–70.

13. Li Y, Matej S, Karp JS. Practical joint reconstruction of activity and attenuation with autonomous scaling for time-of-flight PET. Phys Med Biol 2020. https://doi.org/10.1088/1361-6560/ab8d75.

14. Berg E, Gill H, Marik J, et al. Total-Body PET and highly stable chelators together enable meaningful (89)Zr-antibody PET studies up to 30 days after injection. J Nucl Med 2020;61(3):453–60.

15. Pandit-Taskar N, Postow MA, Hellmann MD, et al. First-in-humans imaging with (89)Zr-Df-IAB22M2C Anti-CD8 minibody in patients with solid malignancies: preliminary pharmacokinetics, biodistribution, and lesion targeting. J Nucl Med 2020; 61(4):512–9.

16. Viswanath V, Pantel AR, Daube Witherspoon ME, et al. Quantifying bias and precision of kinetic parameter estimation on the PennPET Explorer, a long axial field-of-view scanner," in IEEE Transactions on Radiation and Plasma Medical Sciences, doi:10.1109/TRPMS.2020.3021315.

17. Mankoff DA, Pantel AR, Viswanath V, et al. Advances in PET diagnostics for guiding targeted cancer therapy and studying in vivo cancer biology. Curr Pathobiol Rep 2019;7(3):97–108.

Scanner Design Considerations for Long Axial Field-of-View PET Systems

Margaret E. Daube-Witherspoon, PhD[a],*, Simon R. Cherry, PhD[b]

KEYWORDS

- Long axial FOV • Scanner design • Time-of-flight

KEY POINTS

- Long axial field-of-view PET scanners offer the simultaneous advantage of greatly increased body coverage in a single bed position and much higher detection sensitivity than on a standard axial field-of-view PET system.
- Long axial field-of-view PET scanners have been developed and demonstrate the performance possible with longer scanners while also highlighting the challenges associated with these systems.
- For clinical applications, the increased detection efficiency allows some combination of increased signal-to-noise ratio in the images, shorter acquisition times, and lower injected activity.
- For research applications, the dynamics of radiotracers across multiple organ systems or even the entire body is now possible.

INTRODUCTION

PET scanner designs have changed markedly over the past 3 decades, with resulting dramatic improvements in image quality. Many of these advances in scanner technology have had a direct impact on the design of recently developed long (≥70 cm) axial field-of-view (AFOV) PET scanners. This article discusses aspects of scanner design of long AFOV systems and how these choices affect system performance.

Three-dimensional Acquisition

With a few exceptions,[1] most scanners built prior to the early 1990s had lead septa between the detector rings that restricted the contributions of random coincidences and scattered photons (within the object) but also resulted in low geometric sensitivity and long scan times, because only true coincidence events emitted within a series of 2-dimensional slices could be detected. Removing the septa and operating as a fully 3-dimensional (3-D) system led to a 3-times to 5-times increase in the probability of detection of true coincidences (sensitivity) by detecting the oblique lines of response (LORs).[2] With this sensitivity gain, however, came a significant increase in detected random and scattered coincidences that required careful attention to their correction. All current-generation PET scanners operate in 3-D with accurate corrections.

Time-of-Flight Information

The measurement of the difference in arrival times (time-of-flight [TOF]) of the 2 annihilation photons at the detectors and the incorporation of this information into the reconstruction as a means to reduce image noise first was proposed in the early 1980s.[3] Incorporating TOF

a Department of Radiology, University of Pennsylvania, 3620 Hamilton Walk, Room 156H, Philadelphia, PA 19104, USA; b Department of Biomedical Engineering, University of California, 451 Health Sciences Drive, Davis, CA 95616, USA
* Corresponding author.
E-mail address: daubewit@pennmedicine.upenn.edu

PET Clin 16 (2021) 25–39
https://doi.org/10.1016/j.cpet.2020.09.003
1556-8598/21/

information into the reconstruction improves the signal-to-noise properties of the image by restricting the back-projection of each event to the location of most probable annihilation based on the TOF difference, rather than assuming uniform probability along the LOR.[4,5] TOF information effectively enhances the sensitivity of the scanner by improving the signal-to-noise ratio of lesions. The scintillator crystals used at that time in PET scanners (bismuth germanate [BGO] and sodium iodide activated with thallium) did not have adequate timing resolution to be useful in these early TOF systems. Instead, available fast scintillators, such as barium fluoride and cesium fluoride, were used.[6–8] These scintillators, however, have reduced stopping power and light output, so the early TOF-PET systems had overall lower sensitivity and worse spatial and energy resolutions than non-TOF scanners at the time.

Scintillators and Photomultipliers

The introduction of cerium-doped lutetium-based scintillators, such as lutetium oxyorthosilicate (LSO)[9] and lutetium-yttrium oxyorthosilicate (LYSO), allowed for better TOF resolution due to their faster decay constant (40 ns compared with 300 ns for BGO), in addition to a high stopping efficiency that is close to that of BGO. The lutetium-based scintillators cost more to produce than BGO, but, starting in the mid-2000s, fully 3-D TOF-PET scanners based on LSO and LYSO were commercialized with TOF resolutions of 450 picoseconds (ps) to 600 ps.[10,11] These systems used arrays of small crystals coupled to large (25–39 mm diameter) photomultipliers (PMTs) that convert the scintillation light into an electrical signal. More recently, TOF resolutions of 215 ps to 250 ps have been achieved when small crystals are coupled to another advancement in PET technology, silicon PMTs (SiPMs).[12–14] SiPMs are more compact than PMTs and some designs use 1-to-1 coupling of crystals to SiPMs, thereby simplifying the calculation of event positions and reducing light losses that result from light sharing across photodetectors.[15] A vast majority of new commercial PET scanners for human use today use lutetium-based scintillators read out by SiPM photodetectors, although many PMT-based systems still are in clinical use.

State-of-the-Art of PET Systems for Whole-body Imaging

Most commercial PET systems are whole-body devices, with a ring diameter of 75 cm to 90 cm and an intended application of static [^{18}F]-fluorodeoxyglucose (FDG) imaging in oncology. The AFOV ranges from 16 cm to 30 cm, and patients usually are scanned in approximately 8 to 10 overlapping bed positions to cover the organs of interest (head to thighs for most oncology patients) in 10 minutes to 20 minutes, with a dose of 370 MBq to 555 MBq of FDG. For dynamic imaging to capture the temporal behavior of radiotracer delivery, uptake, and clearance, patients typically are imaged in a single bed position over the heart for the first few minutes to capture the blood input function and then either moved to image a single bed position with good temporal sampling or cycled through the scanner to capture more distant lesions with coarse temporal sampling.[16,17]

Table 1 summarizes the current-generation commercial SiPM-based PET scanners. The spatial resolution of these systems ranges between 3 mm and 4.5 mm, full-width at half-maximum. As noted in the table, the sensitivities range from 5 kcps/MBq for the 16-cm AFOV Vereos (Philips; Haifa, Israel) to almost 21 kcps/MBq for the 25-cm AFOV Discovery MI (GE Healthcare; Waukesha, WI).

Although the image quality of a standard AFOV PET scanner generally is excellent, there are several imaging scenarios where a longer AFOV would be advantageous.[22,23] A standard AFOV scanner detects only 0.5% to 2% of the emitted coincident events from a 70-cm long line source (as in the standardized National Electrical Manufacturers Association [NEMA] sensitivity measurement[21]) due to its short axial coverage. This relatively low sensitivity makes it difficult to image radioisotopes with a low positron fraction (eg, ^{89}Zr or ^{90}Y) or radiotracers with slower biological clearance (eg, FDG, where delayed imaging beyond the current 1-hour postinjection would enable imaging lesions with higher contrast). In addition, the 1-min/bed position to 3-min/bed position still results in relatively long total scan durations, with the possibility of patient motion and discomfort; imaging with higher sensitivity enables the total scan time to be reduced significantly. It also opens up the possibility of improved imaging in obese patients as well as imaging with reduced injected activity in situations where radiation dose may be considered limiting (eg, pediatric patients and serial studies to assess treatment response).

HISTORY OF LONG AXIAL FIELD-OF-VIEW SCANNERS
Techniques to Increase Sensitivity

One method to increase the sensitivity is to increase the solid angle of detection of the annihilation photons by reducing the diameter of the detector rings; moving the detectors closer to

Table 1
Performance characteristics[a] of selected commercial silicon photomultiplier-based time-of-flight PET scanners

	Philips Vereos[12]	Siemens Vision[13]	GE Discovery MI[14,18]	United Imaging Healthcare uMI 550[19]	Canon Cartesion Prime[20]
Crystal and size (mm^3)	LYSO 3.86 × 3.86 × 19	LSO 3.2 × 3.2 × 20	LYSO 3.95 × 5.3 × 25	LYSO 2.76 × 2.76 × 16.3	Lu-based 4.2 × 4.2 × 20
Axial FOV (cm)	16.4	26.1	20/25	24	27
Sensitivity (70-cm line) (kcps/MBq)	5.7	16.4	13.7/20.8	10.2	13.5
TOF resolution (ps)	332	210	382	372	257
Spatial resolution (@r = 1 cm)	4.0 mm	3.5 mm	4.3 mm	2.9 mm	2.9 mm

[a] Canon, Canon Medical Systems(Tustin, CA); @r=1 cm, at a radius of 1 cm. a Performance specifications following NEMA standard.[21]

the object allows for more coincidences to be detected.[24] This is one rationale for designing PET scanners that are dedicated to specific organ imaging (eg, brain PET or breast PET systems). This happens, however, at the expense of increased detection of unwanted random and scattered coincidences as well as worse spatial resolution due to parallax errors off-center. For whole-body imaging, there is a limit on how much the ring diameter can be reduced as well: in cases of the thorax and abdomen there is little ability to reduce the bore diameter without making it impossible to scan more obese patients.

Another technique to increase sensitivity is to use longer crystals. The mean stopping distance for 511-keV photons in LSO/LYSO is approximately 11 mm, whereas the length of crystals used in most systems is 18 mm to 20 mm. There are diminishing returns in the gain in efficiency as the crystal length is increased,[25] whereas the detector material cost still increases linearly. Only incremental gains in sensitivity can be achieved by lengthening the crystals beyond the approximately 20 mm typically used in today's scanners. Note that the converse is not the case: using shorter crystals to decrease the cost of a system leads to a measurable loss of sensitivity.[25]

Using a different crystal with a higher stopping power than LSO/LYSO is another way to increase the sensitivity of a scanner. However, 20 mm of BGO, one of the most dense scintillators discovered, has only approximately 1.07 times the coincidence detection efficiency as the same thickness of LSO/LYSO. Once more, these gains are fairly incremental. In addition, with every crystal there are potential trade-offs in energy and timing resolutions, ease of growing, cost, crystal handling, and so forth.

Improving the timing resolution of a scintillator also will lead to increased effective sensitivity and reduced image noise for the same number of detected events because TOF reconstruction can localize the events along the LOR rather than spreading them out uniformly. This has been the rationale for PET scanner manufacturers to continue to improve the TOF resolution of their systems from 600 ps for the Gemini TF (Philips), the first commercial TOF PET scanner, to 215 ps for the latest Vision (Siemens; Chicago, IL). It is possible that further significant gains can be made in this area; however, new detector technology, and/or alternative signal generation mechanisms (eg, prompt luminescence from Cherenkov radiation) likely are required.[26]

The most obvious and effective means of significantly increasing the sensitivity of a PET scanner, however, is to make it longer by adding more detectors along the axial direction. By accepting events along more oblique LORs (larger axial acceptance angle) and covering more of the body with detectors, significant increases in detection sensitivity are possible.[27] This is the driving force behind the recent development of long AFOV PET scanners.

Early Long Axial Field-of-View Designs

There have been several proposed designs for long AFOV scanners to increase the system sensitivity. In the early 2000s, several scanners with extended AFOV were proposed using different detector technologies. Watanabe and colleagues developed a 68.5-cm AFOV system based on BGO detectors[28] with coarse septa between block detector rings to reduce detected scatter, because the energy resolution of BGO is poor (36%), although these septa also reduced the sensitivity advantage of the longer AFOV. Conti and colleagues[29] developed a research PET system with a 53-cm AFOV based on 5 large-panel LSO detectors on a rotating gantry. This system had large dead time losses that led to noisy images and lacked TOF capability. Zhang and Wong[30] proposed a 1-m long scanner composed of BGO crystals in a quadrant-sharing arrangement. Because BGO has a long decay time, it was proposed as a non-TOF system, although the estimated sensitivity was higher than that of a standard AFOV TOF PET scanner. Crespo and colleagues[31] proposed a 2.4-m long system with resistive plate chamber detectors as an inexpensive alternative to scintillators. These detectors have a TOF resolution of 300 ps and excellent spatial discrimination but low stopping power and poor energy resolution that reduce the intrinsic sensitivity of the detectors. In the end, however, each of these designs involved compromises in performance, required the long axial coverage to make up for performance losses, or were not cost effective, and they did not become clinical systems.

Simulation Studies

The interest in long AFOV systems, however, sparked several simulation studies to examine the impact on performance of possible design choices. Eriksson and colleagues[32] looked at the impact of both faster scintillators and large AFOV (up to 2.2 m) on system performance and found advantages for subminute whole-body scan times and dynamic imaging. Poon and colleagues[27] also considered the optimal scanner geometry (AFOV and crystal thickness) for a range of crystal volumes with a coincidence timing window that was allowed to vary with ring difference. Surti and colleagues[25] used simulations to study the optimal use of a given amount of crystal material and found the best lesion detectability was for scanners with long AFOV and short crystals. Later work considering optimal detector designs for a 72-cm long scanner for both lesion detection and quantification showed that improving the TOF resolution led to significant gains in performance, while using smaller crystals or depth-of-interaction (DOI) information to reduce parallax errors provided only small gains in detectability.[33] Schmall and colleagues[34] demonstrated that even for a 2-m long scanner, the axial resolution degradation was small compared with radial parallax errors and could be mitigated with 2-layer DOI information, although DOI adds complexity to the detector design.

DETECTOR TECHNOLOGY CONSIDERATIONS FOR LONG AXIAL FIELD-OF-VIEW SCANNERS

This section focuses on choices and trade-offs in selecting detector technology for long AFOV scanners, where care must be taken to ensure the performance is sufficient to allow the predicted benefits of these systems to be realized in clinical studies, while accounting for the challenges in developing such large, complex systems that relate to cost, reliability, and the need to handle very high total event rates.

Crystal Technology

As with conventional PET scanners, lutetium-based scintillators, such as LSO or LYSO, currently are the material of choice for most long AFOV scanners. These currently are the only materials that can deliver sufficient stopping power and also are bright and fast enough to provide timing resolution of a few hundred picoseconds, energy resolutions of approximately 10% to 14%, and relatively low dead time. The disadvantage, which is not an insignificant one, is that these

materials are quite expensive, and, with the large quantities required for long AFOV scanners (0.5 ton or even more), these systems are expensive. Therefore, alternatives are being studied. One interesting possibility is the use of BGO, which emits both scintillation light and, as exploited only recently, prompt Cherenkov radiation emitted by the energetic electrons produced upon absorption of the annihilation photon. The Cherenkov photons can be used to achieve much better timing resolution than was thought possible with this material.[35,36] Although attractive due to its cost (approximately one-third that of LSO or LYSO), a significant challenge remains for how to reliably detect and trigger on the very faint Cherenkov signals with cost-effective electronics.

Photodetector Technology and Detector Designs

SiPMs have become the photodetector of choice for modern PET scanners, and their detection sensitivity for scintillation light, reliability, low-power consumption, low applied voltage, compact form factor, and relatively low cost all are advantages that are further amplified in the setting of long AFOV PET scanners that use very large numbers of these devices.

There are a couple of choices in how SiPMs are used in conjunction with scintillation crystals. The first is known as 1:1 coupling, in which each scintillator crystal element has its own SiPM readout (**Fig. 1**A). This leads to the best performance in terms of light collection, which in turn leads to good timing and energy resolution. Also, the crystal of interaction is simply identified by knowing which SiPM produced the signal. The downside of this approach is that a PET scanner needs a large number of SiPMs, each with its own channel of readout electronics. Conventional scanners have approximately 50,000 crystal elements. This challenge is exacerbated in long AFOV scanners where the number of crystal elements and, therefore, SiPMs required can exceed 500,000.

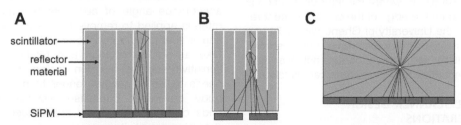

Fig. 1. Schematic cross-section through different types of PET detectors. (*A*) Pixelated with 1:1 coupling; (*B*) pixelated with light sharing using partial reflector coverage along length of crystals; and (*C*) monolithic detector. The red lines indicate sample scintillation light trajectories for a 511-keV photon interaction, demonstrating the light distribution on the SiPMs reading out the scintillator.

An alternative is a light-sharing approach in which an array of scintillation crystals is read out by a smaller number of SiPMs (see **Fig. 1**B). Light produced in each scintillation crystal is allowed to spread across multiple SiPMs (typically by use of a light guide) and the relative signals in neighboring SiPMS then are used to compute the center of the light distribution and thus determine the crystal of interaction. By spreading the light among multiple SiPMs, however, with small gaps between them, the light collection is not as good, and the signals in each SiPM are smaller, compared with 1:1 coupling. Also, the effective area of the detector that is busy while processing an event is larger with this approach, potentially leading to increased overlap of events and dead time at high counting rates. This leads to some degradation in performance, with the benefit, however, of a much-reduced number of SiPMs and channels of electronics. Both these approaches have been implemented successfully in long AFOV PET scanners, as described later.

Alternate Detector Technologies

There is a range of alternate detector technologies being pursued for long AFOV PET scanners, often aimed primarily at reducing cost rather than improving performance relative to existing LYSO/SiPM-based systems. As discussed previously, BGO is being explored as an alternative scintillator material, given its lower cost and higher density that allows using somewhat less material compared with LSO or LYSO for the same detection efficiency. The challenge is to get sufficient timing performance and count rate capability to be competitive with traditional LYSO-based designs. Another approach proposes the use of a monolithic block of scintillator material, read out by an array of SiPMs rather than an array of individual scintillator elements[37] (see **Fig. 1**C). This geometry favors collection of the scintillation light and, therefore, can lead to very good energy and timing resolution. Positioning of each event, however, is more complicated, especially toward the edges of the block, where the light distribution is constrained by the edge of the crystal. Recent results from the University of Ghent, with a 16-mm thick monolithic detector, have demonstrated that excellent performance can be achieved with these detectors when appropriate care is taken.[38]

GENERAL SCANNER DESIGN CONSIDERATIONS
Choice of Axial Field of View

One of the biggest debates as long AFOV PET scanners are being developed is regarding the optimal length of the scanner. There is no right answer, because the question must be framed with respect to the intended application, and currently no comprehensive studies exist that evaluate the cost-to-benefit ratio for a given clinical task as a function of axial scanner length. Therefore, this debate likely will continue unabated for some time to come.

Some of the considerations can be stated clearly. A significant majority of clinical PET studies are for oncology and involve imaging, from eyes to thighs, in order to see distant metastases. Based on anthropometry studies,[39,40] this distance averages approximately 83 cm across the adult population. In the particular case of melanoma, often the entire body from head-to-toe needs to be scanned. The average height (women and men) for the US population is approximately 170 cm, with the 95th percentile at 189 cm for men.

For research studies, and possible future clinical applications of PET, which may involve imaging other systemic diseases (eg, infection) or multiorgan/tissue effects (eg, inflammation), it likely will be important to image at least all the major organs from brain to pelvis (95th percentile length is approximately 97 cm), and in some cases (eg, rheumatoid arthritis) again the entire body may need to be imaged to characterize disease in all the joints. Based on these considerations, the minimum AFOV for single bed position imaging is approximately 85 cm to 90 cm for eyes-to-thighs coverage across the majority of the population, approximately 1 m for coverage of all the vital organs, and close to 2 m for coverage of the entire human body.

Next has to be factored in the sensitivity profile of the PET scanner, which to first order is approximately triangular in shape without attenuation, as shown in **Fig. 2**. If must be accounted for. However, the most oblique LORs traverse a very large amount of tissue and, due to attenuation and scatter, contribute little useful information; with attenuation, the sensitivity profile becomes flatter.[33,34] Therefore, a cut in the axial acceptance angle of approximately 50° to 60° often is applied to remove events at these steep angles that contribute little useful information. To take advantage of high and relatively uniform sensitivity across a given region, the scanner needs to be somewhat longer than the desired body coverage; otherwise, tissues near the ends of the field of view are imaged with low detection sensitivity.

The anthropometry data and the scanner sensitivity profiles, therefore, suggest that to achieve high-sensitivity coverage of all the major

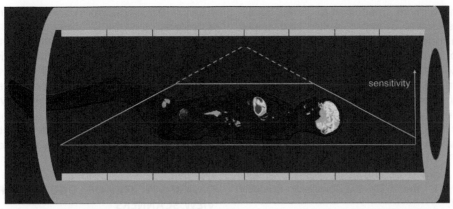

Fig. 2. Schematic showing geometric sensitivity to a point source as a function of axial location for a 2-m long scanner (*dashed line*) and after the axial acceptance angle is restricted to 57° (*solid line*). Profile is superimposed on the image of an average height human subject, demonstrating how an approximately 2-m length ensures very high and uniform sensitivity across all the major organs from brain to pelvis.

organs of the body (brain to prostate/uterus), the scanner would need to have a length of at least approximately 140 cm to image this field in a single bed position (see **Fig. 2**). A shorter length and multibed position imaging may be chosen for cost considerations; however, then the ability to acquire high-quality dynamic data across all the major organs is sacrificed. There remains a range of opinions on the optimal AFOV that largely depend how the value of the increased sensitivity and body coverage as the scanner gets longer are balanced with the trade-off of increasing cost.

One proposed technique to increase the AFOV while controlling costs is to design the scanner with incomplete detector coverage (ie, gaps between detectors in various configurations). A long AFOV TOF-PET scanner with this design would take advantage of the ability of TOF reconstruction to handle missing information better than non-TOF reconstruction.[41,42] Several groups have studied various designs involving incomplete detector coverage,[38,43–49] although few such systems have been built. The tradeoff is a significant loss of sensitivity (often by a factor >2), with axial variations in sensitivity that translate to small differences in noise across the AFOV. The development of these systems largely has been through simulations or extrapolations from standard AFOV systems, although further developments are expected in this area in the future. As discussed later, although not built with missing detectors, the PennPET Explorer scanner currently operates with 7.6-cm axial gaps between rings, thereby demonstrating the feasibility of these designs for total-body PET imaging.

Multimodal Long Axial Field-of-View Scanners

Long AFOV scanners are no different in needing additional information for attenuation and scatter correction that typically come from an integrated CT scanner. Large AFOV coverage benefits from development of low-dose helical CT acquisitions[50] utilizing advanced low-noise x-ray detectors, automatic tube current modulation, optimized beam filtering, and iterative reconstruction as well as denoising methods using deep learning.[51] This is important for low-activity PET applications, where the CT component then becomes the dominant source of radiation dose to the subject.

Another option is to integrate large AFOV PET scanners with MR imaging systems. Although scientifically appealing due to the rich variety of image contrast that then could be assessed by MR imaging, as well as the elimination of the radiation dose from CT, current state-of-the-art MR systems do not have sufficient axial coverage for single bed position imaging of all the major organs. Developing MR imaging systems with a homogeneous magnetic field and the necessary gradients over a meter or more likely would be challenging and expensive. Nonetheless, it is an area that should be studied further.

Technical Design Considerations

There are several technical and engineering considerations in large AFOV scanners. First, the number of components is 5-fold to 10-fold higher than in a conventional PET scanner; therefore, components need to be extremely robust and reliable in order to maintain scanner operations in a busy clinical environment. In addition to careful sourcing and selection of components, tight power regulation and temperature control also are important factors in ensuring scanner stability. Early experience with the 2 long AFOV scanner designs currently in use have demonstrated good reliability of the many detectors and components.

The patient bed also must be designed carefully, especially if a CT scanner is present as part of the system, where deflection of the bed as it moves into the PET field of view, under varying loads, must be avoided or known in order to ensure that the CT and PET are properly spatially registered.

One major difference from conventional PET scanners is the greatly increased length of the tunnel into which the patient is placed. Careful design of the tunnel (eg, lighting and air flow) is desirable to reduce the chance of claustrophobia. Cameras and microphones are helpful for communication with the patient, and, for research studies that may involve on-bed injection and/or blood sampling, access to injection and sampling sites as well as the length and dead space in long tubing require thought and appropriate methods and protocols.

One design simplification in long AFOV scanners is that end shields to reduce scatter from outside the scanner are not necessary if the entire body, or most of the body, is within the field of view of the scanner. Shielding between the CT component and the PET system, however, still may be necessary to avoid the high x-ray flux from CT causing any long-lived luminescence in the PET detectors.

Lastly, the wide range of path lengths through the body dictate the need for variable timing windows. If a body diameter of 40 cm is assumed, the path length that photon pairs travel through the body can range from approximately 40 cm to 70 cm at an axial angle of 60°, requiring that the coincidence timing window is varied according to the path length for best rejection of random coincidences (**Fig. 3**).

DESIGN SPECIFICS OF LONG AXIAL FIELD-OF-VIEW SCANNERS

There currently are 2 operational long AFOV PET scanners: the uEXPLORER, codeveloped by the University of California, Davis (UC Davis), and United Imaging Healthcare (Shanghai, China) and the PennPET Explorer, designed and built at the University of Pennsylvania (UPenn). Both of these efforts were supported through the EXPLORER consortium, which was set up in 2011 to develop long AFOV PET scanners and funded by the National Institutes of Health in 2015. In designing both of these systems, the goal was to maintain the performance of standard AFOV clinical PET scanners (eg, spatial, timing, and energy resolutions) while extending the AFOV in order to explore the potential benefits and applications of these long systems. The optimal AFOV and scanner design is as yet undetermined. Having 2 systems of different designs allows for probing the impact of design characteristics on clinical performance.

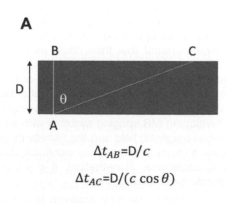

$$\Delta t_{AB} = D/c$$

$$\Delta t_{AC} = D/(c \cos \theta)$$

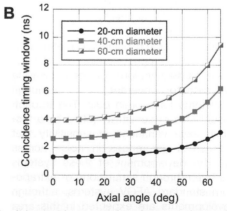

Fig. 3. (A) Illustration of the time needed to capture all valid coincidences arising along a LOR as a function of axial acceptance angle, θ, and object diameter (D). (B) Plot of the coincidence window as a function of angle for different sized objects. It is observed that for very steep angles, the coincidence timing window needed to measure all true coincidences along those LORs increases dramatically; however, these very oblique LORs also are highly attenuated, so few valid coincidences at these angles actually are detected. ΔtAB, transit times for photons traveling between points A and B; ΔtAC, transit times for photons traveling between points A and C; C, speed of light.

Table 2
Performance characteristics of long axial field-of-view time-of-flight–PET scanners

	uEXPLORER[52]	PennPET Explorer[54]
Crystal and size (mm³)	LYSO 2.76 × 2.76 × 18.1	LYSO 3.86 × 3.86 × 19
AFOV (cm)	194	64/112[a]
Sensitivity (70-cm line) (kcps/MBq)	174	54/83
Sensitivity (170-cm line) (kcps/MBq)	147	23/35
TOF resolution	509 ps	256 ps
Spatial resolution (@r = 1 cm)	3 mm	4 mm

[a] Results are reported for the 3/5 ring configurations. @r=1 cm, at a radius of 1 cm.

Table 2 summarizes the performance characteristics of the 2 systems.

uEXPLORER

The uEXPLORER PET/CT scanner (**Fig. 4**) was designed to be the first PET scanner capable of imaging the entire human body at once with an emphasis on extremely high detection sensitivity and spatial resolution.[52] Each detector module consists of a 6 × 7 array of 2.76 mm × 2.76 mm × 18.1 mm LYSO crystals, read out by four 6-mm square SiPMs. These modules are assembled into rectangular panels, which then are arranged in rings to form a scanner with a ring diameter of 78.6 cm and an axial extent of 194 cm. There is a total of 13,440 modules (564,480 crystals) in the entire system. The axial acceptance angle is restricted to 57°, and the timing windows are variable from 4.5 ns to 6.9 ns, depending on the path length across the scanner. The standard energy window is 430 keV to 645 keV. An 80-detector row, 160-slice CT scanner is integrated on the front of the system.

The sensitivity for a 170-cm long line source (which corresponds to the average length of the human body) is 147 kcps/MBq at a radius of 0 cm. For comparison, the sensitivity for a 170-cm long line source on a conventional length scanner would be 2.4 kcps/MBq to 8.6 kcps/MBq, a factor of 17 to 60 lower than the uEXPLORER. The spatial resolution, measured using the standardized NEMA test[21] with simple filtered back-projection reconstruction, is approximately 3 mm and can be improved using more sophisticated iterative reconstruction methods, which are used routinely for clinical scans. TOF resolution, again using NEMA methods, is 509 ps. The system is 510(k) cleared and has been in use for clinical and research studies since August 2018.[53]

PennPET Explorer

The PennPET Explorer scanner (**Fig. 5**) was designed as a scalable system, with an emphasis on high sensitivity with excellent TOF resolution.[54] The PennPET Explorer is based on the detector tile of 64 LYSO crystals currently used in the Philips Vereos PET/CT scanner. Each 8 × 8 array of

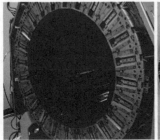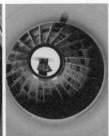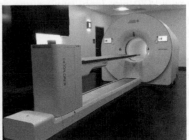

Fig. 4. Photographs of the uEXPLORER total-body PET/CT scanner (*left, middle*) during construction and (*right*) after installation at UC Davis.

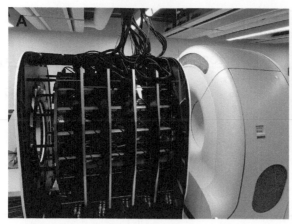
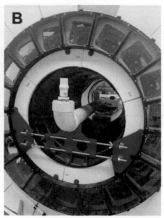

Fig. 5. (*A*) Photograph of PennPET Explorer with 5 detector rings before cosmetic covers have been installed and cabling arrangement completed. An in-line Philips CT (with covers) is to the right of the PET system. The detector rings are mounted on rails and can be moved for maintenance; there is room for the sixth ring at the left end of the imager. (*B*) Photograph of the back of the PennPET Explorer with a 10-cm diameter pipe phantom in place. The electronics for the 18 detector modules are seen behind the acrylic coverings.

3.86 mm × 3.86 mm × 19 mm crystals is coupled to a digital SiPM developed by Philips, Digital Photon Counting. There is 1:1 crystal-sensor coupling. The entire gantry and electronics are water-cooled to allow for superior timing resolution. A detector ring is 76.4 cm in diameter and 22.9 cm axially, comprising 18 modules of 28 detector tiles in a 4 × 7 array. The rings are designed to be stacked axially with a 1-cm physical gap between rings. The prototype 3-ring configuration, for which performance results have been described, was limited to reading out only 5 (of the total 7) rows of tiles in each ring, for a total AFOV of 64-cm and 7.6-cm gaps (corresponding to the 2 inactive rows) between each ring. The transverse FOV is set in software to 57.6 cm. The axial acceptance angle currently is not restricted; the 3-ring prototype had a maximum acceptance angle of ±40°. The scanner is in the process of being extended to 6 rings for a final AFOV of 140 cm, where the maximum acceptance angle will be ±62°.

The sensitivity of the 3-ring prototype PennPET Explorer for a 170-cm long line source is 23 kcps/MBq at a radius of 0 cm; for a 5-ring configuration with an AFOV of 112 cm, the sensitivity has increased to 35 kcps/MBq, a factor of approximately 4-times to 15-times higher than conventional-length scanners. The data readout gaps reduce the total sensitivity by a factor of 2 from what would be achieved with all crystals active. The scatter fraction is 32% and is stable over activity concentrations up to 38 kBq/mL, and the trues rate is linear over this range as well. When cooled to 5°C, the TOF resolution is 256 ps. The spatial resolution is 4.0 mm, using filtered backprojection reconstruction. The scanner has been in use for research studies since August, 2018.[55]

MEASUREMENT OF PERFORMANCE OF LONG AXIAL FIELD-OF-VIEW SYSTEMS

The goal of performance standards for PET is to characterize both intrinsic and overall performance in a reproducible, straightforward way so that systems can be compared meaningfully and performance can be validated against specifications (eg, NEMA NU 2 PET standards[21]). Although measurements of intrinsic performance (ie, spatial resolution, sensitivity, count rate performance, and scatter fraction) are done using activity distributions or reconstruction algorithms that are not clinically relevant, nonetheless, the results are indicative of scanner behavior; for example, a system with low intrinsic sensitivity has higher image noise than one with high sensitivity, although the sensitivity value does not predict the number of acquired events in a clinical scan. This means, however, that the measurements should similarly indicate relative performance for both standard and long AFOV systems, while providing relevant performance metrics that capture system-wide performance.

The NEMA PET scanner performance standards originally were developed in the early 1990s, when it was inconceivable that a scanner would ever be longer than 65 cm, and the tests were designed only to accommodate these shorter systems.[56,57] The spatial resolution is measured with point sources at radial positions of 1 cm and 10 cm, axially positioned at the center of the AFOV and 3/8 of the AFOV from the center. The sensitivity is measured with a 70-cm long line source in a set of 5 aluminum sleeves to measure both total sensitivity and the axial sensitivity profile along the system. Count rate performance and scatter fraction are measured using the same 70-cm long line source but positioned off-center inside a 20-cm diameter polyethylene cylinder. Finally, the image quality phantom is the 18-cm long International Electrotechnical Commission torso phantom positioned with the spheres (diameters: 10–37 mm) at the center of the AFOV with the count rate performance phantom abutted at one end to emulate activity from outside the AFOV of the scanner.

As the scanner AFOV increases, the question arises of how to measure and report the performance of these systems. Simply extending the NEMA phantoms to 2 m long, for example, to cover the largest conceivable PET scanner to date is one possibility. In addition to being extremely cumbersome to fill and handle, however, it is not apparent that these phantoms will provide performance information that is at all relevant to clinical imaging. A typical human is not well-represented by a 20-cm cylinder that is 2 m long; most of the organs of interest are contained within 100 cm to 120 cm, depending on the study, and the average height of a human is approximately 170 cm. Measuring the sensitivity with a source longer than that inflates the number of events that would be present in human imaging, and both UC Davis and UPenn have chosen to measure and report sensitivity for a 170-cm long line source. On the other hand, a 70-cm long line source does not reflect the activity distribution in human imaging, either. As seen in **Table 2**, the sensitivity values for a 170-cm line source are not easily compared with the current NEMA measure with a 70-cm line source. In addition, although a uniform cylinder that extends through the full AFOV is helpful to demonstrate that all corrections work properly throughout the entire scanner, it is cumbersome to handle and difficult to fill uniformly. As seen in **Fig. 5**B, a 10-cm diameter cylinder was used for this purpose on the PennPET Explorer, because it is lighter and more practical than the traditional 20-cm cylinder, although a special apparatus is needed to ensure uniform mixing.

There also are unique performance characteristics of long AFOV systems that warrant measurement. These include axial blurring resulting from the very large axial acceptance angle that can lead to variation in the axial spatial resolution across the AFOV (although simulations[34] and early results[52,54] indicate that the degradation is far smaller than that due to radial parallax errors); increase in multiple scatter events and the impact on the accuracy of the scatter correction, especially at the center of the AFOV; increase in random coincidences and multiple coincidences (>2 photons arriving within the coincidence timing window) and their impact on the maximum activity that should be injected; and sensitivity measured in both air and an attenuating medium because oblique LORs that contribute to the overall increase in total sensitivity when measured in air are more likely to be attenuated by the patient due to their longer pathlengths through the body. In measuring the performance of their long AFOV systems, both UPenn and UC Davis modified and enhanced the NEMA standard measurements to address some of these issues, but further work is needed to reach a consensus on performance measurements that characterize all PET scanners reproducibly and meaningfully.

DATA AND COMPUTATIONAL CHALLENGES WITH LONG AXIAL FIELD-OF-VIEW SYSTEMS

One major consideration related to the use and associated computational infrastructure for long AFOV PET systems derives from the large amounts of data these systems produce and the necessity for robust and reliable procedures for reconstructing, storing, and analyzing these data.

Event Rates and Data Storage

The number of LORs measured by the uEXPLORER scanner, already accounting for the restricted axial acceptance angle, is 92 billion. As the number of possible LORs greatly exceeds the number of events that will be acquired, it, therefore, is most efficient to store the raw data in list mode format rather than binning into projections or sinograms. There also is a trade-off between how much information is retained for each event (for example, is the energy information retained after the energy window has been satisfied?) and the size of the list mode data set.

For a typical clinical scenario (370-MBq injected dose of FDG, 60-minute uptake time), the uEXPLORER registers on the order of 10 million prompt coincidence events per second. A 10-minute scan produces approximately 12 billion prompt events and produces a list mode file of approximately of 200 GB in size. For a 60-minute dynamic acquisition starting from the time of injection, the data set size easily can exceed 1 TB. On the 5-ring PennPET Explorer, where singles data are acquired and processed concurrently in software to form coincidences, an FDG scan with similar injected dose produces approximately 190 GB of singles events for a final coincidence list file that is 70 Gb. It is not certain that the singles list data will be routinely archived, although access to singles information may prove advantageous for data corrections (eg, scatter and randoms). Nevertheless, methods to efficiently move, and potentially archive, these large data sets must be considered.

Image Reconstruction

All modern PET scanners use sophisticated iterative reconstruction methods based on ordered subsets expectation maximization algorithms[58] that permit detailed modeling of the scanner geometry and the statistical nature of the underlying data. There always is a trade-off, however, between the complexity of the modeling and reconstruction time, and nowhere is this more challenging than for long AFOV scanners, which produce high-quality data that would benefit from the most sophisticated modeling approaches, yet at the same time produce large data sets that will be reconstructed into large image volumes, producing severe challenges in terms of computation and memory requirements. For routine clinical purposes, a reconstruction time is required of approximately of a few minutes per scan, and this may require the use of simplifying assumptions within the reconstruction algorithm that may not fully optimize spatial resolution or contrast-to-noise ratio. For research studies, longer reconstruction times may be acceptable; however, these studies also may involve dynamic imaging and produce larger data sets, and reconstruction times (including the need to compute scatter correction files for each frame of a dynamic data set) easily can run into many hours on a high-end computer cluster.

Image Storage and Analysis

Scans from long AFOV PET scanners are often reconstructed into somewhat smaller voxel sizes than on regular scanners, because the higher signal-to-noise ratio supports high-resolution reconstructions. For example, on the uEXPLORER scanner, a typical image matrix size for clinical scans is 256 × 256 × 828 (2.34-mm isotropic voxels); PennPET Explorer images are 288 × 288 × 60 (2-mm isotropic voxels). Although this is not particularly onerous, the

image data set sizes rapidly expand for dynamic studies, exacerbated for long AFOV scanners that can support not only higher spatial resolution but also higher temporal resolution (more frames). For example, a 66-frame dynamic scan on the uEXPLORER results in an image data set size of approximately 7.2 GB that can pose challenges for much of the software developed for analyzing dynamic PET data due to memory limitations.

FURTHER IMPROVEMENTS IN PET SYSTEMS WITH A FOCUS ON LONG AXIAL FIELD-OF-VIEW DESIGNS

Although these first long AFOV systems have verified the large sensitivity gains that were predicted and now are being deployed in a range of clinical and research applications to provide data on the benefits of these sensitivity gains, future improvements clearly are possible. The performance capabilities of the uEXPLORER and PennPET Explorer scanners, both based on existing technology, together with a better understanding of the benefits of long AFOV systems for clinical studies and research investigations, will help form the basis for next-generation systems.

Now that the geometric coverage is close to a maximum; further significant gains in effective sensitivity through instrumentation are going to come only from major improvements in timing resolution. Future approaches or technologies that could push the system timing resolution well below 100 ps would be worthy of pursuit, noting that a timing resolution as good as 20 ps would localize the site of annihilation with sufficient accuracy to eliminate the need for any image reconstruction.[26]

Modest performance improvements also would come from depth-encoding detectors[38] that could reduce or eliminate parallax errors and ensure the spatial resolution is uniform across the field of view as well as new detector materials with better stopping power, especially higher photoelectric cross-sections, which would improve detector efficiency and spatial resolution somewhat.

Electronics, photodetectors, and signal processing are other areas where improvements are possible. For example, the tasks of estimating event position, timing, and energy from detector pulses may be amenable to deep-learning networks, and fast photodetectors possibly with integrated on-chip circuits for optimized timing performance will play an important role in achieving better TOF information. Advanced image reconstruction algorithms that accurately model the physics and statistics of the event formation process, and/or the use of deep-learning approaches during or after image reconstruction,[59] promise further improvements in performance for a given hardware configuration.

Lastly, and justifiably, there will continue to be a focus on detector technologies that can achieve a large AFOV but at a significantly reduced cost. In truth, many of these approaches involve significant sacrifices in sensitivity or other performance parameters, but they still may lead to systems that are adequate for specific and important clinical tasks or research investigations. Approaches being investigated include different detector materials, such as plastic scintillators[60] or resistive plate chambers.[31] As discussed previously, sparse detector configurations also are being pursued, where holes or gaps are introduced to reduce cost[46,47,49] while still providing sufficient data sampling to reconstruct images of the body. One challenge with this approach is that although the cost is approximately linear with detector area, the coincidence efficiency goes as approximately the square of the detector area. Thus, a scanner in which one-fourth of the detectors are removed reduces the cost by approximately 25%, but the coincidence sensitivity is approximately $(0.75)^2 = 0.56$ of its original value, meaning that approximately 44% of the signal will have been lost. This trade-off between cost and sensitivity rapidly becomes unattractive as more detector material is removed.

SUMMARY

Long AFOV PET scanners recently have been built that take advantage of the latest innovations in PET technology. These systems provide extended axial coverage ($\geq$70 cm) that allows coverage of most major organs up to the total body (depending on AFOV) in a single bed position with ultrahigh sensitivity without compromising performance in other areas. The uEXPLORER developed by UC Davis and United Imaging Healthcare and the PennPET Explorer developed at UPenn have demonstrated the performance possible with long AFOV systems while also highlighting the challenges associated with these systems, including design and cost considerations as well as the need for a robust computational infrastructure. As clinical and research experience with long AFOV scanners grows, it is envisioned that long AFOV scanner technology will develop along different paths. Improvements in scanner performance (eg, TOF, energy, and spatial resolutions) will be driven by advances in detection and signal processing technology while systems also will be developed that are more cost-effective using lower cost detectors or sparse detector coverage

to allow for more widespread availability. Long AFOV scanner development still is in its infancy, and its future will depend largely on the observed benefits and unique applications of this very exciting technology.

DISCLOSURE

Dr M.E. Daube-Witherspoon has sponsored research agreements with Siemens Healthcare and Philips Medical Systems. Dr S.R. Cherry has sponsored research agreements with United Imaging Healthcare and Canon Medical Research USA. The University of California, Davis, has a revenue sharing agreement with United Imaging Healthcare.

FUNDING

This work was funded by the National Institutes of Health under grants R01 CA206187 and R01 CA113941.

REFERENCES

1. Karp JS, Muehllehner G, Mankoff DA, et al. Continuous-slice PENN-PET: a positron tomograph with volume imaging capability. J Nucl Med 1990;31: 617–27.
2. Cherry SR, Dahlbom M, Hoffman EJ. PET using a conventional multislice tomograph without septa. J Comput Assist Tomogr 1991;15:655–68.
3. Ter-Pogossian MM, Mullani NA, Ficke DC, et al. Photon time-of-flight-assisted positron emission tomography. J Comput Assist Tomogr 1981;5:227–39.
4. Snyder DL, Thomas LJ, Ter-Pogossian MM. A mathematical model for positron emission tomography systems having time-of-flight measurements. IEEE Trans Nucl Sci 1981;28:3575–83.
5. Politte DG, Snyder DL. Results of a comparative study of a reconstruction procedure for producing improved estimates of radioactivity distributions in time-of-flight emission tomography. IEEE Trans Nucl Sci 1984;NS-31:614–9.
6. Allemand R, Gresset C, Vacher J. Potential advantages of a cesium fluoride scintillator for a time-of-flight positron camera. J Nucl Med 1980;21:153–5.
7. Mullani NA, Ficke C, Ter-Pogossian MM. Cesium fluoride: a new detector for positron emission tomography. IEEE Trans Nucl Sci 1980;NS-27:572–5.
8. Wong WH, Mullani NA, Wardworth G, et al. Characteristics of small barium fluoride (BaF_2) scintillator for high intrinsic resolution time-of-flight positron emission tomography. IEEE Trans Nucl Sci 1984;NS-31: 381–6.
9. Melcher C, Schweitzer JS. Cerium-doped lutetium oxyorthosilicate: a fast, efficient new scintillator. IEEE Trans Nucl Sci 1992;39:1161–6.

10. Surti S, Kuhn A, Werner ME, et al. Performance of Philips Gemini TF PET/CT scanner with special consideration for its time-of-flight imaging capabilities. J Nucl Med 2007;48:471–80.

11. Jakoby BW, Bercier Y, Conti M, et al. Physical and clinical performance of the mCT time-of-flight PET/CT scanner. Phys Med Biol 2011;56:2375–89.

12. Zhang J, Maniawski P, Knopp MV. Performance evaluation of the next generation solid-state digital photon counting PET/CT system. EJNMMI Res 2018;8:97.

13. van Sluis J, de Jong J, Schaar J, et al. Performance characteristics of the digital Biograph Vision PET/CT system. J Nucl Med 2019;60:1031–6.

14. Pan T, Einstein SA, Kappadath SC, et al. Performance evaluation of the 5-ring GE Discovery MI PET/CT system using the National electrical manufacturers association NU 2-2012 standard. Med Phys 2019;46:3025–33.

15. Degenhardt C, et al. The digital silicon photomultiplier: a novel sensor for the detection of scintillation light. In: Yu B, editor. Conference Record of the 2009 IEEE Nuclear science Symposium and Medical imaging Conference :Orlando, FL. Piscataway (NJ): IEEE; 2009. p. 2383-2386.

16. Karakatsanis NA, Lodge MA, Tahari AK, et al. Dynamic whole-body PET parametric imaging: I. Concept, acquisition protocol optimization and clinical application. Phys Med Biol 2013;58:7391.

17. Osborne DR, Acuff S. Whole-body dynamic imaging with continuous bed motion PET/CT. Nucl Med Comm 2016;37:428–31.

18. Hsu DFC, Ilan E, Peterson WT, et al. Studies of a next-generation silicon-photomultiplier-based time-of-flight PET/CT system. J Nucl Med 2017;58:1511–8.

19. Chen S, Hu P, Gu Y, et al. Performance characteristics of the digital uMI550 PET/CT system according to the NEMA NU2-2018 standard. EJNMMI Phys 2020;7:43.

20. Li X, Qi W, Miyahara M, et al. Performance characterization of an SiPM-based time-of-flight Canon PET/CT scanner. J Nucl Med 2020;61S:1505 [abstract].

21. NEMA standards Publication NU 2-2018, performance measurements of positron Emission Tomographs (PET). Rosslyn (VA): National Electrical Manufacturers Association; 2018.

22. Cherry SR, Badawi RD, Karp JS, et al. Total-body imaging: Transforming the role of positron emission tomography. Sci Transl Med 2017;9(381):eaaf6169.

23. Cherry SR, Jones T, Karp JS, et al. Total-body PET: Maximizing sensitivity to create new opportunities for clinical research and patient care. J Nucl Med 2018;59:3–12.

24. Nakanishi K, Hirano Y, Yamamoto S. Comparison of noise equivalent count rates (NECRs) for the PET systems with different ring diameter and electronics. IEEE Trans Radiat Plasma Med Sci 2019;3:371–6.

25. Surti S, Werner ME, Karp JS. Study of PET scanner designs using clinical metrics to optimize the scanner axial FOV and crystal thickness. Phys Med Biol 2013;58:3995–4012.

26. Lecoq P, Morel C, Prior J, et al. Roadmap towards the 10 ps time-of-flight PET challenge. Phys Med Biol 2020. https://doi.org/10.1088/1361-6560/ab9500.

27. Poon JK, Dahlbom ML, Moses WW, et al. Optimal whole-body PET scanner configurations for different volumes of LSO scintillator: a simulation study. Phys Med Biol 2012;57:4077–94.

28. Watanabe M, Shimizu K, Omura T, et al. A high-throughput whole-body PET scanner using flat panel PS-PMTs. IEEE Trans Nucl Sci 2004;53:1136–42.

29. Conti M, Bendriem B, Casey M, et al. Performance of a high sensitivity PET scanner based on LSO panel detectors. IEEE Trans Nucl Sci 2006;53:1136–42.

30. Zhang Y, Wong WH. Design study of a practical-entire-torso PET (PET-PET) with low-cost detector design. In: Conference Record of the 2016 IEEE Nuclear Science Symposium and Medical Imaging Conference :Strasbourg, France. Piscataway, NJ: IEEE; 2016.

31. Crespo P, Reis J, Couceiro M, et al. Whole-body single-bed time-of-flight RPC-PET: simulation of axial and planar sensitivities with NEMA and anthropomorphic phantoms. IEEE Trans Nucl Sci 2012;59:520–9.

32. Eriksson L, Conti M, Melcher CL, et al. Towards sub-minute PET examination times. IEEE Trans Nucl Sci 2011;58:76–81.

33. Surti S, Karp JS. Impact of detector design on imaging performance of a long axial field-of-view, whole-body PET scanner. Phys Med Biol 2015;60:5343–58.

34. Schmall JP, Karp JS, Werner M, et al. Parallax error in long-axial field-of-view PET scanners – a simulation study. Phys Med Biol 2016;61:5443–55.

35. Kwon SI, Gola A, Ferri A, et al. Bismuth germanate coupled to near ultraviolet silicon photomultipliers for time-of-flight PET. Phys Med Biol 2016;61:L38–47.

36. Brunner SE, Schaart DR. BGO as a hybrid scintillator/Cherenkov radiator for cost-effective time-of-flight PET. Phys Med Biol 2017;62:4421–39.

37. Borghi G, Tabacchini V, Bakker R, et al. Sub-3mm, near-200 ps TOF/DOI-PET imaging with monolithic scintillator in a 70 cm diameter tomographic setup. Phys Med Biol 2018;63:155006.

38. Vandenberghe S, Mikhalyova E, Brans B, Defrise M, Lahoutte T, Muylle K, et al. PET 20.0: A cost efficient,

2.00 mm resolution total body monolithic PET with very high sensitivity and an adaptive axial FOV up to 2.00 m. Presented at EANM, Barcelona, Spain. October 12-16, 2019.

39. McDowell MA, Fryat CD, Ogden CL, Flegal KM. Anthropometric reference data for children and adults: United States, 2003-2006. Natl Health Stat Report 2008;10:1-48.

40. Anthropometric Source Book, Volume 2. A Handbook of Anthropometric Data. NASA Reference Publication 1024, 1978.

41. Conti M. Why is TOF PET reconstruction a more robust method in the presence of inconsistent data? Phys Med Biol 2011;56:155–68.

42. Bal G, Panin V, Huff I, Michel C, Young J, Kehren F. Studying effects of missing data for clinical TOF PET. In: Conference Record of 2018 IEEE Nuclear Science Symposium and Medical Imaging Conference: Sydney, Australia. Piscataway, NJ: IEEE; 2018.

43. Yamaya T, Yoshida E, Inadama N, et al. A multiplex 'OpenPET' geometry to extend axial FOV without increasing the number of detectors. IEEE Trans Nucl Sci 2009;56:2644–50.

44. Saloman A, Truhn D, Botnar R, Kiessling F, Schulz V. Sparse crystal setting and large axial FOV for integrated whole-body PET/MR. In: Chmeissani M, editor. Conference Record of 2011 IEEE Nuclear Science Symposium and Medical Imaging Conference: Valencia, Spain. Piscataway, NJ: IEEE; 2011.

45. Zhang J, Knopp MI, Knopp MV. Sparse detector configuration in SiPM digital photon counting PET: a feasibility study. Mol Imaging Biol 2019;21:447–53.

46. Abi Akl M, Bouhali O, Toufique Y, et al. Monte Carlo sensitivity and count rate study of a long axial FOV PET scanner with patient adaptive rings. In: Conference Record of 2019 IEEE Nuclear Science Symposium and Medical Imaging Conference :Manchester, England. Piscataway, NJ: IEEE; 2019.

47. Efthimiou N, Whitehead AC, Stockhoff M, et al. Preliminary investigation of the impact of axial ring splitting on image quality for the cost reduction of total-body PET. In: Conference Record of 2019 IEEE Nuclear Science Symposium and Medical Imaging Conference :Manchester, England. Piscataway, NJ: IEEE; 2019.

48. Zhang Z, Chen B, Perkins AE, et al. Preliminary investigation of optimization-based image reconstruction for TOF PET with sparse configurations. In: Proc. SPIE 11072, 15th Intl Mtg on Fully Three-Dimensional Image Reconstruction in Radiology and Nuclear Medicine, Philadelphia, PA, 2019. https://doi.org/10.1117/12.2534846.

49. Zein SA, Karakatsanis NA, Issa M, et al. Physical performance of a long axial field-of-view PET scanner prototype with sparse rings configuration: a Monte Carlo simulation study. Med Phys 2020. https://doi.org/10.1002/mp.14046.

50. Joyce S, O'Connor OJ, Maher MM, et al. Strategies for dose reduction with specific clinical indications during computed tomography. Radiography 2020; 26:S62–8.

51. Shan H, Padole A, Homayounieh F, et al. Competitive performance of a modularized deep neural network compared to commercial algorithms for low-dose CT image reconstruction. Nat Mach Intell 2019;1:269.

52. Spencer BA, Schmall JP, Berg E, et al. Performance evaluation of the EXPLORER total-body PET/CT scanner based on NEMA NU-2 2018 standard with additional tests of extended geometry In: Conference Record of 2019 IEEE Nuclear Science Symposium and Medical Imaging Conference :Manchester, England. Piscataway, NJ: IEEE; 2019.

53. Badawi RD, Shi H, Hu P, et al. First human imaging studies with the EXPLORER total-body PET scanner. J Nucl Med 2018;60:299–303.

54. Karp JS, Viswanath V, Geagan M, et al. PennPET Explorer: design and preliminary performance of a whole-body imager. J Nucl Med 2019;61:136–43.

55. Pantel AR, Viswanath V, Daube-Witherspoon ME, et al. PennPET Explorer: human imaging on a whole-body imager. J Nucl Med 2019;61:144–51.

56. Karp JS, Daube-Witherspoon ME, Hoffman EJ, et al. Performance standards in positron emission tomography. J Nucl Med 1991;32:2342–50.

57. Daube-Witherspoon ME, Karp JS, Casey ME, et al. PET performance measurements using the NEMA NU 2-2001 standard. J Nucl Med 2002;43: 1398–409.

58. Hudson HM, Larkin RS. Accelerated image reconstruction using ordered subsets of projection data. IEEE Trans Med Imaging 1994;13:601–9.

59. Gong K, Berg E, Cherry SR, et al. Machine learning in PET: from photon detection to quantitative image reconstruction. Proc IEEE 2020;108:51–68.

60. Moskal P, Rundel O, Alfs D, et al. Time resolution of the plastic scintillator strips with matrix photomultiplier readout for J-PET tomograph. Phys Med Biol 2016;65:2025–47.

3D/4D Reconstruction and Quantitative Total Body Imaging

Jinyi Qi, PhD[a],[*],[1], Samuel Matej, PhD[b],[1], Guobao Wang, PhD[c],[1],
Xuezhu Zhang, PhD[a]

KEYWORDS

- PET reconstruction • Direct parametric reconstruction • Time of flight • Long axial FOV
- Kernel reconstruction • Data corrections

KEY POINTS

- Long axial FOV data bring new imaging opportunities and potential of improved reconstruction quality, but also challenges caused by dramatic increase of data sizes and challenges given by the change and variations of data characteristics with increased acceptance angles.
- Good TOF resolution and considerably increased sensitivity of total-body imaging scanners allow novel and improved modeling and ways of processing their data.
- Total-body PET enables simultaneous dynamic imaging of the entire body. 4D reconstruction using the kernel method and/or direct estimation of kinetic parameters can further improve image quality for total-body parametric imaging.

INTRODUCTION

Image reconstruction takes the measured coincidence events as the input and estimates the spatial and temporal distribution of the radioactive tracers within the scanned object. Total-body PET image reconstruction follows a similar procedure to the image reconstruction process for standard whole-body PET scanners. Both analytical and iterative reconstruction methods can be applied. Special considerations need to be taken for the extended axial field of view (AFOV) and large amount of data. Some issues related to the long AFOV include the axial point spread function (PSF) and estimation of correction factors, such as detector normalization factors and those for scattered coincidence events. The large amount of data also requires attention with respect to the computational efficiency of reconstruction

algorithms. One unique aspect of total-body imaging is the simultaneous coverage of the entire human body, which makes it convenient to perform total-body dynamic PET scans. Therefore, four-dimensional (4D) dynamic PET reconstruction and parametric imaging are of great interest in total-body imaging. This article covers some basics of PET image reconstruction and then focuses on three-dimensional (3D) and 4D PET reconstruction for total-body imaging.

LIST-MODE THREE-DIMENSIONAL IMAGE RECONSTRUCTION
Basics

Total-body PET scanners have a huge number of lines of response (LORs). For example, the uEXPLORER scanner (United Imaging Healthcare, Shanghai, China) has more than half a million

[a] Department of Biomedical Engineering, University of California, One Shields Avenue, Davis, CA 95616, USA;
[b] Department of Radiology, University of Pennsylvania, 3620 Hamilton Walk, John Morgan Building, Room 156A, Philadelphia, PA 19104-6061, USA; [c] Department of Radiology, University of California Davis Medical Center, Lawrence J. Ellison Ambulatory Care Center Building, Suite 3100, 4860 Y Street, Sacramento, CA 95817, USA
[1] Equal contributions.
* Corresponding author.
E-mail address: qi@ucdavis.edu

PET Clin 16 (2021) 41–54
https://doi.org/10.1016/j.cpet.2020.09.008

individual crystals, forming more than 90 billion LORs.[1,2] With time-of-flight (TOF) information, the number of elements in a TOF sinogram is more than 1 trillion, which is far greater than the number of coincidence events that could be detected in a regular scan. For example, a 1-hour dynamic scan following a 256 MBq ^{18}F-fluorodeoxyglucose (FDG) injection acquired 61 billion prompt (true + scattered + random) coincidences.[2] Therefore, list-mode-based iterative reconstruction is a natural choice to avoid handling large sinograms.

The data model for total-body image reconstruction is the same as that derived for standard PET image reconstruction.[3–5] The expectation of the ith LOR measurement is related to the radioactivity distribution image $x \in R^{N_v \times 1}$ by

$$\overline{y}_i = (Px + s + r)_i$$

where $P \in R^{N_l \times N_v}$ is the system matrix with the $(i,j)^{th}$ element representing the probability of detecting an event originated from the jth voxel in the ith LOR, $s \in R^{N_l \times 1}$ and $r \in R^{N_l \times 1}$ denote the expectation of the scattered and random coincidences, respectively.[6] N_v and N_l are the total numbers of voxels and LORs, respectively. The list-mode log likelihood function is written as

$$L(x) = \sum_{k=1}^{N_k} \ln(Px + s + r)_{i_k} - \sum_{j=1}^{N_v} \varepsilon_j x_j,$$

$$\varepsilon_j = \sum_{i=1}^{N_l} P_{ij}$$

where N_k is the total number of list-mode events, i_k is the LOR index of the kth event, and ε_j is the overall efficiency of detecting events from the jth voxel.[3]

The maximum likelihood (ML) estimation is obtained by the ML expectation maximization (EM) algorithm[3]

$$\widehat{x}_j^{n+1} = \frac{\widehat{x}_j^n}{\varepsilon_j} \sum_{k=1}^{N_k} \frac{P_{i_k j}}{(Px + s + r)_{i_k}}$$

with x^0 starting from a uniform image.

One of the key components in iterative image reconstruction is the system matrix P. By using a more accurate data-generation model than ideal line integrals used in the filtered back-projection reconstruction method, iterative methods can improve the spatial resolution and the noise properties of reconstructed images. At the same time, however, an accurate model also means higher computation cost and prolonged image reconstruction time. To address this challenge, a factored system matrix is often used.[7,8] Although

a complete factored model includes blurring components in image and sinogram domains,[9] list-mode reconstruction often uses an image domain resolution model,[10] where the system matrix P is factored into

$$P = NAGR$$

where N and A are diagonal matrices containing the normalization factors and object attenuation factors, respectively, for each LOR; G is the geometric projection matrix that is calculated by a ray-tracing algorithm with a TOF kernel; and R is a PSF matrix that models the resolution degradation effects, such as the positron range, photon acollinearity, and detector responses including intercrystal penetration and intercrystal scatter effects.

Many components in the previously mentioned model are estimated in the same way as for standard PET reconstruction. For example, attenuation factors are estimated using a coregistered computed tomography scan with bilinear transformation.[11,12] Random coincidences are estimated using either a delayed window technique or based on singles rates.[13–15] However, other components require special considerations for total-body image reconstruction. In the following sections, we discuss a few unique aspects in the total-body reconstruction with a long AFOV scanner.

Point Spread Function Modeling

The major component in the PSF model is the parallax error caused by annihilation photon crystal penetration. In a standard clinical PET scanner with approximately 20-cm AFOV, the parallax error mostly occurs in the radial direction. For a long AFOV scanner, the parallax error also occurs in the axial direction for the LORs formed between crystals with a large ring difference. As illustrated in Fig. 1, a more oblique LOR (red color) penetrates more adjacent crystals than a less oblique LOR (blue color). Using the uEXPLORER scanner as an example, the axial width of a direct LOR with ring difference of zero is 2.85 mm, which is equal to the crystal pitch, whereas the axial width of an oblique LOR formed by two crystals 180° apart transversely with a polar angle of 57° (the maximum acceptance angle) is 27.6 mm, almost 10 times of that of a direct LOR. Such axial parallax error is not noticeable in standard clinical PET scanner with a 20-cm AFOV. As a result, the PSF in long AFOV scanner is dependent on the radial and axial positions.[16]

To model the spatially variant PSF, point source reconstructions are used. Point source projections are either simulated[17] or measured[7,8] at different

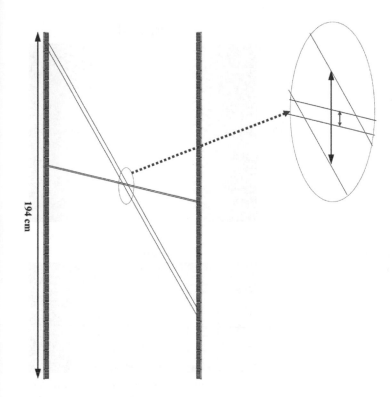

194 cm

radial and axial positions and the data are reconstructed to obtain the PSF models. **Fig. 2** shows reconstructions of a set of simulated point sources inside a simulated 2-m-long scanner[17] at different axial positions on the center axis of the scanner. Clearly, we can observe the degradation in the axial resolution as the point source moves from the axial boundary to the axial center. The resolution degradation effect is less dramatic than the change of the axial width of oblique LORs because the effect of oblique LORs is mitigated by direct LORs passing through the same point. The major effect of the parallax error is still in the radial

direction. **Fig. 3** shows the transaxial profile of a reconstructed point source at 17.2-cm radial offset. Radial elongation is apparent even at this modest radial offset. The full width at half maximum and full width at tenth maximum values of the PSF at selected radial locations are listed in **Table 1** for comparison.

Normalization

Normalization is used in reconstruction to compensate for the variations in detector efficiencies and hardware-related interference

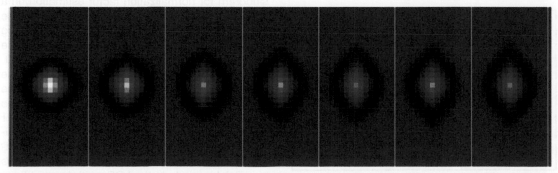

Fig. 2. Sagittal slices of reconstructed point source images on the center axis at different axial positions (left to right): 13 cm, 26 cm, 39 cm, 52 cm, 65 cm, 78 cm, and 91 cm, from the axial edge of the scanner. Vertical axis is the axial direction and horizontal axis is the radial direction.

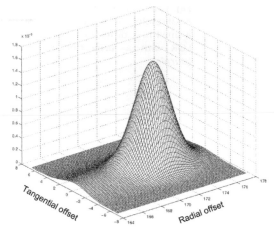

Fig. 3. The transaxial profile of a reconstructed point source at a radial offset of 17.2 cm from the center.

patterns.[18] It can also include any geometric factors that are not modeled in the system matrix P. Normalization factors are computed by comparing measured projections of a physical phantom with known activity distribution and the prediction using the system model. Because of simplifications in the calculation of the system matrix, normalization is often required even for simulated PET scanners with uniform detector response.[17] **Fig. 4** shows a sinogram of a simulated uniform cylinder in a total-body scanner. Although the simulated detectors have uniform response, we can clearly observe pronounced block patterns, which are caused by the combination of intercrystal scatters and the energy-weighted centroid positioning algorithm used in the Monte Carlo simulation. The energy-weighted centroid effectively shifts detected events away from the edge crystals inside a detector block and hence reduces the apparent detection efficiency of edge crystals. In simulations, several geometric symmetries are used to reduce the noise in the normalization

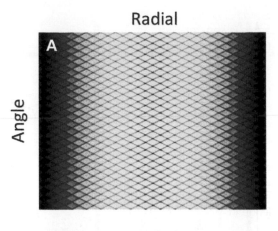

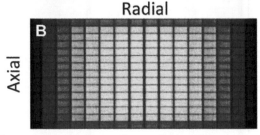

Fig. 4. Sinogram of a uniform cylinder for normalization factor estimation. (*A*) Transaxial view. (*B*) Axial view. Gaps between detector blocks are skipped and only valid LORs shown.

sinogram so that a direct normalization based on the ratio between the measurement and prediction in each LOR can be used.[17] For a real scanner, direct normalization is noisy, so component-based normalization is often preferred to decompose the normalization factors into several components with fewer number of unknowns. The parameters are estimated using either direct calculation[18] or ML estimation.[19]

Regardless whether direct normalization or component-based normalization is used, we need sufficient true coincidence events in each sinogram for normalization factor estimation. In a long AFOV scanner, oblique LORs with a large ring difference have low efficiency in detecting true coincidences because of reduced solid angle and high attenuation of the phantom. As a result, scatter fraction and random fraction increase with increasing oblique angle of the LOR. The combination of these effects makes it difficult to accurately estimate the normalization factors for LORs with extremely large ring differences. Therefore, to avoid noise propagation from the normalization factors into reconstructed images, it is beneficial to exclude the LORs with large oblique angles in the reconstruction, even though this means we are not using all detected events. This

Table 1				
Radial FWHM and FWTM of the point spread function at various radial positions of a simulated 2-m-long EXPLORER				
Radial Offset	0 cm	10 cm	20 cm	30 cm
Radial FWHM	3.0 mm	3.9 mm	5.6 mm	6.8 mm
Radial FWTM	5.4 mm	7.1 mm	10.2 mm	12.3 mm

Abbreviations: FWHM, full width at half maximum; FWTM, full width at tenth maximum.
    Data from Ref.[17]

practical limitation on the maximum acceptance angle is separate from the noise equivalent count rate (NECR) calculation[20] or hardware limitations.[1]

Scatter Estimation and Correction

In total-body imaging with a long axial FOV scanner, photons can have longer paths through the object, resulting in greater chance for multiple-scattering events than that in conventional PET scanners. Although the single scatter simulation or its variant can still be used to estimate the scatter mean,[21] Monte Carlo simulation can model multiple scatters more accurately. The major challenge in Monte Carlo–based scatter estimation is the high computation cost. One way to reduce the simulation time is to compute the scatter sinogram on the detector block level by assuming that the scatter sinogram is smooth after correction for detector efficiencies.[17] Another approach is to use parallel computation with graphical processing unit acceleration. An example of the scatter mean sinogram estimated by the Monte Carlo simulation of an anthropomorphic phantom is shown in **Fig. 5**. Apart from the block boundary effects, the scatter sinograms are fairly smooth in all selected TOF bins.

EFFICIENT RECONSTRUCTION USING DIRECT IMAGE RECONSTRUCTION FOR TIME-OF-FLIGHT DATA FRAMEWORK

Although list-mode reconstruction has the advantage of facilitating straightforward and accurate modeling (in forward projection) for each acquired event, this is at the cost of having to separately calculate forward- and back-projection operations for each individual event, leading to high computational demands. Direct image reconstruction for TOF data (DIRECT)[22] represents an alternative, efficient, reconstruction approach taking advantage of the considerably decreased angular sampling requirement for TOF data. This allows a dramatic decrease in the number of views compared with the classical TOF-sinogram data and thus the ability to process many events

together. It also permits the use of image-like partitioning of the TOF data into histoimages, which in turn allows efficient and highly parallelizable reconstruction operations. Although uExplorer[1] and PennPET Explorer[21] scanners use list-mode reconstruction as their default tool providing practical reconstruction times, high computational efficiency of DIRECT reconstruction approach is especially beneficial for 3D/4D studies using wide acceptance angles and many dynamic or temporal frames.

Direct Image Reconstruction for Time-of-Flight Data Partitioning

The DIRECT framework is based on two key steps: the acquired list-mode events are first sorted into a small set of (transverse and copolar) angular "views" according to the TOF angular sampling requirements,[23,24] and then they are histogrammed into a set of "histoimages" (one histoimage per view; **Fig. 6**). Traditionally, binned TOF events are histogrammed into TOF-sinograms or "histoprojections," which are projections extended in the TOF direction (with their sampling intervals relating to the projection geometry and TOF resolution). Although the histoprojections use also only a limited number of views similarly to DIRECT, the histoprojection data are in a different geometry/space from the reconstructed images. However, in the DIRECT approach the acquired events are histogrammed directly to the "most-likely" voxels of the histoimages. Histoimages are defined by the geometry and desired resolution units, reconstructed image voxels of the desired size. Acquired events and all correction factors are directly placed into the voxels of their respective histoimages, which have a one-to-one correspondence with the reconstructed image voxels, which allows efficient implementation of data correction and reconstruction operations, without the need of any ray-tracing or interpolations within the forward/back projections.

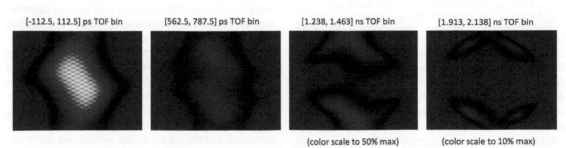

[-112.5, 112.5] ps TOF bin   [562.5, 787.5] ps TOF bin   [1.238, 1.463] ns TOF bin   [1.913, 2.138] ns TOF bin

(color scale to 50% max)   (color scale to 10% max)

Fig. 5. Estimated scatter mean sinogram in four selected TOF bins.

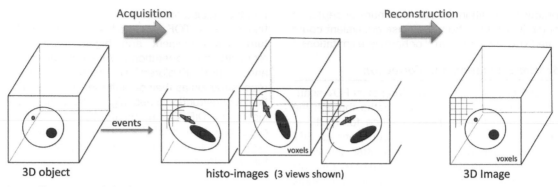

Fig. 6. Illustration of the histoimage partitioning; acquired data are histogrammed into the (most likely) histo-image voxels having one-to-one correspondence with the reconstructed image voxels.

Forward- and Back-Projection Operations in Direct Image Reconstruction for Time-of-Flight Data Framework

Modeling of the acquired data (forward projection) within the histoimage format is simply implemented via a 3D convolution-like operation applied to the current estimate of the image using a specific kernel for each view. Each kernel has an ellipsoidal shape elongated along the view direction, as given by the TOF, detector (LOR), and other resolution effects. Back projection is simply the transpose of forward projection. For spatially invariant detector resolution kernels, fast forward- and back-projection operations is implemented within DIRECT using Fourier-based approaches.[22] For spatially variant and asymmetric kernels, a parallel implementation of the forward- and back-projection operations is efficiently implemented on a graphical processing unit with comparable speeds for practical kernel and image sizes to the Fourier-based implementation with invariant kernels.[25] Correction data (attenuation and normalization factors, and scatter and randoms estimates) are efficiently generated directly in the histoimage geometry.[22,26] Attenuation and sensitivity factors, including gap effects (between detector modules), are accurately and efficiently calculated using Fourier-based approaches.[27]

Direct Image Reconstruction for Time-of-Flight Data Framework Reconstruction

In the classical sinogram-based or histoprojection-based reconstruction approaches the reconstruction operations need to operate between data and image spaces with different geometries, requiring tracing and interpolation operations between the two spaces or different spectral grids in Fourier-based approaches, affecting speed and accuracy of the reconstruction operations. However, in DIRECT approach all operations are voxel-wise multiplications or additions on/between two image structures with the same geometries, without the need of any spatial or spectral interpolations.

In statistical iterative reconstruction algorithms, the corrections, which are generated in the histoimage format, are applied (added or multiplied in) during the forward-projection operation, and the discrepancy and update operations of the algorithm are performed on the image structures. An additional advantage is that the attenuation factors are easily and more accurately applied here before the forward-projection and detector-blurring operations, thus avoiding an approximation often done in conjunction with the image-based resolution modeling where the attenuation factors are usually applied only after the blurring (and geometric projection) operations. Iterative-DIRECT was shown to provide comparable quality and contrast versus noise curves to the list-mode reconstruction for matched resolution models, but with substantially (an order of magnitude) shorter reconstruction times (**Figs. 7** and **8**).[26]

In the analytical algorithm the reconstruction operations are performed again efficiently on the consistent spatial (or spectral) image structures. The analytical reconstruction filter takes into account also the data resolution models (in addition to the TOF resolution). For the analytical algorithm data have to be precorrected before the reconstruction for all of the data imperfections (normalization sensitivity, attenuation, scatter, randoms, dead-time). Gaps in the data in between the detector modules create decreased values in the histoimages, which are, however, nonzero (because of the view grouping), and are therefore straightforwardly corrected by the correspondingly generated geometric sensitivity. However, missing regions in the oblique data (because of the finite detector extent) need to be estimated from the available data, such as by reprojection of a first-

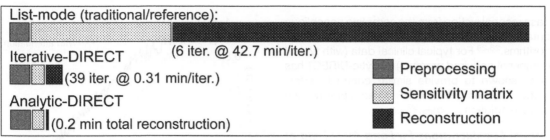

List-mode (traditional/reference):

Iterative-DIRECT   (6 iter. @ 42.7 min/iter.)

(39 iter. @ 0.31 min/iter.)

Analytic-DIRECT

(0.2 min total reconstruction)

◼ Preprocessing
▨ Sensitivity matrix
◼ Reconstruction

Fig. 7. Relative comparison of processing times for iterative- and analytic-DIRECT to traditional list-mode TOF reconstructions at comparable image quality; times are shown for a single CPU reconstruction of one bed position of a typical patient scan.

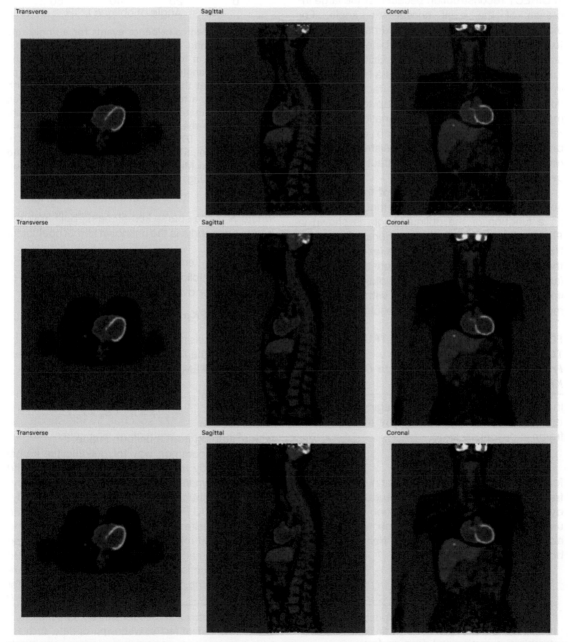

Fig. 8. Comparison of list-mode reconstruction (default tool on PennPET Explorer scanner), iterative-DIRECT (RAMLA), and analytic-DIRECT reconstructions of simulated XCAT phantom data for 70 cm PennPET Explorer scanner.

pass reconstruction from the complete nonoblique data, as in the 3D-RP and 3D-FRP reprojection algorithms.[28,29] For typical clinical data (with typical number of acquired prompts) analytic-DIRECT has been shown to provide similar contrast performance to iterative-DIRECT when applying the same resolution models.[30]

Special Considerations for Long Axial Field of View Data

Similar to the list-mode reconstruction, there are important considerations to be taken into account in DIRECT reconstruction because of the large increase of the axial acceptance angle. For example, many practical approximations related to the oblique data (eg, axial binning/mashing, scatter estimations) have to be revisited and carefully treated. Additionally, there is a large variation in the sensitivity and attenuation factors as function of the oblique angles (with up to an order of magnitude changes) and large variation of the axial resolution. Combination of such data without proper modeling creates inconsistencies in the reconstruction model and also affects the convergence rates.

An example of the variations of the counts (ie, sensitivity) in the data with and without attenuation as a function of the oblique angle is shown in **Fig. 9. Fig. 10** illustrates variations of the axial PSF resolution in the data space (as a function of the oblique angle) and in the reconstructed image (as a function of the axial acceptance angle) in iterative-DIRECT reconstruction without and with modeling of the axially varying resolution.

FOUR-DIMENSIONAL RECONSTRUCTION FOR TOTAL-BODY DYNAMIC PET
Frame-by-Frame Reconstruction Using the Kernel Method

In the setting of dynamic PET imaging, the expectation of the ith LOR measurement in the mth time frame is described by

$$\overline{y}_{i,m} = (\boldsymbol{P}\boldsymbol{x}_m + \boldsymbol{s}_m + \boldsymbol{r}_m)_i,$$

for $m = 1, \cdots, N_m$ with N_m the total number of time frames.[a] Similar to the kernel method for standard dynamic PET image reconstruction,[31–33] we can use a kernel representation to describe the tracer activity in the jth voxel in the mth frame of a total-body dynamic scan,

$$x_{j,m} = (\boldsymbol{K}\alpha_m)_j$$

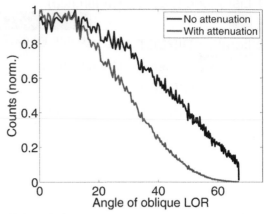

Fig. 9. Recorded coincidence events for a single row of crystals along the axial extent of the simulated scanner 198 cm long (plotted as a function of the LOR oblique angle). Results are shown for a single point source at the center of the imaging FOV with and without attenuation of waterfilled cylinder, 30 cm in diameter and 2 m long. The counts are normalized to the angular bin with the largest number of counts. (From [Jeffrey P Schmall et al 2016 Phys. Med. Biol. 61 5443][16] © Institute of Physics and Engineering in Medicine. Reproduced by permission of IOP Publishing. All rights reserved.)

where $\boldsymbol{K}$ is the sparse kernel matrix built from the image prior and α is the unknown kernel coefficient image.

Using the kernel-based image representation leads to the following kernelized forward projection model for dynamic PET reconstruction:

$$\overline{y}_{i,m} = (\boldsymbol{PK}\alpha_m + \boldsymbol{s}_m + \boldsymbol{r}_m)_i.$$

Based on this model, the ML estimate of α is obtained from the list-mode raw data using the kernelized EM (KEM) algorithm,[31]

$$\widehat{\alpha}_{j,m}^{n+1} = \frac{\widehat{\alpha}_{j,m}^{n}}{\varepsilon_j} \sum_{k=1}^{N_k} \frac{P_{i_k j}}{(\boldsymbol{PK}\alpha_m^n + \boldsymbol{s}_m + \boldsymbol{r}_m)_{i_k}}$$

with α^0 starting from a uniform image.

The most common way for building the kernel matrix $\boldsymbol{K}$ is by use of composite frames derived from the dynamic data before the frame-by-frame reconstruction.[31] For example, a 1-hour dynamic ^{18}F-FDG PET scan can be first rebinned into three composite frames (eg, 10 minutes, 20 minutes, and 30 minutes).[2] From the reconstructed composite images $\{\boldsymbol{x}_m^{reb}\}_{m=1}^3$ (eg, by standard EM reconstruction), three time-activity points are obtained for the jth voxel and form a feature vector

---

[a]Here in the forward projection model, a frame-independent system matrix $\boldsymbol{P}$ is used for conceptual simplicity. In practice, frame-dependent $\boldsymbol{P}_m$ can be used to account for time-dependent factors when appropriate, such as deadtime correction and decay correction.

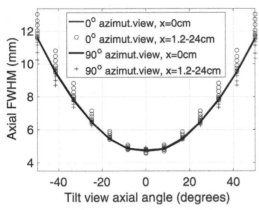

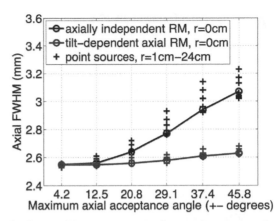

Fig. 10. Axial resolutions of the simulated point-sources for long axial FOV scanner in data and reconstruction spaces. (*Left*) Axial full width at half maximum of PSFs in the histoimage data as a function of oblique angle. (*Right*) Axial full width at half maximum of the point-sources reconstructed with (*red*) and without (*black*) axial tilt-dependent resolution models for gradually increasing maximum acceptance angle of used data. FWHM, full width at half maximum; RM, resolution model.

$f_j = [x^{reb}_{j,1}, x^{reb}_{j,2}, x^{reb}_{j,3}]^T$. The $(j,l)^{th}$ element of the kernel matrix K is then calculated by

$$K_{j,l} = \kappa(f_j, f_l)$$

where $\kappa(\cdot, \cdot)$ denotes the kernel function. One example is the radial Gaussian kernel function

$$\kappa(f_j, f_l) = \exp(-\|f_j - f_l\|^2 / 2\sigma^2)$$

with σ the kernel parameter (eg, $\sigma = 1$).

A total-body image has a large image size (eg, 256 × 256 × 828; with high count density, it is possible for images to be larger still). For practical use, K is commonly built to be sparse. This is achieved by restricting the voxel *l* to be in a neighborhood of the voxel *j*. A typical example is through the k-nearest neighbor search within a 7 × 7 × 7 neighborhood window with k set to be 50.

The KEM reconstruction approach can improve total-body dynamic image significantly as compared with conventional 3D ML EM reconstruction.[2] **Fig. 11** shows a comparison of standard EM reconstruction and the KEM reconstruction for two short frames. Compared with other potential 4D reconstruction approaches, one big advantage of the KEM algorithm is that the reconstruction of a frame is implemented independently from other frames without any direct temporal interaction from each other during the reconstruction. This is particularly beneficial in total-body dynamic PET because a fully 4D reconstruction has a much bigger data size to handle and hence is more computationally intensive than frame-by-frame 3D reconstruction. The kernel method can achieve a balance to bring a significant improvement in image quality while maintaining computational efficiency. For further

improved performance, temporal correlations are also incorporated into the kernel framework to form a spatiotemporal kernel method, which is particularly beneficial to high-temporal resolution dynamic PET imaging.[34]

Direct Estimation of Kinetic Parameters

One of the important purposes of dynamic PET imaging is quantification of tracer kinetics. The conventional framework is to first perform dynamic PET reconstruction and then follow with tracer kinetic modeling in a region of interest or at voxel level.[35,36] This "indirect method" may be suboptimal because information loss can occur in the two separate steps. Alternatively, direct estimation of kinetic parameters is performed by combining the underlying temporal kinetic model and the reconstruction into a single formula, which has the potential to better exploit the available dynamic data.[37–40]

The forward projection model for direct reconstruction is formulated as

$$\bar{y}_{i,m} = [Px_m(\theta) + s_m + r_m]_i,$$

where the dynamic image of the mth frame, x_m, is explicitly expressed as a function of the kinetic parametric images θ,

$$x_m(\theta_j) = \int_{t_{m,s}}^{t_{m,e}} C_T(\tau; \theta_j) e^{-\lambda\tau} d\tau$$

where $t_{m,s}$ and $t_{m,e}$ are the start and end times of time frame m, and λ is the decay constant of the radiotracer. $C_T(t; \theta_j)$ is the tracer concentration in voxel j at time t and is determined by a linear or nonlinear model with the kinetic parameter vector

A   1-s frame at 29-30 s   **B**   2-s frame at 60-62 s

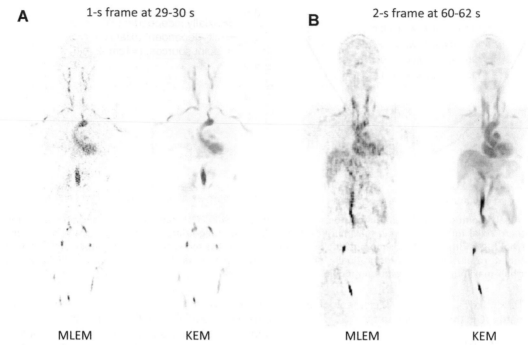

MLEM   KEM   MLEM   KEM

Fig. 11. Comparison of standard ML EM reconstruction with KEM reconstruction for (*A*) a 1-second frame at 29 to 30 seconds postinjection and (*B*) a 2-second frame at 60 to 62 seconds postinjection. The dynamic data were acquired with ^{18}F-FDG for a human subject on the uEXPLORER total-body PET/computed tomography scanner.

θ_j. Examples include B-splines, spectral analysis, Patlak model, one-tissue compartmental model, and irreversible and reversible two-tissue compartmental models.[37,41]

One major challenge for direct reconstruction, in particular for total-body dynamic PET, is the optimization algorithm becomes complicated and not trivial to implement because the 4D dataset is spatiotemporally coupled. This challenge is overcome by using the optimization transfer methods.[40,42] The optimization transfer method with the separable paraboloidal surrogate function[40] can transfer the 4D reconstruction problem into a voxel-wise one-dimensional nonlinear least-square fitting problem at each voxel *j* as defined by

$$\widehat{\theta}_j^{n+1} = \underset{\theta_j}{\arg\min} \sum_{m=1}^{N_m} \widehat{w}_{j,m}^n \left[\widehat{x}_{j,m}^n - x_m(\theta_j) \right]^2$$

where $\{\widehat{x}_{j,m}^n\}_{m=1}^{N_m}$ denotes the intermediate time activity curve (TAC) estimated from the projection data for the jth voxel based on the separable paraboloidal surrogate at reconstruction iteration *n*. $\widehat{w}_{j,m}^n$ are the corresponding weights resulting from the optimization transfer.[40] $x_m(\theta_j)$ represents the model TAC based on the kinetic parameter set θ_j. This one-dimensional fitting problem is easily solved by many existing optimization

algorithms (eg, the Levenberg-Marquardt algorithm) in tracer kinetic modeling.

Alternatively, the optimization transfer method with the EM surrogate function[42] can also transfer the 4D reconstruction into the following equivalent voxel-wise Poisson likelihood-like one-dimensional fitting problem:

$$\widehat{\theta}_j^{n+1} = \underset{\theta_j}{\arg\max} \sum_{m=1}^{N_m} \widehat{x}_{j,m}^n \ln x_m(\theta_j) - x_m(\theta_j),$$

where $\widehat{\boldsymbol{x}}_j^n \triangleq \{\widehat{x}_{j,m}^n\}_{m=1}^{N_m}$ now represents the intermediate TAC estimated from the project data using one-iteration of the standard EM reconstruction update. Such one-dimensional fitting is also solved by different fitting algorithms, including the popular Levenberg-Marquardt algorithm.

One special case of the EM-based optimization transfer method is the nested EM algorithm[43] developed for linear kinetic models. Assume a linear kinetic model,

$$x_m(\theta_j) = (\boldsymbol{B}\theta_j)_m,$$

where $\boldsymbol{B}$ denotes the temporal basis matrix following a specific kinetic model. Then the estimation of θ_j can be obtained from the intermediate TAC $\widehat{\boldsymbol{x}}_j^n$ using the following EM update with N_q subiterations,[43]

$$\widehat{\theta}_j^{n,q+1} = \frac{\widehat{\theta}_j^q}{\boldsymbol{B}^T \boldsymbol{1}} \cdot \left[\boldsymbol{B}^T \frac{\widehat{\boldsymbol{x}}_j^n}{\left(\boldsymbol{B}\theta_j^{n,q}\right)_m} \right], \; q = 0, \cdots, N_q - 1$$

where the vector division is operated element-wise. $\widehat{\theta}_j^{n+1}$ is finally obtained as $\widehat{\theta}_j^{n+1} = \widehat{\theta}_j^{n,N_q}$.

Fig. 12 shows the application of the direct estimation to parametric imaging of the slope (reflecting FDG influx rate) of the Patlak plot for a dynamic ^{18}F-FDG PET scan on the uEXPLORER scanner. As compared with the conventional indirect method, the direct reconstruction demonstrated substantial noise suppression. More quantitative comparisons are found in the recent work of Zhang and colleagues.[2]

SUMMARY AND FUTURE PROSPECTS

Total-body PET provides challenges and opportunities for 3D/4D PET image reconstruction. On the one hand, the large dataset size presents a daunting challenge in computation. Incorporation of the long oblique LORs in reconstruction also requires an accurate model of the response function and proper handling of the correction factors, such as normalization and scatter correction. On the other hand, the high photon-detection sensitivity of total-body PET provides sufficient count density to take advantage of more sophisticated resolution models. Examples include modeling of positron range and photon acollinearity, two factors that put a fundamental limit on PET spatial resolution. Although methods for modeling these two effects have been studied before,[44–46] standard scans on existing whole-body PET scanners are too noisy to exploit these models to enhance the spatial resolution of PET. Total-body PET brings the opportunities to use these models to push the PET resolution beyond these limits. Another opportunity is the combination of total-body PET with machine learning techniques. Although direct reconstruction by neural network[47] for total-body PET may not be feasible with current computing hardware, machine learning is used to improve the image quality

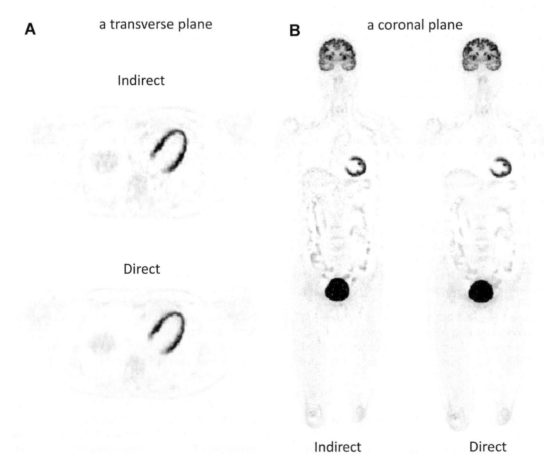

A   a transverse plane   **B**   a coronal plane

Indirect

Direct

Indirect   Direct

Fig. 12. Comparison of the direct method and indirect method for parametric imaging of the slope of the Patlak plot for a human subject ^{18}F-FDG scan on the uEXPLORER scanner. (*A*) Transverse plane. (*B*) Coronal plane.

and/or reduce radiation dose.[47–56] For example, combining the kernel reconstruction with the EXPLORER scanner, researchers have obtained high-quality blood flow images at 100-ms temporal resolution.[57] With the help of deep neural network, it may be possible to generate motion-freeze total-body PET images under a single breath hold. As more total-body PET scanners become operational, we expect to see many new advances in total-body PET image reconstruction.

ACKNOWLEDGMENTS

Dr J. Qi reports support by grants from the National Institute of Biomedical Imaging and Bioengineering (NIBIB) and the National Cancer Institute (NCI) of the National Institutes of Health (NIH) under Award Nos. R01EB000194, R21EB026668, R01CA206187 and funding through a sponsored research agreement by Canon Medical Research USA. Dr G. Wang reports support by grants from NCI and NIBIB under Award Nos. K12 CA138464, R01CA206187, P30CA093373, and R21 EB027346. Dr S. Matej reports support by grants from the National Institute of Biomedical Imaging and Bioengineering and the National Cancer Institute of the National Institutes of Health under Award Nos. R01EB023274, R01CA113941, R01CA196528, and R33CA225310 and funding through a sponsored research agreement by Siemens Medical Solutions USA. Dr S. Matej serves also as a consultant for Siemens Medical Solutions USA.

REFERENCES

1. Badawi RD, Shi H, Hu P, et al. First human imaging studies with the EXPLORER total-body PET scanner. J Nucl Med 2019;60(3):299–303.
2. Zhang X, Xie Z, Berg E, et al. Total-body dynamic reconstruction and parametric imaging on the uEXPLORER. J Nucl Med 2020;61(2):285–91.
3. Huesman RH, Klein GJ, Moses WW, et al. List-mode maximum-likelihood reconstruction applied to positron emission mammography (PEM) with irregular sampling. IEEE Trans Med Imaging 2000;19(5): 532–7.
4. Parra L, Barrett HH. List-mode likelihood: EM algorithm and image quality estimation demonstrated on 2-D PET. IEEE Trans Med Imaging 1998;17(2): 228–35.
5. Barrett HH, White T, Parra LC. List-mode likelihood. J Opt Soc Am A Opt Image Sci Vis 1997;14(11): 2914–23.
6. Qi J, Leahy RM. Iterative reconstruction techniques in emission computed tomography. Phys Med Biol 2006;51(15):R541.
7. Tohme MS, Qi J. Iterative image reconstruction for positron emission tomography based on a detector response function estimated from point source measurements. Phys Med Biol 2009; 54(12):3709.
8. Gong K, Zhou J, Tohme M, et al. Sinogram blurring matrix estimation from point sources measurements with rank-one approximation for fully 3-D PET. IEEE Trans Med Imaging 2017;36(10):2179–88.
9. Zhou J, Qi J. Fast and efficient fully 3D PET image reconstruction using sparse system matrix factorization with GPU acceleration. Phys Med Biol 2011; 56(20):6739.
10. Zhou J, Qi J. Efficient fully 3D list-mode TOF PET image reconstruction using a factorized system matrix with an image domain resolution model. Phys Med Biol 2014;59(3):541.
11. Carney JP, Townsend DW, Rappoport V, et al. Method for transforming CT images for attenuation correction in PET/CT imaging. Med Phys 2006; 33(4):976–83.
12. Kinahan PE, Hasegawa BH, Beyer T. X-ray-based attenuation correction for positron emission tomography/computed tomography scanners. Semin Nucl Med 2003;33(3):166–79.
13. Oliver JF, Rafecas M. Modelling random coincidences in positron emission tomography by using singles and prompts: a comparison study. PLoS One 2016;11(9):e0162096.
14. Oliver JF, Rafecas M. Improving the singles rate method for modeling accidental coincidences in high-resolution PET. Phys Med Biol 2010;55(22): 6951–71.
15. Brasse D, Kinahan PE, Lartizien C, et al. Correction methods for random coincidences in fully 3D whole-body PET: impact on data and image quality. J Nucl Med 2005;46(5):859–67.
16. Schmall JP, Karp JS, Werner M, et al. Parallax error in long-axial field-of-view PET scanners-a simulation study. Phys Med Biol 2016;61(14):5443–55.
17. Zhang X, Zhou J, Cherry SR, et al. Quantitative image reconstruction for total-body PET imaging using the 2-meter long EXPLORER scanner. Phys Med Biol 2017;62(6):2465–85.
18. Badawi RD, Marsden PK. Developments in component-based normalization for 3D PET. Phys Med Biol 1999;44(2):571–94.
19. Bai B, Li Q, Holdsworth CH, et al. Model-based normalization for iterative 3D PET image reconstruction. Phys Med Biol 2002;47(15):2773–84.
20. Poon JK, Dahlbom ML, Moses WW, et al. Optimal whole-body PET scanner configurations for different volumes of LSO scintillator: a simulation study. Phys Med Biol 2012;57(13):4077–94.

21. Karp JS, Viswanath V, Geagan MJ, et al. PennPET explorer: design and preliminary performance of a whole-body imager. J Nucl Med 2020;61(1):136–43.

22. Matej S, Surti S, Jayanthi S, et al. Efficient 3-D TOF PET reconstruction using view-grouped histo-images: DIRECT - Direct Image Reconstruction for TOF. IEEE Trans Med Imaging 2009;28(5):739–51.

23. Politte DG, Hoffman GR, Beecher DE, et al. Image-reconstruction of data from super PETT I: a first-generation time-of-flight positron-emission tomograph (reconstruction from reduced-angle data). IEEE Trans Nucl Sci 1986;33(1):428–34.

24. Vandenberghe S, Daube-Witherspoon ME, Lewitt RM, et al. Fast reconstruction of 3D time-of-flight PET data by axial rebinning and transverse mashing. Phys Med Biol 2006;51(6):1603–21.

25. Ha S, Matej S, Ispiryan M, et al. GPU-accelerated forward and back-projection with spatially varying kernels in 3D DIRECT TOF PET reconstruction. IEEE Trans Nucl Sci 2013;60(1):166–73.

26. Daube-Witherspoon ME, Matej S, Werner ME, et al. Comparison of list-mode and DIRECT approaches for time-of-flight PET reconstruction. IEEE Trans Med Imaging 2012;31(7):1461–71.

27. Matej S, Kazantsev IG. Fourier-based reconstruction for fully 3-D PET: optimization of interpolation parameters. IEEE Trans Med Imaging 2006;25(7):845–54.

28. Kinahan PE, Rogers JG. Analytic 3D image reconstruction using all detected events. IEEE Trans Nucl Sci 1989;36:964–8.

29. Matej S, Lewitt RM. 3D-FRP: direct Fourier reconstruction with Fourier reprojection for fully 3-D PET. IEEE Trans Nucl Sci 2001;48(4):1378–85.

30. Matej S, Daube-Witherspoon ME, Karp JS. Analytic TOF PET reconstruction algorithm within DIRECT data partitioning framework. Phys Med Biol 2016;61(9):3365–86.

31. Wang G, Qi J. PET image reconstruction using kernel method. IEEE Trans Med Imaging 2015;34(1):61–71.

32. Hutchcroft W, Wang G, Chen KT, et al. Anatomically-aided PET reconstruction using the kernel method. Phys Med Biol 2016;61(18):6668–83.

33. Gong K, Cheng-Liao JX, Wang GB, et al. Direct Patlak reconstruction from dynamic PET data using the kernel method with MRI information based on structural similarity. IEEE Trans Med Imaging 2018;37(4):955–65.

34. Wang GB. High temporal-resolution dynamic PET image reconstruction using a new spatiotemporal kernel method. IEEE Trans Med Imaging 2019;38(3):664–74.

35. Rahmim A, Tang J, Zaidi H. Four-dimensional (4D) image reconstruction strategies in dynamic PET: beyond conventional independent frame reconstruction. Med Phys 2009;36(8):3654–70.

36. Reader AJ, Verhaeghe J. 4D image reconstruction for emission tomography. Phys Med Biol 2014;59(22):R371–418.

37. Wang G, Qi J. Direct estimation of kinetic parametric images for dynamic PET. Theranostics 2013;3(10):802–15.

38. Kamasak ME, Bouman CA, Morris ED, et al. Direct reconstruction of kinetic parameter images from dynamic PET data. IEEE Trans Med Imaging 2005;24(5):636–50.

39. Wang G, Fu L, Qi J. Maximum a posteriori reconstruction of the Patlak parametric image from sinograms in dynamic PET. Phys Med Biol 2008;53(3):593–604.

40. Wang G, Qi J. Generalized algorithms for direct reconstruction of parametric images from dynamic PET data. IEEE Trans Med Imaging 2009;28(11):1717–26.

41. Carson RE. Tracer kinetic modeling in PET. In: Bailey DL, Townsend DW, Valk PE, et al, editors. Positron emission tomography. London: Springer; 2005. p. 127–59.

42. Wang G, Qi J. An Optimization Transfer Algorithm for Nonlinear Parametric Image Reconstruction from Dynamic PET Data. IEEE Trans Med Imaging 2012;31(10):1977–98.

43. Wang G, Qi J. Acceleration of the direct reconstruction of linear parametric images using nested algorithms. Phys Med Biol 2010;55(5):1505–17.

44. Bertolli O, Eleftheriou A, Cecchetti M, et al. PET iterative reconstruction incorporating an efficient positron range correction method. Phys Med 2016;32(2):323–30.

45. Fu L, Qi J. A residual correction method for high-resolution PET reconstruction with application to on-the-fly Monte Carlo based model of positron range. Med Phys 2010;37(2):704–13.

46. Alessio A, MacDonald L. Spatially variant positron range modeling derived from CT for PET image reconstruction. IEEE Nucl Sci Symp Conf Rec (1997) 2008;2008:3637–40.

47. Haggstrom I, Schmidtlein CR, Campanella G, et al. DeepPET: a deep encoder-decoder network for directly solving the PET image reconstruction inverse problem. Med Image Anal 2019;54:253–62.

48. Ouyang J, Chen KT, Gong E, et al. Ultra-low-dose PET reconstruction using generative adversarial network with feature matching and task-specific perceptual loss. Med Phys 2019;46(8):3555–64.

49. Liu CC, Qi J. Higher SNR PET image prediction using a deep learning model and MRI image. Phys Med Biol 2019;64(11):115004.

50. Kim K, Wu D, Gong K, et al. Penalized PET reconstruction using deep learning prior and local linear fitting. IEEE Trans Med Imaging 2018;37(6):1478–87.

51. Gong K, Guan J, Liu C-C, et al. PET image denoising using a deep neural network through fine tuning. IEEE Trans Radiat Plasma Med Sci 2018;3(2): 153–61.

52. Gong K, Guan J, Kim K, et al. Iterative PET image reconstruction using convolutional neural network representation. IEEE Trans Med Imaging 2018; 38(3):675–85.

53. Gong K, Catana C, Qi J, et al. PET image reconstruction using deep image prior. IEEE Trans Med Imaging 2018;38(7):1655–65.

54. Xiang L, Qiao Y, Nie D, et al. Deep auto-context convolutional neural networks for standard-dose PET image estimation from low-dose PET/MRI. Neurocomputing 2017;267:406–16.

55. Xie Z, Baikejiang R, Li T, et al. Generative adversarial network based regularized image reconstruction for PET. Phys Med Biol 2020;65(12):125016.

56. Gong K, Berg E, Cherry SR, et al. Machine learning in PET: from photon detection to quantitative image reconstruction. Proceedings of the IEEE 2020; 108(1):51–68.

57. Zhang X, Cherry SR, Xie Z, et al. Subsecond total-body imaging using ultrasensitive positron emission tomography. Proc Natl Acad Sci U S A 2020;117(5): 2265–7.

Analysis of Four-Dimensional Data for Total Body PET Imaging

Varsha Viswanath, PhD[a],*, Rhea Chitalia, BS[b], Austin R. Pantel, MD, MSTR[c],
Joel S. Karp, PhD[a], David A. Mankoff, MD[d]

KEYWORDS

• Dynamic imaging • Parametric imaging • EXPLORER • PennPET explorer • Total body PET

KEY POINTS

• Dynamic imaging on total-body PET scanners will allow us to image multiple organs and lesions simultaneously and select the most apt blood supply as an input function for each lesion.
• The high sensitivity of total-body PET will allow for short (100 ms) temporal frames and low dose (0.5 – 2 mCi) dynamic imaging.
• Using the high temporal sampling and high sensitivity of total-body PET, parametric images of the whole body can be generated, showing higher lesion contrast than traditional SUV images.
• 4D total-body PET can also be leveraged for 4D lesion heterogeneity analysis using machine learning, as well as dual tracer imaging with two 18F-labeled tracers.

INTRODUCTION

In clinical practice, most PET imaging is performed at a single timepoint after tracer injection—that is, "static" PET imaging. In practice, static [18F]-fluorodeoxyglucose (FDG) PET scans are most commonly quantified using a standardized uptake value (SUV), which is simple and robust when done under consistent acquisition protocols and can guide cancer diagnosis and characterization and to determine optimal treatments.[1] Although static PET images quantified with SUVs are valuable for interpreting and diagnosing disease, dynamic information about the rate of uptake of FDG over time and the delivery of tracer can offer complementary insights for clinical decision making. For example, dynamic FDG data of patients with breast cancer has been shown to improve the ability to measure cancer response to treatment compared with static imaging at 60 minutes after injection, especially for low uptake tumors.[2] Dynamic PET imaging also plays a key role in developing new radiotracers to measure their dynamic biodistribution after injection. Dynamic imaging of such radiotracers is necessary to understand the biochemistry of new tracers, which in turn informs which kinetic parameters are likely to be of clinical significance. This information can then be used to design static imaging protocols that are more practical for routine clinical implementation.

Parameters of interest can be determined either via compartmental models or graphical methods. A few review articles that go into more detail can be found,[3,4] but a brief overview of relevant material is included here. Compartmental models represent the biochemistry of the

[a] Department of Radiology, University of Pennsylvania, John Morgan Building, 3620 Hamilton Walk, Room 150, Philadelphia, PA 19103, USA; [b] Department of Radiology, University of Pennsylvania, Richards Building, 3700 Hamilton Walk, Room D700, Philadelphia, PA 19103, USA; [c] Department of Radiology, University of Pennsylvania, Hospital of the University of Pennsylvania, 1 Donner Building, 3400 Spruce Street, Philadelphia, PA 19104-4283, USA; [d] Department of Radiology, Abramson Cancer Center, University of Pennsylvania, Hospital of the University of Pennsylvania, 1 Donner Building, 3400 Spruce Street, Philadelphia, PA 19104-4283, USA
* Corresponding author.
E-mail address: Varsha.Viswanath@pennmedicine.upenn.edu

PET Clin 16 (2021) 55–64
https://doi.org/10.1016/j.cpet.2020.09.009
1556-8598/21/© 2020 The Authors. Published by Elsevier Inc. This is an open access article under the CC BY-NC-ND license (http://creativecommons.org/licenses/by-nc-nd/4.0/).

radiotracer as a series of key transport or biochemical reaction steps, simplified into 1 or more tissue compartments fed by a measured tracer time activity curve. Kinetic parameters typically reflect the flux of tracer into and out of these compartments, often related to the enzymatic conversion of the tracers. For example, FDG is modeled using an irreversible 2-tissue compartment model, where tracer flows reversibly from the blood into the first tissue compartment (tissue FDG) and then is converted by hexokinase into FDG-6-phosphate and trapped in the second tissue compartment.[5] The flux (K_i) through hexokinase is a valuable kinetic parameter that provides information similar to SUV, but more specifically reflects use of the key enzyme, hexokinase, which is the rate-limiting step for glycolysis. Kinetic parameters of interest for other tracers, especially those with reversible binding or transport, include delivery of tracer from the blood to the tissue (K_1), the tissue volume of distribution of the tracer, or the binding potential of radiotracers designed to be ligands that bind to receptors. Compartmental models are very powerful to tease out information about the underlying processes in tracer uptake. The disadvantage of compartmental models, however, is that they estimate many parameters simultaneously and require nonlinear optimization, which may limit precision and accuracy. Graphical methods transform dynamic data such that a linear fit can be performed and the slope of the fit equals a clinically relevant kinetic parameter. For example, the Patlak graphical analysis can be applied to tracers with irreversible trapping such as FDG, and the slope of the fit equals the flux of the tracer through the key enzymatic step.[6] The slope of the standard Logan graphical analysis method equals the volume of distribution for a reversibly transported or bound tracer.[7] This method also enables the use of a reference tissue instead of the blood clearance function, where the slope from the so-called Logan reference region graphical analysis equals 1 plus the binding potential.[8]

Because dynamic imaging data are acquired continuously, standard apparent field of view scanners limit the axial extent, and thus the number of lesions or organs that can be imaged in a single session. Total body PET scanners allow for simultaneous dynamic imaging of multiple organs or lesions in the body, opening the door for applications such as regular dynamic clinical FDG PET imaging, rigorous analysis of new radiotracers, probing new systems of biology, and developing complex new modeling methods that can leverage dynamic whole body, 4-dimensional data (TB 4D PET). In this review, we explore some of the capabilities, applications and approaches relevant to TB 4D PET, including region-specific blood input functions, tracer kinetics late after injection, low-dose dynamic imaging, novel approaches to 4D image analysis and parametric image generation, and dual tracer injections.

BLOOD SAMPLING FROM MULTIPLE LOCATIONS

Standard kinetic modeling for PET relies on measuring the blood input function, the time-course of radiotracer available in the blood, to properly fit data to compartmental models and estimate important kinetic parameters. The gold standard for measuring the blood input function is arterial sampling, which is invasive and uncomfortable for patients. Instead, an image-derived input function (IDIF) can be measured by placing a volume of interest on a nearby arterial blood pool. An IDIF has the advantage of being noninvasive and inherently scaled similarly to the tissue or lesion time–activity curves, because both are measured from the reconstructed images; however, because dynamic imaging on standard apparent field of view scanners is typically done in a single bed position, the IDIF is sometimes measured from small arteries, such as the carotid artery for neurologic tracers or the iliac arteries for prostate tracers. These IDIFs suffer from partial volume effects, which underestimate activity levels in smaller structures and can lead to mixing of data form adjacent structures—for example, neighboring arteries and veins. These can lead to problematic artifacts, for example, blunting the peak of the blood clearance (model input) function when the more time-dispersed venous peak blends with the arterial peak of the blood clearance function. On a total body PET scanner, the IDIF can be measured from a number of different blood pools (**Fig. 1**) and the most relevant large vessel IDIF can be used for kinetic modeling. Thus far, dynamic FDG data of normal human subjects has been acquired on both the PennPET Explorer and the United Imaging uEXPLORER and time–activity curves from various blood vessels and organs are shown in **Fig. 1**.

Another important factor is temporal sampling to capture the full dynamics of the blood clearance function; however, sampling is often limited by low count statistics. Dynamic datasets on standard apparent field of view scanners typically sample early frames at 5 to 10 seconds, with the goal of sampling finely enough to capture the peak of

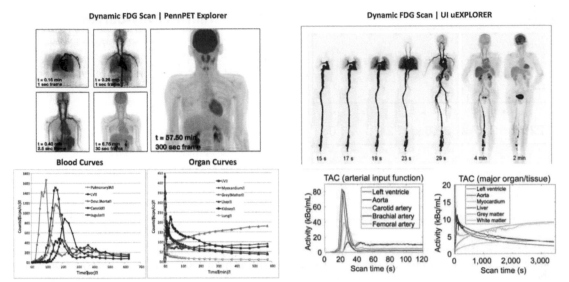

Fig. 1. Dynamic studies from both the PennPET Explorer (*left*) and United Imaging uExplorer (*right*) showing blood time–activity curves from many sources and organ time–activity curves from organs in the FOV. (*From* R. D. Badawi, H. Shi, P. Hu, S. Chen, T. Xu, P. M. Price *et al.*, "First human imaging studies with the EXPLORER total-body PET scanner," *J Nucl Med,* vol. 60, no. 3, pp. 299-303, 2019; and A. R. Pantel, V. Viswanath, M. E. Daube-Witherspoon, J. G. Dubroff, G. Muehllehner, M. J. Parma *et al.*, "PennPET Explorer: Human imaging on a whole-body imager," *J Nucl Med,* vol. 61, no. 1, pp. 144-151, 2019; and X. Zhang, Z. Xie, E. Berg, M. S. Judenhofer, W. Liu, T. Xu *et al.*, "Total-body dynamic reconstruction and parametric imaging on the uEXPLORER," *Journal of Nuclear Medicine,* vol. 61, no. 2, pp. 285-291, 2020.)

the IDIF without limiting the number of counts per frame and therefore increasing the image noise. The high sensitivity of total body PET has enabled faster temporal sampling of the early portion of the dynamic data. The earliest time frames of the raw time–activity curves in **Fig. 1** are sampled at 1 second and show little to no noise in the curves, implying that finer sampling could be possible. Although a 2 to 3 times sensitivity gain is expected from the larger solid angle of acceptance of coincident gammas owing to increasing the axial length of the scanner, this sensitivity advantage extends over a large axial range as the axial field-of-view increases; therefore, 1-second temporal sampling is feasible for regular use on 4DTB datasets for radiotracer distributed over multiple organs. In fact, using a specialized algorithm[9] to minimize image noise, 100-m frames were reconstructed and resultant time–activity curves from the left ventricle, aorta, and myocardium, clearly showed the cardiac cycle (**Fig. 2**).

MEASURING KINETICS OVER A PROLONGED TIME PERIOD AFTER INJECTION

In addition to leveraging the high sensitivity of total body PET to reconstruct short (0.1–1.0 second) images, the sensitivity can also be used to image as late as 10 half-lives (<0.1% of the dose) and acquire

quantitatively accurate images.[10] This property may be particularly helpful to characterize tracers with slow washout kinetics, as is the case for FDG in organs with significant phosphatase activity. Phosphatase converts FDG-6-phosphate back to FDG and can impact the visualization of tumor sites and the interpretation of static uptake measures such as SUV.[11] For cancer imaging, where few tumors have phosphatase activity, delayed imaging times may be helpful to separate tumors from FDG-avid normal tissues such as the brain. Spence and colleagues[12] have previously shown the ability to visualize FDG in brain tumors and measure the time–activity curves of FDG in the normal brain and brain tumors at 3 to 5 hours after injection, demonstrating this concept. Whole body PET can capture data much later. Data acquired out to 18 to 24 hours (9.8–13.1 half-lives) on the PennPET Explorer show similar behavior in the brain while also noting that myocardial uptake does not drastically decrease, even at the last time points (**Fig. 3**),[13] highlighting differences in normal tissue phosphatase activity and FDG washout that are difficult to measure on standard PET devices. These data can be fit by a reversible 2-tissue compartment kinetic model quantify k_4 in the brain, heart, and other organs for a more thorough understanding of the behavior of FDG. In addition, it is well-known that the contrast of many tumors increases over time

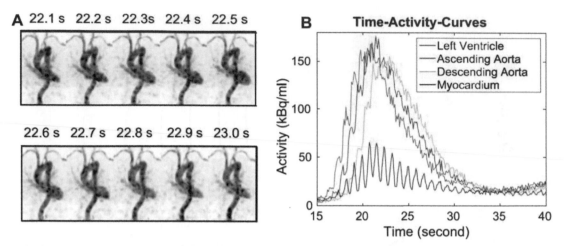

Fig. 2. (A) Reconstruction dynamic PET images (maximum intensity projection) of 10 consecutive 100-m frames from 22 seconds after injection. (B) Dynamic time–activity curves from 100-m frames. (*Courtesy of* Dr. Ramsey D. Badawi.)

owing to trapping in the lesions and washout of FDG in background tissues.[14] The high sensitivity of total body PET will make imaging at a later time point clinically feasible without loss of image quality. In addition, factors such as late efflux of tracers from certain tissues can be studied and could be considered when making decisions on the approach to acquiring and interpreting the static images most commonly used in the clinic.

The ability to image at low activity levels and still recover quantitatively accurate information will be valuable for studies of tracers using isotopes with longer half-lives, many of which have mixed emission schemes, and where radiation considerations limit the injected activity dose. For example, antibodies labeled with ^{89}Zr, a long-lived isotope with a 20% β+ fraction, are used for applications, such as cell tracking, that require imaging times on the order of days or even weeks.[15,16] For theranostic applications, activity late after injection is important for radiation dosimetry studies, but owing to limitations of current scanners, uptake after 2 to 3 half-lives is typically extrapolated and not measured.[17] Accurate delineation of the "tail" of radiotracer clearance could have a significant impact on estimates of dosimetry, especially important in applications of theranostic dosing. The increased sensitivity may also enable previously challenging clinical tasks. The estimation of radiation dose of ^{90}Y spheres for liver-directed therapy is currently challenging to image owing to the low β+ fraction of ^{90}Y (0.0034%).[18] Total body PET may be able to image and reconstruct quantitatively accurate images after ^{90}Y radioembolization to ensure delivery of therapy to the tumor site.

LOW-DOSE DYNAMIC IMAGING

The increased sensitivity of total body PET scanners can also be leveraged for low-dose dynamic imaging. This property is especially valuable when testing new radiotracers, which can have radiotracer production limitations or organ dose limits, and simultaneously limits the dose to the patient. Viswanath and colleagues[19] conducted a study where dynamic lesions were embedded into a dynamic dataset of a normal human subject injected with 15 mCi of FDG and imaged from 0 to 60 minutes on the PennPET Explorer. Dynamic lesion embedding is a method where separately acquired sphere data in the location of the desired lesion are combined frame by frame with normal human subject dynamic data to create a synthetic dynamic dataset with lesions that have the desired dynamic time course. Lesions were embedded with known kinetic parameters and data were subsampled to assess how low the injected dose could be decreased while still recovering the kinetic parameters. Results showed that estimation of the FDG flux constant (K_{FDG}) when using the Patlak graphical analysis,[6] could be accurate estimated at an emulated dose of 0.5 mCi for high flux spheres and 5 mCi for low flux spheres (**Fig. 4**). Compartmental analysis, which provides additional insight into tracer delivery and distribution, may also be facilitated by the improved count statistics of TB PET. Estimation of K_{FDG} using a 2-tissue compartment model, assuming irreversible trapping ($k_4 = 0$) showed a systematic positive bias, but the K_{FDG} could be estimated at emulated doses of 0.5 to 1.0 mCi with 10% precision. The FDG blood-to-tissue delivery parameter, K_1, as

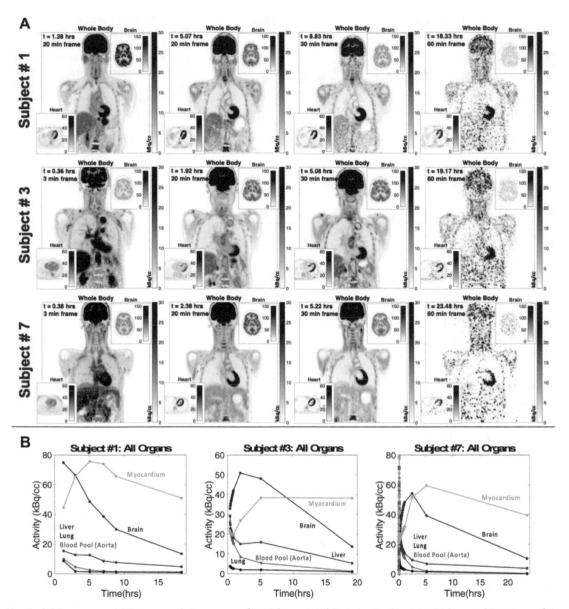

Fig. 3. (A) Images and (B) time–activity curves of FDG human subjects imaged out to 24 hours. (*Courtesy of* Dr. Ramsey D. Badawi.)

estimated from an irreversible 2-tissue compartment model ($k_4 = 0$), showed a systematic negative bias for low and medium flux spheres across all emulated activities. High flux spheres had little bias and less than 10% precision, even at an emulated dose of 0.5 mCi. This work shows imaging with 0.5 to 1.0 mCi on total body PET scanners will allow for accurate quantitation of K_{FDG}, or flux of other ^{18}F-labeled tracers; however, the large bias of K_1 for low and medium flux spheres implies that the early time frames (1 second in duration) introduced too much noise into the image, and thus the time–activity curve, so a dual-binning

reconstruction approach may be best for total body PET. Short (1 second) time bins would be reconstructed early on to accurately capture the blood peaks, which as shown in **Fig. 1** had little noise, and longer (5 seconds) time bins would be reconstructed to measure the tissue or lesion time–activity curves. Although this methodology has not been tested, dynamic GATE simulations of ^{18}F]fluorothymidine in a phantom on a model of the PennPET Explorer were used to do a similar analysis, but with 5-second frames early on, and results showed much less bias in K_1 estimation that decreased for higher doses.[20] Further analysis

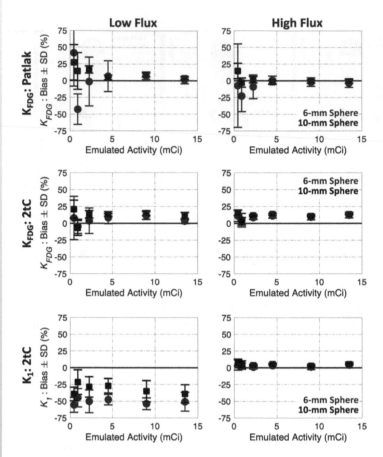

Fig. 4. Bias and precision of K_{FDG}, as estimated using both Patlak (*top*) and a 2-tissue compartment (*middle*), and K_1 (*bottom*) for both low and high flux spheres. (*From* V. Viswanath, A. R. Pantel, M. E. Daube-Witherspoon, R. Doot, M. Muzi, D. A. Mankoff et al., "Quantifying bias and precision of kinetic parameter estimation on the PennPET Explorer, a long axial field-of-view scanner," *IEEE TRPMS*, 2020.)

can help define optimal approaches for demanding tasks of dynamic image analysis such as low-dose imaging and parametric image generation.

PARAMETRIC IMAGE RECONSTRUCTION

The combination of increased sensitivity of total body PET and the ability to dynamically image the whole body at once offers the opportunity to reconstruction parametric images of flux, delivery, volume of distribution, and other kinetic parameters of interest. There are a number of different approaches that have been tested, including voxel-based dynamic image analysis as well as approaches that inherently consider the 4D nature of the dataset.[4] For voxel-based applications for dynamic FDG data, parametric flux image generation has been most successful using the Patlak graphical analysis to calculate flux (Patlak slope) and distribution volume (Patlak intercept). This application has been implemented on dynamic PET data by Zhang and colleagues[9] using their kernel method to minimize

noise in resultant parametric images.[21,22] Additionally, a novel approach to embedding the graphical analysis in the reconstruction process has shown good preliminary results from Li and colleagues using a nested Patlak fit within iterations of a DIRECT reconstruction[23,24] (**Fig. 5**). Such images may be especially useful for detection of small or low uptake lesions, especially in the liver where high parenchymal uptake result in difficulty detecting lesions; however, images show that the liver has a low K_i, so liver lesions, which have been shown to have a K_i of 0.08 ± 0.04,[25,26] should be much easier to detect on parametric flux images. The higher contrast of lesions on parametric K_{FDG} images from the uEXPLORER has been shown by Wang and colleagues[27] in chest, kidney, and thigh lesions. They report a 3x increase in lesion contrast on flux images, estimated using a 2-tissue compartment model, compared with SUV images.

As an alternative to voxel-based, 2-dimensional (uptake, time) analytical approaches, methods that use the full 4D dataset may provide improvements

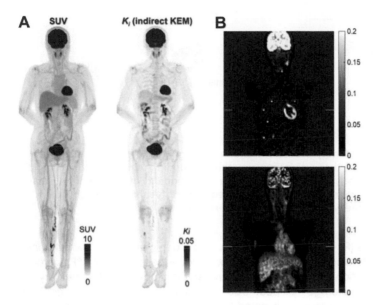

Fig. 5. (*A*) Parametric flux image from the uEXPLORER using Patlak (Reprinted with permission from[21]). (*B*) Parametric image reconstruction using Patlak of dynamic FDG data from the PennPET Explorer with dynamically embedded lesions showing maps of flux from the Patlak slope (*top*) and distribution volume from the Patlak intercept (*bottom*). (Y. Li, V. Viswanath, M. E. Daube-Witherspoon, J. S. Karp, and S. Matej, Nested Parametric Image Reconstruction using Time-of-Flight PET Histoimages, 2020 IEEE Nucl. Sci. Symp. Med. Imag. Conf., 2020, Boston, MA.)

in both efficiency and precision by using the extensive kinetic information and robust counting statistics available in 4D datasets. These methods may be useful for 4D datasets acquired on TB PET scanners. These approaches segment 4D images to generate at set of 1-dimensional dynamic (uptake, time) basis functions, which can then be kinetically analyzed by compartmental analysis or other parameter estimation techniques. Parametric images are then generated by recombining the kinetic estimates derived from the basis functions using the segmentation kernel. Well-tested approaches include mixture analysis,[28] factor analysis,[29] and other novel methods.[30] Prior studies have supported the ability to combine these methods with compartmental analysis[31]; however, alternative approaches may have advantages that include speed, efficiency, and more robust linear estimation approaches. In addition to graphical methods such as previously described Patlak analysis, alternative model-free approaches to describe and analyze dynamic data include spectral analysis[32,33] and wavelet analysis.[30] Another approach uses the residue formulation developed for nonimaging studies[34] to estimate tracer delivery retention (flux or volume of distribution), and has the advantage—in addition to being efficient and robust—of generating linear parameter estimates, facilitating use with parametric imaging methods such as mixture analysis.[35,36] This approach can be combined with methods to estimate the IDIF for a complete package that is, broadly applicable to 4D PET, including whole body PET scans.[37]

FOUR-DIMENSIONAL LESION HETEROGENEITY

In addition to using dynamic information to characterize a tumor, machine learning-based algorithms can be employed to leverage 4D information to quantify tumor heterogeneity. Dynamic imaging simulations of the PET proliferation tracer, [18F]fluorothymidine,[38] by GATE simulations of a modified IQ phantom imaged on the 70-cm PennPET Explorer were used to design a 4D segmentation algorithm, that used both spatial and temporal components of voxel behavior to identify subregions with discrete 4-D behavior within lesions (**Fig. 6**). An initial version of this approach was applied to dynamic FDG data of 50 patients with breast cancer, among whom 17 women had events of cancer recurrence. Identifying subregions within breast lesions allowed for the development of a novel imaging signature of 4D functional tumor heterogeneity by quantifying the degree of separation between identified functionally discrete subregions. Compared with a baseline Cox regression model of known prognostic factors such as age, hormone receptor status, baseline tumor size, and kinetic PET markers including SUV, K_1, and K_i, the addition of the functional tumor heterogeneity imaging signature demonstrated greater discriminatory capacity when predicting disease free survival.[39] In addition, dichotomizing patients into low- and high-risk groups based on the functional tumor heterogeneity imaging signature and baseline prognostic factors demonstrated significant separation

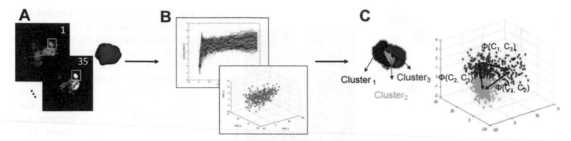

Fig. 6. A 4D segmentation algorithm to identify subregions within solid tumors. (*A*) The primary lesion is segmented from a set of dynamic scans using time activity curves within a bounding region identified by radiologist. (*B*) Functional principal component analysis is used to reduce the dimensionality of the tumor time activity curves. (*C*) A Markov random field–based segmentation approach is used to identify subregions within the tumor from which an functional tumor heterogeneity imaging signature is extracted.

($P<.05$) of Kaplan–Meier survival curves (R. Chitalia, V. Viswanath, A. R. Pantel, L. Peterson, E. Cohen, M. Muzi and colleagues., "Functional 4-D clustering for characterizing intra tumor heterogeneity: evaluation in dynamic FDG-PET as a prognostic biomarker for breast cancer," 2020 (in preparation)).

Characterizing 4D functional tumor heterogeneity based on spatial and temporal information has the potential to be expanded beyond dynamic FDG imaging of disease, which will be much easier to implement on total body PET scanners owing to the decreased noise in individual image frames and resultant voxel time–activity curves. Because this work is independent of the compartmental model used in current dynamic PET analyses, it can be applied to analyze kinetics in studies using tracers in development as well as additional clinical radiotracers like DOTATATE or PSMA. In addition, such machine learning-based approaches can be applied to semidynamic datasets where data are acquired from 40 to 60 minutes after injection, parsed into 1-minute frames, and analyzed for heterogeneity.

DUAL TRACER IMAGING

Because the high sensitivity of total body PET enables low-dose dynamic imaging, this advantage can then be parlayed into dual tracer or even multi-tracer dynamic imaging in a single imaging session, where tracers can be injected at successively higher doses to effectively swamp any residual radiation from prior injections. All data would be collected dynamically, but for abbreviated scan durations (eg, 0–30 minutes instead of 0–60 minutes) to minimize the overall time the patient had to lie on the bed. Dual tracer imaging would allow for characterization of tumors using tracers that reveal complementary information about tumor markers and potential

treatments. This is depicted in **Fig. 7** where, based on prior work, a low-dose (3 mCi) of [^{18}F]fluoroglutamine, a tracer that measures the delivery and pool size of glutamine to tumors,[40] could be injected followed by a higher dose (15 mCi) injection of FDG. This pairing of tracers is especially valuable when imaging triple negative breast cancer, which may use glutamine as an energy source, in addition to glucose, resulting in a small [^{18}F]fluoroglutamine pool size, and thus low uptake on imaging. The efficacy of subsequent treatment with a glutaminase inhibitor can be seen on [^{18}F]fluoroglutamine imaging with an increase in pool size, and thus uptake, that would not be evident on FDG only imaging (V. Viswanath, R. Zhou, H. Lee, S. Li, A. Cragin, R. K. Doot and colleagues., "Kinetic modeling of [18F] (2S,4R)4-fluoroglutamine in mouse models of breast cancer to estimate glutamine pool size as an indicator of

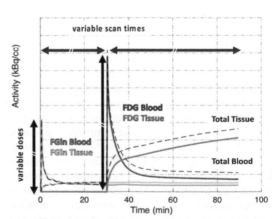

Fig. 7. Example of a dual tracer study (Reprinted with permission from paper). (*From* D. A. Mankoff, A. R. Pantel, V. Viswanath, J. S. Karp, "Advances in PET Diagnostics for Guiding Targeted Cancer Therapy and Studying In Vivo Cancer Biology," *Current Pathobiology Reports,* vol. 7, no. 3, pp. 97-108, 2019; with permission.)

tumor glutamine metabolism," *J Nucl Med,* 2020 (in preparation)).[40,41]

SUMMARY

Both the high sensitivity and extended axial length of total body PET imaging enables total body 4D PET data acquisition. The high sensitivity can be leveraged for low dose imaging, abbreviated dynamic acquisitions, finely sampled dynamic data, collecting kinetic data from 10 or more half-lives, and dual tracer imaging, while total body coverage enables the measurement of IDIFs from various locations and the reconstruction of total body parametric images. Total body PET will be a key resource for implementing dynamic or semi-dynamic acquisitions in routine clinical practice and enable rigorous testing of new radiotracers to expand the clinical usefulness of PET.

ACKNOWLEDGMENTS

The authors would like to thank the following funding sources: NIH R01-CA206187, R33-CA225310, R01-CA113941, and KL2-TR001879.

DISCLOSURE

The authors have nothing to disclose.

REFERENCES

1. Farwell MD, Pryma DA, Mankoff DA. PET/CT imaging in cancer: current applications and future directions. Cancer 2014;120(22):3433–45.
2. Doot RK. Getting the most out of 18F-FDG PET scans: the predictive value of 18F-FDG PET–derived blood flow estimates for breast cancer. J Nucl Med 2016;57(11):1667–8.
3. Dimitrakopoulou-Strauss A, Pan L, Sachpekidis C. Kinetic modeling and parametric imaging with dynamic PET for oncological applications: general considerations, current clinical applications, and future perspectives. Eur J Nucl Med Mol Imaging 2020. https://doi.org/10.1007/s00259-020-04843-6.
4. Muzi M, O'Sullivan F, Mankoff DA, et al. Quantitative assessment of dynamic PET imaging data in cancer imaging. Magn Reson Imaging 2012;30(9):1203–15.
5. Phelps M, Huang S, Hoffman E, et al. Tomographic measurement of local cerebral glucose metabolic rate in humans with (F-18) 2-fluoro-2-deoxy-D-glucose: validation of method. Ann Neurol 1979; 6(5):371–88.
6. Patlak CS, Blasberg RG. Graphical evaluation of blood-to-brain transfer constants from multiple-time uptake data. Generalizations. J Cereb Blood Flow Metab 1985;5(4):584–90.
7. Logan J, Fowler JS, Volkow ND, et al. Graphical analysis of reversible radioligand binding from time—activity measurements applied to [N-11C-methyl]-(−)-cocaine PET studies in human subjects. J Cereb Blood Flow Metab 1990;10(5):740–7.
8. Logan J, Fowler JS, Volkow ND, et al. Distribution volume ratios without blood sampling from graphical analysis of PET data. J Cereb Blood Flow Metab 1996;16(5):834–40.
9. Zhang X, Zhou J, Cherry SR, et al. Quantitative image reconstruction for total-body PET imaging using the 2-meter long EXPLORER scanner. Phys Med Biol 2017;62(6):2465.
10. Pantel AR, Viswanath V, Daube-Witherspoon ME, et al. PennPET Explorer: human imaging on a whole-body imager. J Nucl Med 2019;61(1):144–51.
11. Mankoff DA, Muzi M, Krohn KA. Quantitative positron emission tomography imaging to measure tumor response to therapy: what is the best method? Mol Imaging Biol 2003;5(5):281–5.
12. Spence AM, Muzi M, Mankoff DA, et al. 18F-FDG PET of gliomas at delayed intervals: improved distinction between tumor and normal gray matter. J Nucl Med 2004;45(10):1653–9.
13. Viswanath V, Pantel AR, Daube-Witherspoon ME, et al. "Quantifying the k4 of fluorodeoxyglucose in normal organs using the PennPET Explorer, a long axial field of view PET scanner," in biomedical engineering society conference, Philadelphia (PA): 2019.
14. Dirisamer A, Halpern BS, Schima W, et al. Dual-time-point FDG-PET/CT for the detection of hepatic metastases. Mol Imaging Biol 2008;10(6):335–40.
15. Sellmyer MA, Richman SA, Lohith K, et al. Imaging CAR T cell trafficking with eDHFR as a PET reporter gene. Mol Ther 2020;28(1):42–51.
16. Pandit-Taskar N, Postow MA, Hellmann MD, et al. First-in-humans imaging with 89Zr-Df-IAB22M2C Anti-CD8 minibody in patients with solid malignancies: preliminary pharmacokinetics, biodistribution, and lesion targeting. J Nucl Med 2020; 61(4):512–9.
17. Li T, Ao EC, Lambert B, et al. Quantitative imaging for targeted radionuclide therapy dosimetry-technical review. Theranostics 2017;7(18):4551.
18. Taebi A, Roudsari B, Vu C, et al. Hepatic arterial tree segmentation: towards patient-specific dosimetry for liver cancer radioembolization. J Nucl Med 2019;60(supplement 1):122.
19. Viswanath V, Pantel AR, Daube-Witherspoon ME, et al. Quantifying bias and precision of kinetic parameter estimation on the PennPET Explorer, a long axial field-of-view scanner. IEEE Trans Radiat Plasma Med Sci 2020 (Accepted).
20. Viswanath V, Pantel AR, Daube-Witherspoon ME, et al. "Dynamic imaging on the 70-cm PennPET Explorer using GATE simulations.," in 2018 total body

PET conference, Ghent, Belgium. EJNMMI Phy 2018;5(Suppl 1):19 [Abstract: A21].

21. Zhang X, Xie Z, Berg E, et al. Total-body dynamic reconstruction and parametric imaging on the uEXPLORER. J Nucl Med 2020;61(2):285–91.

22. Zhang X, Xie Z, Berg E, et al. Total-body parametric imaging using kernel and direct reconstruction on the uEXPLORER. J Nucl Med 2019;60(supplement 1):456.

23. Matej S, Surti S, Jayanthi S, et al. Efficient 3-D TOF PET reconstruction using view-grouped histo-images: DIRECT—direct image reconstruction for TOF. IEEE Trans Med Imaging 2009;28(5):739–51.

24. Li Y, Viswanath V, Daube-Witherspoon ME, et al, "Nested parametric image reconstruction using time-of-flight PET histoimages," in IEEE NSS/MIC, Boston (MA): 2020.

25. Graham M, Peterson L, Hayward R. Comparison of simplified quantitative analyses of FDG uptake. Nucl Med Biol 2000;27(7):647–55.

26. Dimitrakopoulou-Strauss A, Strauss LG, Burger C, et al. Prognostic aspects of 18F-FDG PET kinetics in patients with metastatic colorectal carcinoma receiving FOLFOX chemotherapy. J Nucl Med 2004;45(9):1480–7.

27. Wang G, Parikh M, Nardo L, et al. Total-body dynamic PET of metastatic cancer: first patient results. J Nucl Med 2020;61(supplement 1):208.

28. O'Sullivan F. Imaging radiotracer model parameters in PET: a mixture analysis approach. IEEE Trans Med Imaging 1993;12(3):399–412.

29. Wu H-M, Hoh CK, Buxton DB, et al. Quantification of myocardial blood flow using dynamic nitrogen-13-. ammonia PET studies. J Nucl Med 1995;36:2087–93.

30. Alpert NM, Reilhac A, Chio TC, et al. Optimization of dynamic measurement of receptor kinetics by wavelet denoising. Neuroimage 2006;30(2):444–51.

31. Eary JF, Mankoff DA, Spence AM, et al. 2-[C-11] thymidine imaging of malignant brain tumors. Cancer Res 1999;59(3):615–21.

32. Cunningham VJ, Jones T. Spectral analysis of dynamic PET studies. J Cereb Blood Flow Metab 1993;13(1):15–23.

33. Veronese M, Rizzo G, Bertoldo A, et al. Spectral analysis of dynamic PET studies: a review of 20 years of method developments and applications. Comput Math Methods Med 2016;2016:7187541.

34. Meier P, Zierler KL. On the theory of the indicator-dilution method for measurement of blood flow and volume. J Appl Phys 1954;6(12):731–44.

35. O'sullivan F, Muzi M, Spence AM, et al. Nonparametric residue analysis of dynamic PET data with application to cerebral FDG studies in normals. J Am Stat Assoc 2009;104(486):556–71.

36. O'Sullivan F, Muzi M, Mankoff DA, et al. Voxel-level mapping of tracer kinetics in PET studies: a statistical approach emphasizing tissue life tables. Ann Appl Stat 2014;8(2):1065.

37. Huang J, O'Sullivan F. An analysis of whole body tracer kinetics in dynamic PET studies with application to image-based blood input function extraction. IEEE Trans Med Imaging 2014;33(5):1093–108.

38. Bading JR, Shields AF. Imaging of cell proliferation: status and prospects. J Nucl Med 2008;49(2):64S.

39. Chitalia R, Viswanath V, Pantel AR, et al. 4D radiomic biomarker of functional tumor heterogeneity to predict breast cancer recurrence in pretreatment dynamic FDG-PET. American Society of Clinical Oncology; 2020.

40. Zhou R, Pantel AR, Li S, et al. [18F](2S, 4R) 4-fluoro-glutamine PET detects glutamine pool size changes in triple-negative breast cancer in response to glutaminase inhibition. Cancer Res 2017;77(6):1476–84.

41. Mankoff DA, Pantel AR, Viswanath V, et al. Advances in PET diagnostics for guiding targeted cancer therapy and studying in vivo cancer biology. Curr Pathobiol Rep 2019;7(3):97–108.

Oncologic Applications of Long Axial Field-of-View PET/Computed Tomography

Lorenzo Nardo, MD, PhD[a], Austin R. Pantel, MD, MSTR[b],*

KEYWORDS

- PET • Whole-body imager • EXPLORER • Human imaging • Oncology

KEY POINTS

- Human imaging on the uEXPLORER at U.C. Davis and the PennPET EXPLORER at the University of Pennsylvania have demonstrated superb image quality.
- The increased sensitivity of these instruments enables imaging with less injected activity or shorter scans or delayed imaging. These new capabilities can uniquely benefit oncologic imaging.
- The increased sensitivity of EXPLORER PET and new imaging paradigms create new challenges in imaging interpretation that must be overcome for optimal integration into the clinical workflow.
- The ability to image lesser activities can be leveraged for research studies, including dosimetry and cell tracking applications, and even dual-tracer imaging.

INTRODUCTION

The increased axial coverage of long axial field-of-view (AFOV) PET scanners enable whole-body PET imaging in a single-bed position. The resultant marked increase in physical sensitivity produces images of higher quality than conventional PET scanners. These sensitivity gains can be leveraged in several oncologic applications, both in research and in the clinic.

The EXPLORER Consortium has developed 2 long AFOV for human use, these being the uEXPLORER (currently installed at the University of California, Davis and at several sites in China) and the PennPET EXPLORER at the University of Pennsylvania. Performance testing of both devices and initial human studies have already been published.[1–3] Recent updates regarding development and/or application of these scanners are discussed in other chapters in this edition of the PET Clinics (Lorenzo Nardo and colleagues' article, "Clinical Implementation of Total-Body PET/CT at University of California, Davis"; and Xiuli Sui and colleagues' article, "Total Body PET/CT Highlights in Clinical Practice Experiences from Zhongshan Hospital, Fudan University," in this issue for the uEXPLORER and Austin R. Pantel and colleagues' article, "Update on the PennPET Explorer: A Whole-Body Imager with Scalable Axial Field-of-View," in this issue for the PennPET EXPLORER). At the current time, the uEXPLORER is being used for both research and clinical imaging. The PennPET EXPLORER is being expanded to its final configuration for research investigations.

Human imaging on both of these long AFOV scanners have demonstrated many of the theoretic benefits of increased photon detection

Funding: NIH R01-CA206187, R01-CA113941, R01CA249422, R01-CA225874, and KL2TR001879.
[a] Department of Radiology, U.C. Davis, 4860 Y Street Suite 3100, Sacramento, CA 95817, USA; [b] Department of Radiology, University of Pennsylvania, 3400 Spruce Street, 1 Silverstein, Suite 130, Philadelphia, PA 19104, USA
* Corresponding author.
E-mail address: austin.pantel@pennmedicine.upenn.edu

PET Clin 16 (2021) 65–73
https://doi.org/10.1016/j.cpet.2020.09.010

sensitivity: (1) total-body diagnostic quality images have been obtained in approximately 1 minute, increasing the tolerability of imaging; (2) diagnostic quality images have been realized with significantly reduced quantities of radiotracer, decreasing the overall radiation exposure of patients; (3) delayed acquisitions that may improve the visualization of tumor by increasing the ratio between tumor uptake and background; (4) increased image quality has demonstrated sites of uptake previously unseen on conventional PET that may result in early detection of tumor/recurrence.

The implementation of this technology is not without risks. The interpretation of findings that were not visualized on conventional PET/CT scanners, or were visualized but have different quantitative levels of uptake, must be studied to avoid "overcalling." New interpretation paradigms may be necessary as not to decrease the specificity of whole-body PET imaging.

This work reviews the advantages and challenges posed by the implementation of total body PET/CT in oncology. Exemplary whole-body PET images provide the motivation for this discussion. Early lessons and future directions are also discussed in this evolving field.

SHORTER SCAN TIME

Exploiting the increased physical sensitivity of long AFOV, whole-body PET scanners can produce diagnostic images in as short as 1 minute. Initial human studies on the uEXPLORER and the PennPET EXPLORER explored the effects of decreased scan time by simulating shorter studies using listmode data.[2,3] Both scanners demonstrated the ability to generate images with acceptable image quality in approximately half a minute.

Fast acquisition time can benefit both adult and pediatric patients. The inherent stress of PET imaging often necessitates anesthesia for pediatric patients with inherent risks of the anesthesia itself, as well as the need for invasive monitoring. Further, anesthesia requires additional staff and equipment.[4] This increase in imaging complexity also adds to imaging cost and may even delay necessary imaging. Decreasing the anesthetic requirement or the elimination of anesthesia altogether could clearly benefit pediatric imaging. In addition, shorter imaging time would aid in the imaging oncologic patients who may have difficulty and pain when lying flat on the scanner table, such as patients with widespread osseous metastatic disease. For these patients, lying flat for 20 to 30 minutes presents a significant barrier to

imaging, and imaging may be degraded from motion if the patient is uncomfortable. Faster imaging on a long AFOV device may increase the accessibility for these patient populations.

Shorter imaging frames may also benefit characterizing disease with radiotracers with time-varying kinetics. For example, ^{18}F-fluciclovine uptake in tumors usually peaks early and decreases over time, whereas bladder uptake increases over time from urinary excretion.[5] Urinary activity layers in the dependent aspect of the urinary bladder over time. Urine activity can be misinterpreted as a recurrent tumor if localizing to the prostate bed, especially when confounded by motion artifact and/or suboptimal anatomic delineation from a low-dose correlative computed tomography (CT). The use of a series of short time frame images, for example, 2-minute frame duration, obtained from the 20-minute dataset may help avoid this pitfall and show that the bladder uptake follows the ureters uptake in time. However, uptake in the same region before radiotracer excretion may be suspicious for recurrent tumor.

Fast acquisition on long AFOV PET imagers may enable breath-hold examinations. Even with state-of-the art PET scanners, imaging the chest occurs over minutes, precluding breath-hold imaging. Imaging in the setting of shallow respiration leads to respiratory motion artifact and partial volume averaging, both decreasing apparent uptake of lung nodules. Further, coregistration with the CT suffers. Breath-hold PET has been shown to mitigate these effects.[6,7] Prior simulation scans have demonstrated the possibility of pushing the limit of acquisition time to less than half a minute.[1,3] Breath-hold PET should be accompanied by breath-hold CT obtained in the same phase of respiration for anatomic registration and attenuation correction. This application may improve the characterization and detection of small lung nodules. The clinical implications of such an improvement would have to be studied in the context of current treatment paradigms.

LOW DOSE

The increased sensitivity of whole-body PET can allow for a decrease in the injected activity while preserving image quality. On the uEXPLORER, images have been acquired with 18.5 MBq (0.5 mCi) of fluorodeoxyglucose (FDG), about 1/20th of the standard injected activity, that are considered to be of high quality. Examples of PET/CT images obtained using 18.5 MBq (0.5 mCi) are shown in **Fig. 1**. As shown in this

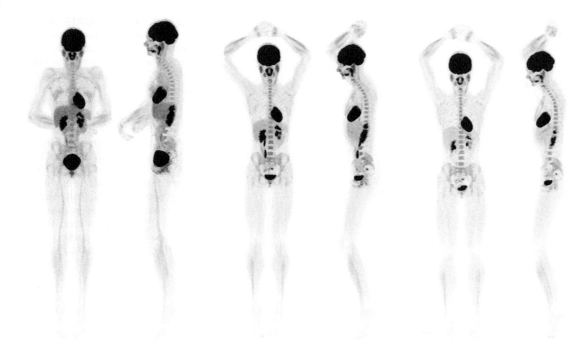

Fig. 1. A 43-year-old healthy female participant, injected with 18.5 MBq of ^{18}F-FDG. Anterior and left lateral MIP views from three 20-minute datasets are presented: 40 to 60 minutes (*left*), 90 to 110 minutes (*center*), and 180 to 200 minutes (*right*). Images, scaled to the same window level, demonstrate the normal radiotracer biodistribution with high image quality. MIP, maximum intensity projection.

image, the expected biodistribution of FDG can be reliably traced even 3 hours after injection of such a small amount of activity. On the prototype PennPET Explorer with a 64 cm AFOV, ^{68}Ga-DOTATATE PET images of a patient with metastatic neuroendocrine tumor obtained 3.5 hours after injection of the radiotracer were comparable with images obtained on a standard-of-care PET scanner obtained 65 minutes after injection (**Fig. 2**). At the time of scanning on the PennPET Explorer, the activity was one-fifth that at the time of the clinical scan and corresponded to an injected activity of 30 MBq if a standard uptake of an hour was used.[2]

Beyond merely a technologic achievement, imaging with less injected activity may have important clinical applications, especially in the pediatric, adolescent, and young adult population. Decreasing radiation dose is receiving increasing attention for these developing age groups. For example, lymphoma is the third most common childhood malignancy and PET/CT is widely accepted in its diagnosis-treatment paradigm.[8] Typically, a patient undergoes at least 3 FDG-PET/CTs. For example, a routine clinical protocol for Hodgkin lymphoma includes one PET/CT at staging, one after 2 cycles of chemotherapy and one after completion of treatment.

The patient may receive one or more additional PET/CT scans when there are concerns for persistent or recurrent disease. Decreasing the injected activity from 370 MBq (10 mCi) to 18.5 MBq (0.5 mCi) for 3 PET/CT studies decreases the exposure related to FDG injection from 21 mSv to approximately 1.1 mSv. Furthermore, decreasing the radiation dose per scan may increase the utilization of PET/CT in long-term follow-up of these patients to screen for recurrence, which is not generally routine practice at this time.[8] The role of total-body PET/CT for pediatric imaging is further explored in a review article by Nardo and colleagues.[9]

In addition to reducing radiation exposure in pediatric imaging, unnecessary exposure to radiation in the adult population should also be avoided. Several campaigns in both the United States and Europe are dedicated to educating physicians about adhering to "as low as reasonably acceptable" principles, in the pediatric and adult population. For example, the "Image Wisely" campaign is a joint initiative supported by several radiological societies that aims to lower the amount of radiation used in medically necessary imaging studies and eliminate unnecessary procedures in adult imaging.[10] Similarly, "Image Gently" exists for pediatric radiology.[11] The use of decreased injected

A

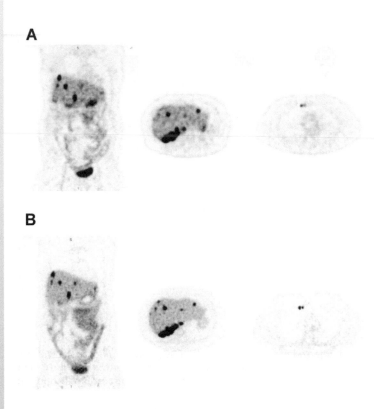

B

Fig. 2. (*A*) 68Ga-DOTATATE PET images (coronal and transverse) of a subject with metastatic neuroendocrine tumor imaged on a standard-of-care PET scanner 65 minutes after radiotracer injection. (*B*) Coronal and transverse images from same subject on PennPET acquired 3.5 hours after injection (20-minute scan). Although the scan on the PennPET Explorer was obtained 2.5 hours after the standard-of-care commercial scan (greater than two-half lives), image quality is comparable. This research was originally published in JNM. Pantel et al. PennPET Explorer: Human Imaging on a Whole-Body Imager. 2020;**61**(1):144-51. © SNMMI.

activity in total body PET/CT with low-dose protocols is in keeping with the pledge that many radiologists have made to these campaigns. The implementation of low-dose PET/CT may also allow PET/CT to be used as a screening tool for patients with hereditary cancer syndromes, such as BRCA+ breast and ovarian cancers, Li-Fraumeni, or Lynch syndromes, where the risk of developing cancer is several times higher than that of the nonaffected population.[12]

Imaging with lower activity can also be of benefit when using radiotracers with limited supply, for example, as shown with 68Ga-DOTATATE on the PennPET Explorer study described earlier. Given production difficulty with 68Ga-DOTATATE, imaging each patient with a lesser dose may increase the availability of this study for patients.[2] Similarly, imaging with lower activity may benefit research radiotracers with difficult productions or dose limitations.

DELAYED IMAGING

As an alternate to imaging with less injected activity at typical uptake times, the high sensitivity of long AFOV scanners enables imaging at delayed time points using the standard injected activity. Indeed, imaging on the PennPET EXPLORER was shown to be possible as late as 24 hours after the injection of 500 MBq (13.5 mCi) of FDG. Imaging at approximatively 4 hours demonstrated diagnostic image quality.[2] Depending on radiotracer kinetics, delayed imaging may prove valuable. For instance, given trapping of FDG in malignancy owing to increased hexokinase activity and washout of background tissue, lesion contrast increases over time. Imaging a clinical patient with metastatic colon cancer demonstrated this on the prototype PennPET Explorer with 64 cm AFOV (**Fig. 3**). An epiphrenic lymph node was only seen on delayed imaging 2.75 and 4.2 after injection; this lymph node was not visualized by conventional PET 1 hour after injection. Washout of tracer from normal tissues increased contrast in this lymph node, which, in combination with increased sensitivity from the PennPET Explorer, enabled detection.[2] Several clinical studies have shown increased sensitivity with FDG in detecting disease by using delayed imaging.[13,14] Delineation of normal tissue and tumor may also benefit from delayed imaging, as has been shown with FDG-PET in glioma imaging.[15]

TOTAL BODY IMAGING

The 194 cm AFOV of the uEXPLORER scanner allows total body coverage in more than 90% of the population. This opens the door to performing total body dynamic imaging, providing simultaneous time activities curves for organs/lesions not contained within the view of conventional PET/CT. These datasets, inclusive of entire body kinetics, can be reconstructed and analyzed to create parametric images that may offer complementary information to typical standardized uptake value–scaled images. For example, utilization rate (K_i) images of FDG can be provided to the radiologist to visualize glucose utilization in the target lesion not confounded by nonspecific uptake. These images are now available at UC Davis, and their clinical value is being evaluated and compared with the routine static acquisition images. As expected, it is challenging to implement such protocols in clinical routine due to limited scanner time. However, if significant clinical utility is demonstrated, then workflows may be developed to allow these protocols to be routinely used.

INCREASED DETECTION CHALLENGES

The improved image quality of total body PET may result in the detection of radiotracer uptake in small structures that cannot be seen on conventional PET/CT scanners. This ability arises from to the significant gain in signal, which allows reconstruction without the need for filtering to reduce noise, and from the excellent intrinsic spatial resolution of these devices. The visualization of such small structures presents challenges in the interpretation of total body PET images.

The interpretation of PET signal must be made in the context of disease pathophysiology versus normal physiology. Correlation with other imaging modalities is often helpful. For example, with total body PET/CT scanners, the visualization of a small lymph node with uptake measuring 2 to 3 times more than liver background may be interpreted as a normal finding rather than lymphoproliferative or metastatic disease (**Fig. 4**). Mild reactive uptake in cervical lymph nodes, particular submandibular lymph nodes, is a common finding on conventional PET/CT and offers a challenge to the reader in terms of reporting the significance. Total body PET only accentuates these findings, although it is possible that delayed imaging may help. Normal anatomic features—for example, preservation of the fatty hilum—may also support a benign cause. In another context, though, radiotracer uptake in a small lymph node may indicate disease. For example, uptake in a small pelvic lymph node on an ^{18}F-fluiclvoine study in a patient with biochemical recurrence of prostate cancer may likely represent a site of recurrent disease. In this case, total body PET provides a clear advantage.

With increasing experience interpreting studies from total body PET scanners, uptake in normal physiologic structures becomes apparent or more prominent. For example, the celiac ganglia and parasympathetic chain are seen more frequently in total body ^{18}F-fluciclovine studies (**Fig. 5**); on FDG studies, the adrenal glands, pituitary gland, and gray matter of the spinal cord are often prominent.[16] The radiologist must appreciate that these structures are normal, as misinterpreting these findings may lead to unnecessary follow-ups or procedures exposing the patients to further risk, such as radiation exposure.

The high spatial resolution of the uEXPLORER enables more accurate quantification of radiotracer uptake in small lesions. For example, ground glass opacities and small pulmonary nodule may now be visualized with uptake levels that are exceeding the radiologist expectations. These findings, though, may still correlate with benign findings.

FUTURE DIRECTIONS

The long AFOV and technical advantages of the total body PET can be exploited for many research purposes in oncology, far beyond the applications described earlier.

Dosimetry studies of novel radiotracers can benefit from a long AFOV PET scanner. The ability to image lower activities afforded by increased sensitivity can be used to image at later time periods after radiotracer injection to better estimate the organ time-activity curve. For example, images on the PennPET Explorer with FDG were obtained out to 10 half-lives postinjection,[2] permitting studies of the biodistribution of FDG over extended time-periods in healthy volunteers. Such increases in data could improve estimates of cumulative activity and thus the absorbed dose.

Total body PET also allows for the generation of vastly improved images when using radiotracers with unfavorable dosimetry such as those labeled with [89]Zr,[17] which for safety reasons can only be injected in small quantities. This technique is particularly valuable when imaging antibodies, antibody fragments and such, which must be labeled with long-lived isotopes due to their slow kinetics. This has profound positive implications

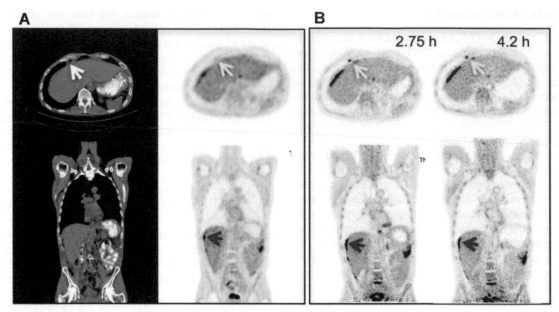

Fig. 3. (*A*) Standard-of-care ^{18}F-FDG PET/CT images (transverse and coronal) from a patient with metastatic colon cancer. (*B*) PennPET image acquired 2.75 and 4.2 hours after injection (10-minute scans) demonstrate better delineation of perihepatic disease (*red arrow*) compared with standard-of-care PET. An epiphrenic lymph node (*yellow arrow*) is also only seen on the delayed PennPET images. This research was originally published in JNM. Pantel et al. PennPET Explorer: Human Imaging on a Whole-Body Imager. 2020;**61**(1):144-51. © SNMMI.

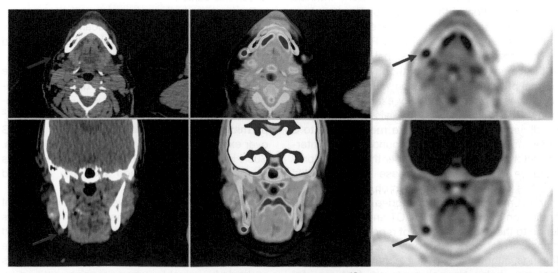

Fig. 4. A 53-year-old healthy female subject, injected with 389 MBq of ^{18}F-FDG. The shown images from a 20-minute acquisition obtained 90 minute after injection. The arrow indicates a small right submandibular lymph node with a tiny fatty hilum. This lymph node was approximatively 3 times more FDG avid than liver background. The finding was followed clinically and demonstrated to be a reactive lymph node.

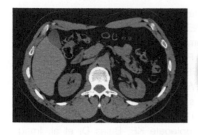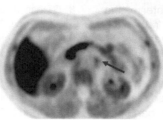

Fig. 5. A 56-year-old man with biochemical recurrence of prostate cancer. Ten-minute images were reconstructed starting from 4-minute postinjection of 306 MBq of ^{18}F-Fluciclovine. The red arrow demonstrates uptake within the left celiac ganglia with radiotracer uptake similar or higher than bone marrow; this finding should not be misinterpreted as a metastatic retroperitoneal lymph node.

for immunoPET, which in turn may benefit oncologic science, drug development, and personalized medicine.[18] PET imaging of cell-based therapies is a related application of interest. A critical concern when directly labeling cells for PET applications is toxicity to the cells, whereas a limiting factor when using reporter-gene approaches is detecting the cell signal over the background. In both cases, the sensitivity gain from total body PET is likely to deliver important advantages.

Long AFOV PET can enable sequential imaging of 2 PET tracers. By imaging a lower dose of a first tracer and subsequently imaging a higher dose of a second tracer, 2 PET tracers may be imaged in 1 image session.[19] Such a protocol is analogous to ventilation-perfusion imaging with two ^{99m}Tc-based radiotracers where the counts from the second tracer overwhelm the first. Oncologic applications are numerous, with a simple example being the use of NaF followed by FDG.[20] The ability to image the first radiotracer on the PennPET Explorer—with doses as low as 18.5 to 74 MBq (0.5–2 mCi)[21]—permits such a protocol. More details on this potential use of a long AFOV scanner are provided in Varsha Viswanath and colleagues' article, "Analysis of 4D Data for Total-Body PET Imaging," in this issue.

Another unmet challenge in oncology is the ability to quantitatively understand, track, and predict side effects and off-target impacts of drug therapies and impacts of concurrent symptoms such as cachexia. Total body PET, by allowing simultaneous interrogation and parametric imaging of all organs, allows assessment of multiorgan function and multiorgan interactions. This facilitates a "systems biology" approach to understanding the pathophysiology of cancer and may open numerous doorways to future avenues of productive research. Related to this may be the possibility of better understanding the abscopal effect, whereby treatment of one site of disease leads to response in untreated sites.[22]

One of the earliest uses of PET was to study perfusion. Total body PET offers the possibility, for the first time, of quantitatively measuring perfusion across the entire body, allowing measurement of perfusion for metastatic disease. This may have important applications in, for example, determining whether particular lesions may be expected to respond well to radiation therapy[23] or to track response to antiangiogenic therapy.[24]

Finally, there may be future applications of total-body PET in cancer prevention. By interrogating the mind-body connection with repeat studies at low dose in healthy subjects, there is the opportunity to understand how different kinds of stress (psychological, dietary, etc) can affect the inflammatory and oncogenic milieu of the body. This in turn could lead to quantitative measurements of the mechanistic impacts of lifestyle changes, which may reduce cancer risk.

SUMMARY

The initial implementation of total body PET/CT at UC Davis and at the University of Pennsylvania has demonstrated improved image quality and opened the doors to many new applications in oncology. In the research setting, total body PET/CT can aid in the development of new radiopharmaceuticals and serves as a valuable tool to elucidate underlying biology. In the clinical setting, several new applications have been already successfully used, including low-dose imaging, delayed imaging, faster imaging, and the use of parametric maps.

These applications, both in research and in the clinic, will drive the future development and adoption of long AFOV PET. Particularly, the ideal AFOV will likely depend on desired use. Both the PennPET Explorer, tested initially in a prototype configuration of 64 cm and more recently with 112 cm, and the uExplorer with a 2 m AFOV produce images superior to commercial PET scanners. As the AFOV increases beyond a 70 cm AFOV, though, the peak sensitivity at the center of the scanner does not markedly improve; rather the axial extent of maximal sensitivity increased.[25] For applications where maximum sensitivity must be maintained over a large area of the body, such as early biodistribution studies of novel radiotracers, an AFOV of 1.4 m or greater may be necessary. For targeted studies of particular body regions, such as imaging the abdomen/pelvis for prostate cancer or dynamic imaging of the breasts with novel radiotracers, scanners with an AFOV of 1 m or less may be most cost-effective. As the indications for the scanners continue to evolve, so should the scanners themselves, pushing the current boundaries of modern PET imaging.

DISCLOSURE

Support for development of the PennPET EX-PLORER was received from Philips Healthcare and from the Department of Radiology at the University of Pennsylvania. L. Nardo is the principle investigator of a service agreement with United Imaging Healthcare. UC Davis has a revenue-sharing agreement with United Imaging Healthcare that is based on uEXPLORER sales.

REFERENCES

1. Karp JS, Viswanath V, Geagan MJ, et al. PennPET explorer: design and preliminary performance of a whole-body imager. J Nucl Med 2020;61(1):136–43.
2. Pantel AR, Viswanath V, Daube-Witherspoon ME, et al. PennPET explorer: human imaging on a whole-body imager. J Nucl Med 2020;61(1):144–51.
3. Badawi RD, Shi H, Hu P, et al. First human imaging studies with the EXPLORER total-body PET scanner. J Nucl Med 2019;60(3):299–303.
4. Arlachov Y, Ganatra RH. Sedation/anaesthesia in paediatric radiology. Br J Radiol 2012;85(1019): e1018–31.
5. Sorensen J, Owenius R, Lax M, et al. Regional distribution and kinetics of [18F]fluciclovine (anti-[18F]FACBC), a tracer of amino acid transport, in subjects with primary prostate cancer. Eur J Nucl Med Mol Imaging 2013;40(3):394–402.
6. Torizuka T, Tanizaki Y, Kanno T, et al. Single 20-second acquisition of deep-inspiration breath-hold PET/CT: clinical feasibility for lung cancer. J Nucl Med 2009;50(10):1579–84.
7. Balamoutoff N, Serrano B, Hugonnet F, et al. Added value of a single fast 20-second deep-inspiration breath-hold acquisition in FDG PET/CT in the assessment of lung nodules. Radiology 2018; 286(1):260–70.
8. Gillman J, States LJ, Servaes S. PET in pediatric lymphoma. PET Clin 2020;15(3):299–307.
9. Nardo L, Schmall JP, Werner TJ, et al. Potential roles of total-body PET/computed tomography in pediatric imaging. PET Clin 2020;15(3):271–9.
10. Mayo-Smith WW, Morin RL. Image wisely: the beginning, current status, and future opportunities. J Am Coll Radiol 2017;14(3):442–3.
11. Goske MJ, Applegate KE, Bulas D, et al. Image gently: progress and challenges in CT education and advocacy. Pediatr Radiol 2011;41(Suppl 2): 461–6.
12. Tiwari R, Singh AK, Somwaru AS, et al. Radiologist's primer on imaging of common hereditary cancer syndromes. Radiographics 2019;39(3):759–78.
13. Kubota K, Itoh M, Ozaki K, et al. Advantage of delayed whole-body FDG-PET imaging for tumour detection. Eur J Nucl Med 2001;28(6):696–703.
14. Mayerhoefer ME, Giraudo C, Senn D, et al. Does delayed-time-point imaging improve 18F-FDG-PET in patients with MALT lymphoma?: observations in a series of 13 patients. Clin Nucl Med 2016;41(2): 101–5.
15. Spence AM, Muzi M, Mankoff DA, et al. 18F-FDG PET of gliomas at delayed intervals: improved distinction between tumor and normal gray matter. J Nucl Med 2004;45(10):1653–9.
16. Adbelhafez Yasser G. ECR 2020 book of abstracts: Vienna, Austria. 15 March 2020. Insights Imaging 2020;11(1):34.
17. Beckford Vera D, Schulte B, Henrich T, et al. First-in-human total-body PET imaging of HIV with 89Zr-VRC01 on the EXPLORER. J Nucl Med 2020; 61(supplement 1):545.
18. Wei W, Jiang D, Ehlerding EB, et al. Noninvasive PET imaging of T cells. Trends Cancer 2018;4(5): 359–73.
19. Mankoff DA, Pantel AR, Viswanath V, et al. Advances in PET diagnostics for guiding targeted cancer therapy and studying in vivo cancer biology. Curr Pathobiol Rep 2019;7(3):97–108.
20. Lin FI, Rao JE, Mittra ES, et al. Prospective comparison of combined 18F-FDG and 18F-NaF PET/CT vs. 18F-FDG PET/CT imaging for detection of malignancy. Eur J Nucl Med Mol Imaging 2012;39(2):262–70.
21. Viswanath V, Pantel A, Daube-Witherspoon M, et al. Quantifying bias and precision of kinetic parameter estimation on the PennPET Explorer, a long axial field-of-view scanner. IEEE Trans Radiat Plasma Med Sci 2020;1. https://doi.org/10.1109/TRPMS. 2020.3021315.
22. Rodríguez-Ruiz ME, Vanpouille-Box C, Melero I, et al. Immunological mechanisms responsible for radiation-induced abscopal effect. Trends Immunol 2018;39(8):644–55.
23. Capaldi DP, Banks TI, Hristov DH, et al. Parametric response mapping of co-registered PET and

perfusion CT to identify radioresistant sub-volumes in locally advanced cervical carcinoma. Int J Radiat Oncol Biol Phys 2019;105(1):S226.

24. Bao X, Wang M-W, Luo J-M, et al. Optimization of early response monitoring and prediction of cancer antiangiogenesis therapy via noninvasive PET molecular imaging strategies of multifactorial bioparameters. Theranostics 2016;6(12): 2084–98.

25. Surti S, Pantel AR, Karp JS. Total body PET: why, how, what for? IEEE Trans Radiat Plasma Med Sci 2020;4(3):283–92.

Total-body PET Imaging
A New Frontier for the Assessment of Metabolic Disease and Obesity

Maria Chondronikola, PhD, RDN[a,b], Souvik Sarkar, MD, PhD[b,c],*

KEYWORDS

- PET • Metabolic syndrome • Nonalcoholic fatty liver disease • Adipose tissue • Skeletal muscle

KEY POINTS

- The high prevalence of obesity and its related metabolic diseases accentuate the urgency for the discovery and implementation of effective prevention and treatment strategies.
- The mechanisms underlying the multiorgan pathophysiology of obesity are not fully understood.
- Dynamic PET with ^{18}F-fluorodeoxyglucose can be used to determine metabolic processes relevant to metabolic disease.
- Total-body PET imaging provides for the first time the opportunity to assess the systemic effects of metabolic disease with tissue-specific resolution at the whole-body level.
- Total-body PET imaging can be used not only to create important new knowledge but also to facilitate the development of precision medicine approaches for diagnosis and treatment of obesity and metabolic disease.

INTRODUCTION

Obesity and its related metabolic diseases (type 2 diabetes, cardiovascular disease, hepatic steatosis, cancer, and so forth) constitute a major public health issue because of their high prevalence,[1] impact on the well-being of the population,[2,3] and financial burden to the health care systems.[4,5] Lifestyle modifications (including nutrition and exercise) constitute the first-line approach for the prevention and treatment of the obesity-related metabolic diseases. In addition, an armamentarium of pharmacologic approaches is available for the treatment of obesity-related metabolic complications. However, many patients with obesity-related metabolic perturbations fail to achieve their treatment goals.[6–8] Therefore, there is a need to better understand the pathophysiology of obesity and to establish new effective and safe approaches for the prevention and treatment of obesity-related metabolic complications.

Functional medical imaging technologies are currently the new frontier in the assessment of metabolic function and health. Their competitive advantage stems from the ability to noninvasively quantify different metabolic processes at tissue-specific levels in vivo. Alternatively, an assessment of these metabolic processes would either require implementation of invasive procedures or would not otherwise be feasible. The recently launched total-body PET scanner EXPLORER[9–11] and development of dynamic total-body PET technologies applicable to EXPLORER[12–15] enables, for the first time, the performance of simultaneous dynamic imaging of all body tissues and organs. This total-body PET provides a new level of detail and capability to diagnose multiple organ involvement in obesity-related metabolic dysfunction. The technical aspects of the total-body PET imaging and estimation of the different kinetic parameters are reviewed elsewhere in this issue. This

[a] Department of Nutrition, University of California Davis, One Shields Avenue, Davis, CA 95616, USA; [b] Harokopio University of Athens, El Venizelou 70, Kallithea 17676, Greece; [c] Division of Gastroenterology and Hepatology, University of California Davis, Davis, CA, USA
* Corresponding author. 4150 V Street, PSSB 3500, Sacramento, CA 95817.
E-mail address: ssarkar@ucdavis.edu

PET Clin 16 (2021) 75–87
https://doi.org/10.1016/j.cpet.2020.09.001

article discusses how total-body PET can be used to (1) improve the current knowledge of the pathophysiology of obesity, and (2) contribute to the development of precision medicine approaches for the improved diagnosis, treatment, and prevention of obesity-related metabolic dysfunction.

UNDERSTANDING OBESITY AND ITS RELATED METABOLIC ABNORMALITIES

Obesity is associated with the development of several chronic diseases (including cardiovascular disease, type 2 diabetes, hepatitis steatosis, cancer, and chronic kidney disease) and accelerated aging.[16,17] In the light of the recent novel coronavirus (severe acute respiratory syndrome-coronavirus-2) pandemic, preliminary data suggest that obesity is associated with increased rates of severe COVID19 (coronavirus disease 2019),[18] suggesting the people with obesity may also be more vulnerable to developing infectious diseases-related complications. Excessive adiposity (particularly abdominal obesity) is a risk factor for development of metabolic abnormalities such as insulin resistance, hyperglycemia, and atherogenic hyperlipidemia (low high-density lipoprotein cholesterol and high triglyceride levels) and high blood pressure.[19] The term metabolic syndrome encompasses the cluster of the previously mentioned metabolic abnormalities frequently observed in obesity.[20] However, some individuals with excessive adiposity seem to be protected from the metabolic complications of obesity,[21] whereas some lean individuals are prone to the development of metabolic abnormalities even in the absence of obesity.[22]

Metabolic syndrome is a systemic condition that affects multiple organs. Insulin resistance is considered to be a major contributor for the development of metabolic syndrome and the other obesity-related metabolic perturbations.[23–25] Insulin is a key metabolic regulator that acts in multiple organs (**Fig. 1**). In people with normal insulin sensitivity, insulin stimulates glucose uptake in skeletal muscle and suppresses adipose tissue lipolysis and hepatic endogenous glucose production.[26] In people with insulin resistance and metabolic syndrome, the peripheral tissues are less sensitive to the action of insulin leading to (1) impaired insulin-stimulated glucose uptake in skeletal muscle, (2) impaired suppression of lipolysis in adipose tissue, and (3) decreased suppression of hepatic endogenous glucose production in the liver. Liver and skeletal muscle insulin resistance results in increase in blood glucose levels. Adipose insulin resistance results in increased levels of circulating free fatty acids (FFAs), leading

to the accumulation of excessive amounts of intrahepatic triglycerides causing fatty liver disease and ectopic fat accumulation in other tissues.[27–30] Further, insulin resistance leads to increased compensatory insulin secretion from the beta cells of the pancreas to maintain euglycemia.[31] The increased insulin signaling stimulates increased de novo lipogenesis to the liver, which further promotes the accumulation of intrahepatic triglycerides.[32] In addition, insulin resistance is also associated with inability of the muscle to adequately metabolize fats, which further accentuates adipose tissue insulin resistance and ectopic fat deposition to the liver and nonadipose organs.[24,33,34] Altered glucose and lipid metabolism leads to activation of downstream inflammatory pathways thought to contribute to the deleterious effects of fatty liver disease and the other obesity-related metabolic perturbations.[27–30]

APPROACHES FOR THE ASSESSMENT OF METABOLIC FUNCTION IN CLINICAL PRACTICE AND RESEARCH

The methods currently used for the diagnosis of obesity-related metabolic perturbations include the assessment of various circulating biomarkers of metabolic health (eg, plasma/serum glucose, insulin, lipid and cholesterol concentrations, glycosylated hemoglobin A1c) mostly after overnight fasting. Functional assessments of metabolic health (eg, oral glucose tolerance test) are implemented less often and their use is reserved for the assessment of metabolic health only in high-risk groups of the population (eg, women at risk of gestational diabetes).[35] In clinical metabolic research, functional assessment of whole-body and tissue-specific metabolic health can be performed by using 1 or a combination of the following methods: (1) intravenous infusions of stable isotope tracers with or without the concurrent infusion of various hormones (eg, insulin, glucagon, somatostatin),[26,36–38] (2) meal tolerance tests,[39,40] (3) arteriovenous catheterization of specific organs (eg, liver, adipose tissue depots, or muscle groups),[41–43] (4) microdialysis (usually in skeletal muscle and fat depots),[44] and (5) biopsies of target tissues followed by the implementation of molecular biology and biochemical assessments.[37,45,46]

Although the previously mentioned traditional methods to quantitatively assess metabolic function and health have greatly increased the current understanding of the pathophysiology of obesity-related metabolic diseases and improved clinical practice, they have limitations. The diagnostic

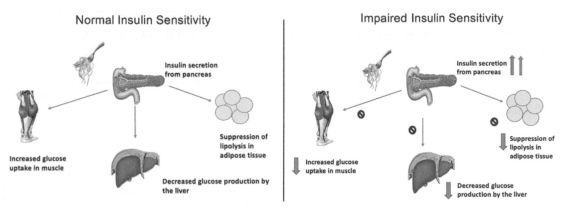

Fig. 1. Effects of insulin in skeletal muscle, adipose tissue, and liver in people with normal insulin sensitivity and insulin resistance.

methods used in clinical practice are nonspecific and not particularly sensitive. In contrast, the approaches used in clinical research only are more than minimally invasive, labor intensive, and time consuming. Further, because of the limited access to tissue samples other than subcutaneous adipose tissue and skeletal muscle, most obesity metabolic research has focused on those 2 tissues. The assessment of metabolic function of other organs, such as the liver and pancreas, has been possible primarily by quantifying the concentrations of their secreted factors and applying mathematical modeling approaches.[47,48] Considering the limitations of the traditional approaches for the assessment of metabolic function, the need for novel methods that can improve patient care and accelerated clinical metabolic research efforts becomes apparent.

STANDARD PET VERSUS TOTAL-BODY PET FOR THE ASSESSMENT OF METABOLIC HEALTH

Although a strong focus of PET imaging remains in oncology, PET imaging technology has also been developed to assist in diagnosis and prognosis in metabolic diseases that can involve multiple target organs. At this time, PET imaging is not routinely used for diagnosis of metabolic diseases. Use of the widely accessible radiotracer 2-deoxy-2-[18F] fluoro-D-glucose (FDG) is well known as an effective method for imaging glucose metabolism related to glycolysis in cells.[49] Impaired glucose homeostasis is one of the hallmarks of obesity-related metabolic dysfunction, making FDG highly relevant for the diagnosis and study of obesity-related metabolic disorders. Current clinical usage of FDG is mainly limited to static PET protocols that examine tracer spatial distribution at a late time point after injection, providing standardized

uptake value as a semiquantitative measure of glucose use.[50,51] Although it suffers from the lack of detailed kinetic data, static PET allows the imaging of the entire body, albeit with a time lag of image capture between organs. Studies have shown the utility of static FDG-PET imaging for studying physiologic processes affected by obesity and metabolic syndrome.[36,52–56] However, this static means of using FDG-PET may not enable its full potential in metabolic processes.

Dynamic FDG-PET acquires FDG activity images at multiple time points to monitor both the spatial and temporal distributions, enabling the ability to exploit the kinetic characteristics of FDG uptake by tracer kinetic modeling.[57] These kinetic parameters derived from dynamic FDG-PET represent the underlying molecular processes of FDG uptake and trapping in the metabolic tissues and organs that may better characterize the physiologic processes leading to disease. The FDG measures of glucose uptake and transport can be harnessed to determine subtle changes that may be reflective of an early disease process. PET imaging also allows use of other markers of metabolic disease. Fatty acid metabolism can be investigated using FFA radiotracers such as ^{11}C-palmitate[58] or 14(R,S)-[18F]fluoro-6-thia-heptadecanoic acid (FTHA).[59] **Table 1** summarizes additional tracers that can be used to quantify metabolic processes or processes that affect metabolic function. Furthermore, dynamic PET imaging allows use of a combination of tracers to determine specific changes in metabolic function in health and disease.

Although dynamic PET imaging created a window of opportunity to develop state-of-the-art diagnostic technologies relevant to obesity and its related metabolic diseases, it limits the ability to image multiple organs simultaneously in standard PET scanners that are ∼15 to 30 cm across.

Table 1
Summary of the most common PET radioligands for the assessment of the obesity-related metabolic dysfunction

Radioligand	Function	Outcome
FDG	Glucose analogue	Assessment of glucose disposal
^{11}C-palmitate or FTHA	Free fatty acid analogue	Assessment of FFA metabolism
^{11}C-acetate	Substrate for Krebs cycle	Assessment of blood flow and oxidation of circulating substrates
^{18}F-fluciclovine	Leucine analogue	Leucine disposal
^{11}C-PBR28	Ligand for benzodiazepine receptors (expressed in mitochondria)	Index of mitochondrial content
^{18}F-dopamine	Dopamine analogue	Sympathetic innervation
^{11}C-MRB	Ligand for norepinephrine transporter	Sympathetic innervation
^{11}C-HED	Norepinephrine analogue	Sympathetic innervation
^{15}O-H$_2$O, ^{15}O-CO, ^{15}O-O$_2$	H$_2$O, CO, O$_2$ analogues	Tissue perfusion and blood volume
FDGal	Galactose analogue (exclusively cleared by liver)	Index of liver metabolic function
[N-methyl-11C]cholylsarcosine	Conjugated bile acid analogue	Hepatic excretory function
[^{18}F]FMPEP-d$_2$	Ligand for the cannabinoid CB1 receptor	Assessment of endocannabinoid system

This is not exhaustive list of PET tracers that can be used for the assessment of obesity-related metabolic dysfunction.

Abbreviations: ^{11}C-HED, [11C]-meta-hydroxyephedrine; ^{11}C-MRB, (S; S)-11C-O-methylreboxetine; ^{11}C-PBR28, N-Acetyl-N-(2-[11C]methoxybenzyl)-2-phenoxy-5-pyridinamine; FDGal, 2-[^{18}F]fluoro-2-deoxy-D-galactose, [^{18}F]FMPEP-d$_2$, (3R,5R)-5-(3-[18F]Fluoromethoxy-d2)phenyl)-3-((R)-1-phenyl-ethylamino)-1-(4-trifluoromethyl-phenyl)-pyrrolidin-2-one.

Total-body PET enables the simultaneous performance of dynamic metabolic imaging at the whole-body level, profoundly increasing the amount of information that can be extracted for a single scan (radiomics).[9–11] Further, the development of dynamic total-body PET methods allows assessment of metabolic function at the whole-body level with tissue-specific resolution.[12–15] In addition, the increased signal-to-noise ratio, decreased exposure to ionizing radiation, and shorter acquisition times compared with the standard PET imaging approaches[10] make the use of total-body PET attractive even for investigations that may not require assessment of kinetics in all tissues.

OBESITY AND METABOLISM RESEARCH AREAS THAT COULD BENEFIT FROM TOTAL-BODY PET
Nonalcoholic Fatty Liver Disease

The liver is one of the key organs affected in obesity, with nonalcoholic fatty liver disease (NAFLD) as its manifestation. NAFLD is characterized by a spectrum of liver disorder from fat deposition in the hepatocytes (steatosis) to florid inflammation, termed nonalcoholic steatohepatitis (NASH), and fibrosis.[29,60,61] Inflammation or NASH is the key driver to fibrosis, with risk of progression to cirrhosis and its complications of portal hypertension and hepatocellular carcinoma.[29,60–63] Fibrosis remains the key determinant of worse disease outcome in patients with NAFLD.[64] The pathophysiology and progression of NAFLD remains an area of intense research, with multiple new therapeutic agents under investigation to reduce inflammation and regress fibrosis.[65,66] There is a limited availability of noninvasive tests that can detect liver inflammation. Liver biopsy remains the primary method to define liver inflammation and carries risks for significant complications.[60,61] Dynamic FDG-PET/CT has the ability to help detect liver steatosis and inflammation[12,67] and provides a tool to define these essential aspects of NAFLD with noninvasive means.

In a subset of patients with NAFLD, inflammation develops with progressive fibrosis and impairment of liver function. The dysmetabolic effect extends far beyond the liver and manifests as chronic kidney disease and cardiovascular disease, besides other extrahepatic manifestations.[68–71] For example, a major cause of comorbidity in patients with NAFLD is cardiovascular disease. Worsening steatosis or fibrosis in NAFLD are directly linked to higher risks for cardiac disease independent of associated metabolic syndrome.[68,72,73] Specifically, patients with NAFLD have lower early diastolic relaxation (e') and higher left ventricular filling pressure (E/e' ratio), which has been linked to lower myocardial glucose uptake.[74] There remains a missing link in the detailed understanding of changes in glucose signals in these tissues that lead to the adverse effects of NAFLD. Dynamic total-body FDG-PET provides a unique way to study simultaneous glucose uptake change in liver, adipose tissue, muscle, and myocardium.

Chronic kidney disease has also been associated with worsening NAFLD. Studies have shown deteriorating kidney function with worsening NAFLD independent of confounding risks such as type 2 diabetes or hypertension.[68,69] Besides the need to understand the epidemiology, there is a growing need to understand the pathophysiology of the downstream effects of NAFLD on the kidney. Insulin resistance is thought to be a key cause of the kidney disease either directly or indirectly through worsening liver disease. Altered glucose transport and metabolism may be one of the early steps affected in this process. Data from our group, in patients with varying degrees of NAFLD defined by liver biopsy, showed altered glucose uptake with worsening of liver disease.[75] FDG influx rate or kidney K_i was significantly increased with worse liver steatosis, but decreased as liver inflammation worsened[75] (and unpublished data).

Total-body PET studies in people with NAFLD are expected to have significant clinical impact to allow detection of concomitant cardiovascular and/or kidney disease in these patients. There remains a significant knowledge gap within the NAFLD field, not only of the pathophysiology of NAFLD but also of the mechanism of extrahepatic disease development in relation to NAFLD. Closing this knowledge gap is of clinical significance with the development of therapies that may improve the liver disease but may have unintended consequences on other organs.

Skeletal Muscle

Skeletal muscle is one of the largest tissues in the human body and it plays a major role in the maintenance of metabolic health.[76] Abnormalities in skeletal muscle metabolism not only influence metabolic health but they may also affect physical function.[77] Because of its large size and high capacity for nutrient use and energy production, skeletal muscle has been extensively studied for its role in metabolic health and is a major target for lifestyle and pharmacologic interventions against obesity-related metabolic disorders.

In the fasting state, lipids are the primary substrate (90% of substrate use) for skeletal muscle,[78,79] whereas, on food ingestion, skeletal muscle switches its substrate preference from fatty acids to glucose. During postprandial or insulin-stimulated conditions, skeletal muscle is thought to be responsible for 70% to 80% of the glucose clearance, which can be used for glycogen synthesis or oxidation.[80–82] The contribution of skeletal muscle in glucose and lipid metabolism further increases during exercise.[83,84] In people with metabolically abnormal obesity, hyperlipidemia and hyperglycemia are thought to induce molecular changes to skeletal muscle signaling, mitochondrial energetics, and accumulation of reactive lipid molecules that further impair the capacity of the skeletal muscle to oxidize and/or store nutrients.[76]

The role of skeletal muscle in metabolic health has been established using traditional clinical research methods (including skeletal muscle samples biopsies, microdialysis, and arteriovenous catheterization of leg or arm skeletal muscle in conjunction with the infusion of stable isotope tracers).[41,46] Although these methods have greatly advanced knowledge of muscle metabolism, they are more than minimally invasive and they require access to specially trained personnel and clinical infrastructure. Further, some of those methods can be particularly challenging to implement in some patient populations (eg, the elderly, patients with compromised veins or sarcopenic obesity). Dynamic PET/CT imaging has been used to less invasively assess muscle metabolic function in terms of glucose uptake in fasting and insulin-stimulated conditions, FFA uptake, oxidation, and perfusion.[85,86] A limitation of this approach is that the assessment of muscle metabolism is limited to the small sample of muscle included in the 15 to 30 cm of the field of view. These results are then sometimes used to estimate the contribution of muscle to whole-body metabolism. However, skeletal muscle is a heterogeneous tissue and the assumption that all muscles are metabolically equivalent is not accurate.[87] Total-body PET can become an important tool for muscle metabolism research because it can (1) directly assess the metabolic processes of interest (ie, glucose uptake) in all the different muscle groups, enabling more accurate quantification of the total contribution of skeletal muscle to metabolic regulation at the whole-body level; (2) unveil important information with regard to the crosstalk between skeletal muscle and other tissues (adipose tissue, brain, heart muscle, and so forth); and (3) inform about potential off-target effects of interventions that are currently focused on muscle metabolism.

White Adipose Tissue

Adipose tissue has been probably the most vilified tissue in the human body (with the exception of malignant tissues) because of its association with obesity and its related metabolic diseases. Adipose tissue is one of the largest organs in the human body.[88] In people with obesity, adipose tissue can comprise 50% or more of the total body weight. For many years, the prominent view was that adipose tissue is a metabolically inert connective tissue that contains lipid droplets. Over the years, it became apparent that adipose tissue is an important organ for the maintenance of metabolic homeostasis and nutritional status.[88] Its main function is the storage of excess energy in the form of intracellular triglycerides in the postprandial period and mobilization of fatty acids that can be used for energy production during fasting.[88] Further research established the role of adipose tissue as an endocrine organ secreting various peptides that affect metabolic regulation in other tissues (eg, leptin, adiponectin, tumor necrosis factor alpha).[89]

Obesity and weight gain lead to accumulation of adipose tissue. However, increased amounts of adipose tissue per se is probably not the primary factor responsible for the obesity-related metabolic dysfunction. Results from studies in animal models support that genetically engineered rodents can become extremely obese while maintaining a normal metabolic function.[90] Consistently, evidence from experimental studies in humans supports that about 7% of people with obesity seem to be protected from its related metabolic perturbations,[21] whereas removal of adipose tissue using liposuction does not improve metabolic health in people with obesity.[91] These results suggest that adipose tissue function may be more important than mass for the maintenance of metabolic health. Current evidence supports that the differences in adipose tissue insulin sensitivity, lipogenesis, adipocyte size, adipose tissue resident immune cell populations and their secreted inflammatory factors, and extracellular matrix formation are associated with metabolic health in people with obesity,[21] suggesting that restoring adipose tissue function can be an important goal toward improving metabolic health in people with obesity even in the absence of weight loss.

At this point it is also important to emphasize that adipose tissue is a heterogeneous tissue. The various adipose tissue depots (eg, visceral, subcutaneous, white, brown, pericardial) have different metabolic properties in terms of physiologic function and histopathology.[89,92] The different adipose tissue depots have been distinctly associated with the risk of developing metabolic disease. For example, increased waist circumference has been linked with a higher risk for the development of metabolic syndrome,[93,94] whereas accumulation of subcutaneous adipose tissue in the lower body is thought to be protective against the development of the obesity-related metabolic perturbations.[95] Visceral adiposity has also been associated with insulin resistance and metabolic syndrome.[96] The mechanisms underlying the association of visceral adiposity with obesity-related metabolic dysfunction are unclear.[96]

In clinical practice, the body mass index is used as a nonspecific marker of adiposity, whereas waist circumference and waist-to-hip ratio are used as markers of central adiposity. In clinical research, different imaging methods (dual emission x-ray absorptiometry, magnetic resonance imaging, CT) and other modalities (eg, bioelectrical impedance, waist circumference assessment) are used for assessment of adipose tissue mass and distribution (eg, subcutaneous, intra-abdominal).[97] Infusion of stable isotope tracers (ie, glycerol and palmitate) has been used to assess whole-body adipose tissue lipolysis and insulin sensitivity.[37] However, this approach does not permit the characterization of the metabolic function of specific adipose tissue depots. Adipose tissue biopsies have been used for the molecular and functional assessment of specific adipose tissue depots ex vivo and they have predominantly focused on the abdominal or the gluteal subcutaneous depots, which are easy to access.[98] Some studies have used dynamic PET to characterize the metabolic properties of specific adipose tissue depots that were included in the 15 to 30 cm of a conventional PET/CT scanner.[99,100] The currently available approaches for the assessment of adipose tissue function do not permit the thorough assessment of all the different adipose tissue depots and evaluation of their functional heterogeneity. Total-body PET allows, for the first time, the simultaneous assessment of different metabolic or other physiologic processes (eg, glucose or FFA uptake, perfusion, oxygen extraction) in all the different adipose tissue depots. The results of these studies will increase the current

understanding of the role of the various adipose tissue depots in metabolic health. Moreover, total-body PET can help to assess the plasticity of adipose tissue in response to existing therapeutic interventions (eg, weight loss, bariatric surgery, medications), environmental stimuli (exercise, cold exposure, diet manipulation), or different disease states (eg, type 2 diabetes, cardiovascular disease, NAFLD). Total-body PET in conjunction with FDG can be used to provide important information on the role of adipose tissue as a metabolic sink for glucose. Additional radioligands (described in **Table 1**) can be also used to answer important questions with regard to the contribution of the different adipose tissue depots to nutrient use, the link between the central nervous system (CNS) and metabolic function in adipose tissue, and the role of adipose tissue vascularization and perfusion in the regulation of adipose tissue metabolism and systemic health.

Brown Adipose Tissue

Brown adipose tissue (BAT) is a recently rediscovered tissue in humans,[101–103] observed en passant in oncologic FDG-PET/CT scans some 20 years ago,[104] that has attracted significant interest as a potential emerging target against obesity and its related metabolic diseases because of its high capacity for glucose and lipid disposal and oxidation. Human BAT is located the supraclavicular, cervical, auxiliary, spinal, perirenal, and posterior abdominal areas.[56,105] BAT is different from the classic subcutaneous white adipose tissue. It has higher inner... tion and vascularization, multiple lipid droplet... a high number of mitochondria, which cont... levels of uncoupling protein 1 (UCP1).[106] ... mitochondrial protein that uncoupl... phosphorylation from ATP produc... increased thermogenesis. P... independent mechanisms ha... contribute to some of the... BAT.[107–109] In humans, ... bolic activity (assess... associated with incr... acid mobilization... tivity.[110] Moreove... that white adipose ti... similar to the brown adip... to adrenergic or other stin... burn injury and beta3-adrene... This process is also known as bro... of the white adipose tissue. Brown... thermogenic adipocytes in white adip... have attracted significant attention as emer... gets against conditions related to energy in... ance, including, for example, obesity. Howeve...

the study of BAT metabolism is still in its infancy and there are several open questions that remain to be answered with regard to the role of BAT and thermogenic adipocytes in metabolic function and health.

Considering that FDG-PET/CT is the most popular method and the current gold standard for the assessment of BAT,[111] total-body PET is expected to greatly accelerate the progress in this research area. The higher signal-to-noise ratio of the total-body PET allows the more accurate and reproducible quantification of BAT. The whole-bod... coverage allows the performance of dynamic... aging in all the BAT depots, which has n... feasible previously. The potentially lowe... of radiation exposure involved with ... total-body PET enables the in... perform multiple imaging session... tients to better characterize th... strate preferences for BA... combination with the a... (including the selection... likely to help addres... gard to (1) the di... metabolism of ... other nutrien... other met... bution ... studi... ma...

studies in humans. The examination of GI metabolism in vivo is particularly challenging because it requires deployment of endoscopic approaches with or without intestinal biopsies.[114] For assessment of the gut microbiome, fecal analysis of the microbial population is performed using various molecular biology approaches, and often microbial colonies are transplanted in gnotobiotic mice to assess the potential metabolic effects of the different microbial populations.[115] However, this approach does not necessarily recapitulate the functional importance of the different microbial populations in human metabolism in vivo.

At present, there are several open questions with regard to the role of the lower GI tract in metabolic health. Further, it is important to better understand whether and how the lower GI tract can be targeted for the prevention and treatment of obesity-related metabolic dysfunction. The deployment of total-body PET in conjunction with use of the appropriate radioligands is expected address some of those questions and to unveil ntly unknown effects of existing lifestyle and interventions in gut metabolism. For liver-secreted bile acids have increasen noted to play a larger role beyond the gut (enterohepatic circulation). Through on the gut microbiome and nuclear rectly or indirectly, they also modulate tabolic signals.[116–118] Combination tracers such as 2-[^{18}F]fluoro-2-ose[119] and bile-acid tracers (eg, holylsarcosine)[120] may also open study the role of the gut-liver-olic health.

tem

e most avid consumers of % and 20% of the total re-.[121] Apart from its direct ucose metabolism, the in the coordination of other peripheral tis-insulin-sensitive tis-y-related metabolic sociated with the ease and other t present, there he role of the process and systemic dis-ne by Iozzo n the ability rstand the e and its ic total-

body PET imaging with appropriate kinetic modeling techniques and well-controlled studies can effectively help clinicians to understand the role of the brain in regulating the metabolic axis.

LIMITATIONS AND FUTURE RESEARCH OPPORTUNITIES

Total-body dynamic PET imaging opens new possibilities for investigational and clinical applications in metabolic diseases. A lot of challenges remain that open areas of future research. Dynamic PET dictates the need for tissue-specific kinetic modeling, which becomes especially relevant when trying to study multiple organs simultaneously. It also increases the need to understand and develop network models that will improve understanding of multiorgan interactions in systemic disease. If multiple tracers are used to study glucose and lipid metabolism, the network model needs to account for both. Blood flow to the organs may be altered as tissue inflammation worsens; this will need to be accounted for either with flow tracers or advanced modeling. It will be greatly beneficial if these multiple tracers can be incorporated at significantly lower doses while obtaining quantifiable data, thus significantly reducing the radiation dose. For tracers with low first-pass extraction or important late-time-point kinetics, a limitation of total-body dynamic PET imaging is the long imaging time, which may be 60 minutes or more, in order to accurately determine the kinetic parameters. Newer modeling and advancement of understanding of related physiology will help reduce the time needed to capture relevant disease data. As with any PET/CT scanner, exposure to ionizing radiation is a consideration. Total-body PET enables efficient capture of tracer data and can allow significantly lower tracer and radiation doses, which will enable research and clinical studies in pretherapeutic and posttherapeutic states in the same patient. Lower radiation doses will also enable applications in children, a population at very high risk of obesity and its complications.

To summarize, total-body PET imaging with the multitude of metabolic tracers coupled with advanced modeling techniques has provided the metabolic diseases field with state-of-the-art tools to define physiologic processes in health and disease.

CLINICS CARE POINTS

- Metabolic syndrome is a systemic disease affecting multiple tissues and metabolic processes.

- The current methods that are clinically used for the assessment of metabolic health provide only a crude evaluation of the metabolic function.
- Total-body PET imaging can not only increase the current knowledge in the pathophysiology of human obesity, but also facilitate the development of targeted intervention against metabolic disease.

ACKNOWLEDGMENTS

Dr. Chondronikola is supported by the by the National Center for Advancing Translational Sciences (NCATS), National Institutes of Health (NIH), through grant UL1 TR001860 and the USDA National Institute of Food and Agriculture, Hatch project number CA-D-NTR-2618-H.

REFERENCES

1. Hales CM, Carroll MD, Fryar CD, et al. Prevalence of obesity and severe obesity among adults: United States, 2017–2018. NCHS Data Brief, no 360. Hyattsville (MD): National Center for Health Statistics; 2020.
2. Jia H, Lubetkin EI. The impact of obesity on health-related quality-of-life in the general adult US population. J Public Health 2005;27(2):156–64.
3. Kolotkin RL, Andersen JR. A systematic review of reviews: exploring the relationship between obesity, weight loss and health-related quality of life. Clin Obes 2017;7(5):273–89.
4. Hong Y-R, Huo J, Desai R, et al. Excess costs and economic burden of obesity-related cancers in the United States. Value Health 2019;22(12):1378–86.
5. Leung MYM, Carlsson NP, Colditz GA, et al. The burden of obesity on diabetes in the United States: medical expenditure panel survey, 2008 to 2012. Value Health 2017;20(1):77–84.
6. Fox KM, Tai M-H, Kostev K, et al. Treatment patterns and low-density lipoprotein cholesterol (LDL-C) goal attainment among patients receiving high- or moderate-intensity statins. Clin Res Cardiol 2018;107(5):380–8.
7. Avramopoulos I, Moulis A, Nikas N. Glycaemic control, treatment satisfaction and quality of life in type 2 diabetes patients in Greece: the PANORAMA study Greek results. World J Diabetes 2015;6(1):208–16.
8. Khunti K, Wolden ML, Thorsted BL, et al. Clinical inertia in people with type 2 diabetes: a retrospective cohort study of more than 80,000 people. Diabetes Care 2013;36(11):3411–7.
9. Cherry SR, Badawi RD, Karp JS, et al. Total-body imaging: transforming the role of positron emission tomography. Sci Transl Med 2017;9(381):eaaf6169.
10. Badawi RD, Shi H, Hu P, et al. First human imaging studies with the EXPLORER total-body PET scanner. J Nucl Med 2019;60(3):299–303.
11. Cherry SR, Jones T, Karp JS, et al. Total-body PET: maximizing sensitivity to create new opportunities for clinical research and patient care. J Nucl Med 2018;59(1):3–12.
12. Wang G, Corwin MT, Olson KA, et al. Dynamic PET of human liver inflammation: impact of kinetic modeling with optimization-derived dual-blood input function. Phys Med Biol 2018;63(15):155004.
13. Zhang X, Xie Z, Berg E, et al. Total-body dynamic reconstruction and parametric imaging on the uEXPLORER. J Nucl Med 2020;61(2):285–91.
14. Zhang X, Zhou J, Cherry SR, et al. Quantitative image reconstruction for total-body PET imaging using the 2-meter long EXPLORER scanner. Phys Med Biol 2017;62(6):2465–85.
15. Zuo YSS, Corwin MT, Olson K, et al. Structural and practical identifiability of dual-input kinetic modeling in dynamic PET of liver inflammation. Phys Med Biol 2019;64(17):175023.
16. Minamino T, Orimo M, Shimizu I, et al. A crucial role for adipose tissue p53 in the regulation of insulin resistance. Nat Med 2009;15(9):1082–7.
17. Pi-Sunyer X. The medical risks of obesity. Postgrad Med 2009;121(6):21–33.
18. Stefan N, Birkenfeld AL, Schulze MB, et al. Obesity and impaired metabolic health in patients with COVID-19. Nat Rev Endocrinol 2020;16(7):341–2.
19. Alberti KGMM, Zimmet P, Shaw J. The metabolic syndrome—a new worldwide definition. Lancet 2005;366(9491):1059–62.
20. Alberti KG, Eckel RH, Grundy SM, et al. Harmonizing the metabolic syndrome: a joint interim statement of the International diabetes Federation task Force on epidemiology and prevention; National heart, Lung, and blood Institute; American heart association; World heart Federation; International Atherosclerosis society; and International association for the study of obesity. Circulation 2009;120(16):1640–5.
21. Smith GI, Mittendorfer B, Klein S. Metabolically healthy obesity: Facts and fantasies. J Clin Invest 2019;129(10):3978–89.
22. Ding C, Chan Z, Magkos F. Lean, but not healthy: the 'metabolically obese, normal-weight' phenotype. Curr Opin Clin Nutr Metab Care 2016;19(6):408–17.
23. Birkenfeld AL, Shulman GI. Nonalcoholic fatty liver disease, hepatic insulin resistance, and type 2 diabetes. Hepatology 2014;59(2):713–23.
24. Perry RJ, Samuel VT, Petersen KF, et al. The role of hepatic lipids in hepatic insulin resistance and type 2 diabetes. Nature 2014;510(7503):84–91.

25. Bugianesi E, Moscatiello S, Ciaravella MF, et al. Insulin resistance in nonalcoholic fatty liver disease. Curr Pharm Des 2010;16(17):1941–51.

26. Conte C, Fabbrini E, Kars M, et al. Multiorgan insulin sensitivity in lean and obese subjects. Diabetes Care 2012;35(6):1316–21.

27. Bechmann LP, Hannivoort RA, Gerken G, et al. The interaction of hepatic lipid and glucose metabolism in liver diseases. J Hepatol 2012;56(4):952–64.

28. Cusi K. Role of obesity and lipotoxicity in the development of nonalcoholic steatohepatitis: pathophysiology and clinical implications. Gastroenterology 2012;142(4):711–25.e6.

29. Rinella ME. Nonalcoholic fatty liver disease: a systematic review. JAMA 2015;313(22):2263–73.

30. Parekh S, Anania FA. Abnormal lipid and glucose metabolism in obesity: implications for nonalcoholic fatty liver disease. Gastroenterology 2007; 132(6):2191–207.

31. Ramlo-Halsted BA, Edelman SV. The natural history of type 2 diabetes. Implications for clinical practice. Prim Care 1999;26(4):771–89.

32. Smith GI, Shankaran M, Yoshino M, et al. Insulin resistance drives hepatic de novo lipogenesis in nonalcoholic fatty liver disease. J Clin Invest 2019;130(3):1453–60.

33. Goedeke L, Perry RJ, Shulman GI. Emerging pharmacological targets for the treatment of nonalcoholic fatty liver disease, insulin resistance, and type 2 diabetes. Annu Rev Pharmacol Toxicol 2019;59:65–87.

34. Samuel VT, Shulman GI. Nonalcoholic fatty liver disease as a nexus of metabolic and hepatic diseases. Cell Metab 2018;27(1):22–41.

35. 2. Classification and diagnosis of diabetes: Standards of medical care in diabetes—2020. Diabetes Care 2020;43(Supplement 1): S14–31.

36. Chondronikola M, Volpi E, Borsheim E, et al. Brown adipose tissue improves whole-body glucose homeostasis and insulin sensitivity in humans. Diabetes 2014;63(12):4089–99.

37. Chondronikola M, Volpi E, Borsheim E, et al. Brown adipose tissue activation is linked to distinct systemic effects on lipid metabolism in humans. Cell Metab 2016;23(6):1200–6.

38. Magkos F, Fraterrigo G, Yoshino J, et al. Effects of moderate and subsequent progressive weight loss on metabolic function and adipose tissue biology in humans with obesity. Cell Metab 2016;23(4): 591–601.

39. Steil GM, Hwu C-m, Janowski R, et al. Evaluation of insulin sensitivity and β-cell function indexes obtained from minimal model analysis of a meal tolerance test. Diabetes 2004;53(5):1201–7.

40. Caumo A, Bergman RN, Cobelli C. Insulin sensitivity from meal tolerance tests in normal subjects:

a minimal model index. J Clin Endocrinol Metab 2000;85(11):4396–402.

41. Katsanos CS, Chinkes DL, Sheffield-Moore M, et al. Method for the determination of the arteriovenous muscle protein balance during non-steady-state blood and muscle amino acid concentrations. Am J Physiol Endocrinol Metab 2005;289(6):E1064–70.

42. Horowitz JF, Coppack SW, Klein S. Whole-body and adipose tissue glucose metabolism in response to short-term fasting in lean and obese women. Am J Clin Nutr 2001;73(3):517–22.

43. Sidossis LS, Mittendorfer B, Walser E, et al. Hyperglycemia-induced inhibition of splanchnic fatty acid oxidation increases hepatic triacylglycerol secretion. Am J Physiol 1998;275(5 Pt 1): E798–805.

44. Weir G, Ramage LE, Akyol M, et al. Substantial metabolic activity of human brown adipose tissue during warm conditions and cold-induced lipolysis of local triglycerides. Cell Metab 2018;27(6): 1348–55.e4.

45. Chondronikola M, Annamalai P, Chao T, et al. A percutaneous needle biopsy technique for sampling the supraclavicular brown adipose tissue depot of humans. Int J Obes (Lond) 2015;39(10): 1561–4.

46. Gallo A, Abraham A, Katzberg HD, et al. Muscle biopsy technical safety and quality using a self-contained, vacuum-assisted biopsy technique. Neuromuscul Disord 2018;28(5):450–3.

47. Smith GI, Polidori DC, Yoshino M, et al. Influence of adiposity, insulin resistance, and intrahepatic triglyceride content on insulin kinetics. J Clin Invest 2020;130(6):3305–14.

48. Fabbrini E, Mohammed BS, Magkos F, et al. Alterations in adipose tissue and hepatic lipid kinetics in obese men and women with nonalcoholic fatty liver disease. Gastroenterology 2008;134(2): 424–31.

49. Gambhir SS. Molecular imaging of cancer with positron emission tomography. Nat Rev Cancer 2002;2(9):683–93.

50. Ben-Haim S, Ell P. (18)F-FDG PET and PET/CT in the evaluation of cancer treatment response. J Nucl Med 2009;50(1):88–99.

51. Boellaard R, Delgado-Bolton R, Oyen WJG, et al. Fdg PET/CT: EANM procedure guidelines for tumour imaging: version 2.0. Eur J Nucl Med Mol Imaging 2015;42(2):328–54.

52. Abele JT, Fung CI. Effect of hepatic steatosis on liver FDG uptake measured in mean standard uptake values. Radiology 2010;254(3):917–24.

53. Keiding S. Bringing physiology into PET of the liver. J Nucl Med 2012;53(3):425–33.

54. Keramida G, Hunter J, Peters AM. Hepatic glucose utilisation in hepatic steatosis and obesity. Biosci Rep 2016;36(6):e00402.

55. Iozzo P, Geisler F, Oikonen V, et al. Insulin stimulates liver glucose uptake in humans: an 18F-FDG PET Study. J Nucl Med 2003;44(5):682–9.

56. Leitner BP, Huang S, Brychta RJ, et al. Mapping of human brown adipose tissue in lean and obese young men. Proc Natl Acad Sci U S A 2017; 114(32):8649–54.

57. Schmidt KC, Turkheimer FE. Kinetic modeling in positron emission tomography. Q J Nucl Med 2002;46(1):70–85.

58. Sochor H, Schelbert H, Schwaiger M, et al. Studies of fatty acid metabolism with positron emission tomography in patients with cardiomyopathy. Eur J Nucl Med 1986;12(1):S66–9.

59. Guiducci L, Grönroos T, Järvisalo MJ, et al. Biodistribution of the fatty acid analogue 18F-FTHA: plasma and tissue partitioning between lipid pools during fasting and hyperinsulinemia. J Nucl Med 2007;48(3):455–62.

60. Loomba R, Sanyal AJ. The global NAFLD epidemic. Nat Rev Gastroenterol Hepatol 2013; 10(11):686–90.

61. Chalasani N, Younossi Z, Lavine JE, et al. The diagnosis and management of nonalcoholic fatty liver disease: practice guidance from the American Association for the Study of Liver Diseases. Hepatology 2018;67(1):328–57.

62. Harrison SA. NASH, from diagnosis to treatment: where do we stand? Hepatology 2015;62(6): 1652–5.

63. Friedman SL, Neuschwander-Tetri BA, Rinella M, et al. Mechanisms of NAFLD development and therapeutic strategies. Nat Med 2018;24(7):908–22.

64. Angulo P, Kleiner DE, Dam-Larsen S, et al. Liver fibrosis, but no other histologic features, is associated with long-term outcomes of patients with nonalcoholic fatty liver disease. Gastroenterology 2015;149(2):389–97.e10.

65. Filozof C, Goldstein BJ, Williams RN, et al. Nonalcoholic steatohepatitis: limited available treatment options but promising drugs in development and recent progress towards a regulatory approval pathway. Drugs 2015;75(12):1373–92.

66. Yilmaz Y. Biomarkers for early detection of nonalcoholic steatohepatitis: implications for drug development and clinical trials. Curr Drug Targets 2013;14(11):1357–66.

67. Sarkar S, Corwin MT, Olson KA, et al. Pilot study to diagnose nonalcoholic steatohepatitis with dynamic (18)F-FDG PET. AJR Am J Roentgenol 2019;212(3):529–37.

68. Armstrong MJ, Adams LA, Canbay A, et al. Extrahepatic complications of nonalcoholic fatty liver disease. Hepatology 2014;59(3):1174–97.

69. Ganzetti G, Campanati A, Offidani A. Non-alcoholic fatty liver disease and psoriasis: so far, so near. World J Hepatol 2015;7(3):315–26.

70. Targher G, Chonchol M, Zoppini G, et al. Risk of chronic kidney disease in patients with nonalcoholic fatty liver disease: is there a link? J Hepatol 2011;54(5):1020–9.

71. Younossi ZM, Stepanova M, Anstee QM, et al. Reduced patient-reported outcome scores associate with level of fibrosis in patients with nonalcoholic steatohepatitis. Clin Gastroenterol Hepatol 2019;17(12):2552–60.e10.

72. Anstee QM, Mantovani A, Tilg H, et al. Risk of cardiomyopathy and cardiac arrhythmias in patients with nonalcoholic fatty liver disease. Nat Rev Gastroenterol Hepatol 2018;15(7):425–39.

73. Lee YH, Kim KJ, Yoo ME, et al. Association of nonalcoholic steatohepatitis with subclinical myocardial dysfunction in non-cirrhotic patients. J Hepatol 2017;68(4):764–72.

74. Tang K, Zheng X, Lin J, et al. Association between non-alcoholic fatty liver disease and myocardial glucose uptake measured by (18)F-fluorodeoxyglucose positron emission tomography. J Nucl Cardiol 2018. https://doi.org/10.1007/s12350-018-1446-x.

75. Kuo A, Liu CH, Spencer B, et al. THU-321-Fluorodeoxyglucose perfusion and uptake in abdominal organs is associated with hepatic disease state in patients with nonalcoholic fatty liver disease. J Hepatol 2019;70(1):e301–2.

76. Orešič M, Vidal-Puig A. A systems biology approach to study metabolic syndrome. Switzerland: Springer International Publishing; 2013.

77. Kestenbaum B, Gamboa J, Liu S, et al. Impaired skeletal muscle mitochondrial bioenergetics and physical performance in chronic kidney disease. JCI insight 2020;5(5):e133289.

78. Dagenais GR, Tancredi RG, Zierler KL. Free fatty acid oxidation by forearm muscle at rest, and evidence for an intramuscular lipid pool in the human forearm. J Clin Invest 1976;58(2): 421–31.

79. Kelley DE, Simoneau JA. Impaired free fatty acid utilization by skeletal muscle in non-insulin-dependent diabetes mellitus. J Clin Invest 1994; 94(6):2349–56.

80. DeFronzo RA, Gunnarsson R, Björkman O, et al. Effects of insulin on peripheral and splanchnic glucose metabolism in noninsulin-dependent (type II) diabetes mellitus. J Clin Invest 1985; 76(1):149–55.

81. DeFronzo RA, Jacot E, Jequier E, et al. The effect of insulin on the disposal of intravenous glucose. Results from indirect calorimetry and hepatic and femoral venous catheterization. Diabetes 1981; 30(12):1000–7.

82. Nuutila P, Koivisto VA, Knuuti J, et al. Glucose-free fatty acid cycle operates in human heart and

skeletal muscle in vivo. J Clin Invest 1992;89(6): 1767–74.

83. Kiens B. Skeletal muscle lipid metabolism in exercise and insulin resistance. Physiol Rev 2006; 86(1):205–43.

84. Rose AJ, Richter EA. Skeletal muscle glucose uptake during exercise: how is it regulated? Physiology (Bethesda) 2005;20:260–70.

85. Hällsten K, Yki-Järvinen H, Peltoniemi P, et al. Insulin-and exercise-stimulated skeletal muscle blood flow and glucose uptake in obese men. Obes Res 2003;11(2):257–65.

86. Turpeinen AK, Takala TO, Nuutila P, et al. Impaired free fatty acid uptake in skeletal muscle but not in myocardium in patients with impaired glucose tolerance: studies with PET and 14(R,S)-[18F]fluoro-6-thia-heptadecanoic acid. Diabetes 1999; 48(6):1245–50.

87. Schiaffino S, Reggiani C. Fiber types in mammalian skeletal muscles. Physiol Rev 2011;91(4): 1447–531.

88. Rosen Evan D, Spiegelman Bruce M. What we talk about when we talk about fat. Cell 2014;156(1): 20–44.

89. Oikonomou EK, Antoniades C. The role of adipose tissue in cardiovascular health and disease. Nat Rev Cardiol 2019;16(2):83–99.

90. Kusminski CM, Holland WL, Sun K, et al. MitoNEET-driven alterations in adipocyte mitochondrial activity reveal a crucial adaptive process that preserves insulin sensitivity in obesity. Nat Med 2012;18(10): 1539–49.

91. Klein S, Fontana L, Young VL, et al. Absence of an effect of liposuction on insulin action and risk factors for coronary heart disease. N Engl J Med 2004;350(25):2549–57.

92. Cinti S. The adipose organ at a glance. Dis Model Mech 2012;5(5):588–94.

93. Canoy D, Luben R, Welch A, et al. Fat distribution, body mass index and blood pressure in 22,090 men and women in the Norfolk cohort of the European Prospective Investigation into Cancer and Nutrition (EPIC-Norfolk) study. J Hypertens 2004; 22(11):2067–74.

94. Meisinger C, Döring A, Thorand B, et al. Body fat distribution and risk of type 2 diabetes in the general population: are there differences between men and women? The MONICA/KORA Augsburg cohort study. Am J Clin Nutr 2006;84(3):483–9.

95. Manolopoulos KN, Karpe F, Frayn KN. Gluteofemoral body fat as a determinant of metabolic health. Int J Obes 2010;34(6):949–59.

96. Bergman RN, Kim SP, Catalano KJ, et al. Why visceral fat is bad: mechanisms of the metabolic syndrome. Obesity 2006;14(S2):16S–9S.

97. Hu FB. Measurements of adiposity and body composition. Obesity epidemiology 2008;53–83.

https://doi.org/10.1093/acprof:oso/9780195312911. 001.0001.

98. Karastergiou K, Fried SK, Xie H, et al. Distinct developmental signatures of human abdominal and gluteal subcutaneous adipose tissue depots. J Clin Endocrinol Metab 2013;98(1):362–71.

99. Ferrannini E, Iozzo P, Virtanen KA, et al. Adipose tissue and skeletal muscle insulin-mediated glucose uptake in insulin resistance: role of blood flow and diabetes. Am J Clin Nutr 2018;108(4): 749–58.

100. Honka M-J, Latva-Rasku A, Bucci M, et al. Insulin-stimulated glucose uptake in skeletal muscle, adipose tissue and liver: a positron emission tomography study. Eur J Endocrinol 2018;178(5):523–31.

101. Cypess AM, Lehman S, Williams G, et al. Identification and importance of brown adipose tissue in adult humans. N Engl J Med 2009;360(15): 1509–17.

102. Virtanen KA, Lidell ME, Orava J, et al. Functional brown adipose tissue in healthy adults. N Engl J Med 2009;360(15):1518–25.

103. van Marken Lichtenbelt WD, Vanhommerig JW, Smulders NM, et al. Cold-activated brown adipose tissue in healthy men. N Engl J Med 2009;360(15): 1500–8.

104. Hany TF, Gharehpapagh E, Kamel EM, et al. Brown adipose tissue: a factor to consider in symmetrical tracer uptake in the neck and upper chest region. Eur J Nucl Med Mol Imaging 2002; 29(10):1393–8.

105. Cypess AM, White AP, Vernochet C, et al. Anatomical localization, gene expression profiling and functional characterization of adult human neck brown fat. Nat Med 2013;19(5):635–9.

106. Cannon B, Nedergaard J. Brown adipose tissue: function and physiological significance. Physiol Rev 2004;84(1):277–359.

107. Kazak L, Chouchani ET, Jedrychowski MP, et al. A creatine-driven substrate cycle enhances energy expenditure and thermogenesis in beige fat. Cell 2015;163(3):643–55.

108. Houstěk J, Cannon B, Lindberg O. Gylcerol-3-phosphate shuttle and its function in intermediary metabolism of hamster brown-adipose tissue. Eur J Biochem 1975;54(1):11–8.

109. Nugroho DB, Ikeda K, Barinda AJ, et al. Neuregulin-4 is an angiogenic factor that is critically involved in the maintenance of adipose tissue vasculature. Biochem Biophys Res Commun 2018;503(1):378–84.

110. Chondronikola M, Sidossis LS. Brown and beige fat: from molecules to physiology. Biochim Biophys Acta 2019;1864(1):91–103.

111. Chen KY, Cypess AM, Laughlin MR, et al. Brown adipose reporting criteria in imaging STudies (BARCIST 1.0): Recommendations for

standardized FDG-PET/CT experiments in humans. Cell Metab 2016;24(2):210–22.

112. Stanford KI, Middelbeek RJ, Townsend KL, et al. Brown adipose tissue regulates glucose homeostasis and insulin sensitivity. J Clin Invest 2013;123(1): 215–23.

113. Fujisaka S, Ussar S, Clish C, et al. Antibiotic effects on gut microbiota and metabolism are host dependent. J Clin Invest 2016;126(12):4430–43.

114. Xiao C, Stahel P, Carreiro AL, et al. Oral glucose mobilizes triglyceride stores from the human intestine. Cell Mol Gastroenterol Hepatol 2019;7(2): 313–37.

115. Turnbaugh PJ, Ridaura VK, Faith JJ, et al. The effect of diet on the human gut microbiome: a metagenomic analysis in humanized gnotobiotic mice. Sci Transl Med 2009;1(6):6ra14–16ra14.

116. Arab JP, Arrese M, Shah VH. Gut microbiota in non-alcoholic fatty liver disease and alcohol-related liver disease: current concepts and perspectives. Hepatol Res 2020;50(4):407–18.

117. Chiang JYL, Ferrell JM. Bile acids as metabolic regulators and nutrient sensors. Annu Rev Nutr 2019;39:175–200.

118. Chiang JYL, Ferrell JM. Bile acid receptors FXR and TGR5 signaling in fatty liver diseases and therapy. Am J Physiol Gastrointest Liver Physiol 2020; 318(3):G554–73.

119. Nho K, Kueider-Paisley A, MahmoudianDehkordi S, et al. Altered bile acid profile in mild cognitive impairment and Alzheimer's disease: relationship to neuroimaging and CSF biomarkers. Alzheimers Dement 2019;15(2):232–44.

120. Orntoft N, Frisch K, Ott P, et al. Functional assessment of hepatobiliary secretion by (11)C-cholylsarcosine positron emission tomography. Biochim Biophys Acta Mol Basis Dis 2018;1864(4 Pt B): 1240–4.

121. Bélanger M, Allaman I, Magistretti Pierre J. Brain energy metabolism: focus on astrocyte-neuron metabolic cooperation. Cell Metab 2011;14(6): 724–38.

122. Myers MG, Olson DP. Central nervous system control of metabolism. Nature 2012;491(7424):357–63.

123. Tschritter O, Preissl H, Hennige AM, et al. The cerebrocortical response to hyperinsulinemia is reduced in overweight humans: a magnetoencephalographic study. Proc Natl Acad Sci U S A 2006;103(32):12103–8.

124. Naderali EK, Ratcliffe SH, Dale MC. Obesity and Alzheimer's disease: a link between body weight and cognitive function in old age. Am J Alzheimers Dis Other Demen 2009;24(6):445–9.

125. Ashrafian H, Harling L, Darzi A, et al. Neurodegenerative disease and obesity: what is the role of weight loss and bariatric interventions? Metab Brain Dis 2013;28(3):341–53.

126. Iozzo P, Guzzardi MA. Imaging of brain glucose uptake by PET in obesity and cognitive dysfunction: life-course perspective. Endocr Connect 2019;8(11):R169–83.

Total-Body PET Imaging in Infectious Diseases

Timothy J. Henrich, MD[a],*, Terry Jones, DSc[b], Denis Beckford-Vera, PhD[c],
Patricia M. Price, MD[d], Henry F. VanBrocklin, PhD[c]

KEYWORDS

- Total-body PET • Infectious diseases • Human immunodeficiency syndrome • COVID-19 • T cells

KEY POINTS

- Total-body Positron Emission Tomography (PET) enables very high sensitivity imaging with dramatically improved signal to noise ratio.
- Total-body PET can be leveraged to decrease the amount of radiotracer required, thereby permitting more frequent imaging or longer imaging periods during radiotracer decay.
- Novel approaches to PET imaging in infectious disease are limited by traditional imaging technologies which may be overcome by total-body PET strategies.

ROLE OF PET IMAGING IN INFECTIOUS DISEASES CLINICAL CARE AND PATHOGENESIS RESEARCH

PET imaging has an important role in infectious disease pathogenesis-based research and clinical care.[1,2] [18F]fluorodeoxyglucose (FDG) is preferentially taken up by inflammatory cells and macrophages in the tissue,[3,4] and has been the mainstay of molecular imaging in viral, bacterial, and fungal infections.[5,6] However, the role of FDG PET imaging is somewhat limited in its role in the diagnosis and treatment of various infectious pathogens given the nonspecific nature of tracer uptake and limitations of sensitivity, especially in the setting of concomitant malignancies and disorders of immune regulation and inflammation.[7] As a result, novel infectious disease molecular imaging strategies are on the forefront of clinical and pathogenesis-based research. These approaches are broad, and include immunoPET incorporating antibodies or antibody fragments/minibodies targeting pathogen-specific antigens or cells responsible for immune responses and drugs that target various pathogen-specific metabolic or enzymatic pathways.[1,2,8] The recent COVID-19 pandemic has prioritized investigation of communicable diseases and so it is timely that PET research should contribute to the global response. Molecular imaging in infectious diseases and associated morbidities involves the following general foci:

1. Pathogenesis-based research to determine the location and extent of infection, associated innate and adaptive immune responses, and inflammation (detrimental and beneficial). Imaging of associated comorbidities, including multiple organ inflammation (eg, vascular, central nervous system, pulmonary inflammation), is also a critical component of this pathogenesis-based research that has direct

Funding Sources: NIH/NIAID UM1AI126611 (Delaney AIDS Research Enterprise; DARE); R01AI152932 R01 (T.J. Henrich; H.F. VanBrocklin). The content is solely the responsibility of the authors and does not necessarily represent the official views of the National Institutes of Health. Grant support for raltegravir PET imaging provided by Merck.

[a] Division of Experimental Medicine, University of California San Francisco, 1001 Potrero Avenue, Building 3, Room 525A, San Francisco, CA 94110, USA; [b] Department of Radiology, University of California Davis Medical Center, Sacramento, CA, USA; [c] Department of Radiology and Biomedical Imaging, University of California San Francisco, San Francisco, CA, USA; [d] Department of Surgery and Cancer, Imperial College, London, UK
* Corresponding author.
E-mail address: Timothy.Henrich@ucsf.edu

PET Clin 16 (2021) 89–97
https://doi.org/10.1016/j.cpet.2020.09.011

clinical relevance, especially the setting of acute or chronic viral diseases, such as COVID-19 and human immunodeficiency virus (HIV).[1,2,7,9]

2. Diagnostic studies to determine specific pathogens or groups of pathogens (eg, HIV, Enterobacteriaceae, *Mycobacterium tuberculosis*) using novel immunoPET tracers that directly engage pathogen antigens/proteins directly or other drugs that target unique metabolic or enzymatic pathways.[2,7,10–13]

3. Determining responses to antimicrobial and antiviral therapies. These responses may include direct pathogen burden and location, longitudinal assessment of immunologic, inflammatory responses, and associated comorbidities.[1]

4. Imaging of host cellular receptors and other targets of infectious pathogens. These are diverse and may include, for example, imaging density and distribution of angiotensin-converting enzyme-2 receptors used by SARS-CoV-2 for cell entry and replication, and CD4 and other viral coreceptors used by HIV to engage host cells.[10,14]

5. Total-body tissue distribution and pharmacokinetic (PK)/pharmacodynamics (PD) of various antimicrobial drugs and other anti-infective small molecule or biologic agents.

6. Metabolic disturbances or other clinical factors that may lead to increased susceptibility or morbidity from various infection pathogens.

A classic example of how decades of molecular imaging experience has been applied to studying various aspects of chronic (and acute) viral infections is PET imaging in people with HIV and animal models of HIV or simian immunodeficiency virus (SIV) infection. In addition to its profound disruption of the cellular immune system and loss of CD4 T cells over time in untreated infection, HIV infection has been associated with increased cardiovascular disease, metabolic dysregulation, neurologic disorders, and various hematologic and solid-tumor malignancies,[15,16] even in the setting of otherwise suppressive antiretroviral therapy (ART). As a result, PET imaging has been used to (1) localize and characterize tissue measures of inflammation and cardiac disease using FDG; (2) characterize neurologic outcomes of viral infection including neuroimaging of various metabolic pathways, dopamine transport, and cellular activation; (3) determine ART-related toxicities; (4) quantify changes in various immune cell types, such as CD4+ T-cell distribution; and (5) directly visualize areas of persistent HIV infection in the setting of otherwise suppressive ART, as we have recently reviewed.[7]

Clearly, these types of PET studies can and are being applied to other viral and bacterial infections, with a more recent surge of interest in various imaging modalities to characterize SARS-CoV-2 infection and related immune responses and inflammatory morbidity.[17,18] Nonetheless, major limitations using standard PET imaging technologies have been identified (described later), and novel molecular imaging approaches for the clinical and pathogenesis-based research of various infectious pathogens are urgently needed.[1,2] High-sensitivity, total-body PET imaging strategies have major potential to overcome these challenges and revolutionize noninvasive infectious disease research.

ADVANTAGES OF TOTAL-BODY PET IMAGING

The most advanced form of molecular imaging of the human body, total-body PET, is being introduced into clinical use.[19–22] Less than 1% of the photons emitted during traditional PET scanning are detected given the limited axial field of view and body length (typically <25 cm) that can be imaged at one time. The field of view in total-body PET platforms, such as uEXPLORER or PennPET Explorer, is extended over the entire individual (1–2 m) by using a large number of parallel detectors that simultaneously detect photon emission.[21,23–26] These platforms accept more coincident positron decays that may be used to maximize sensitivity while introducing only slightly degraded axial spatial resolution and a small increase in scatter fraction. As a result, early data suggest that total-body PET provides a greater than 40-fold gain in effective sensitivity and a greater than six-fold increase in signal-to-noise ratio compared with standard PET.[27] These dramatically enhanced performance characteristics allow for decreased PET scanning times acquiring data "total-body wide" and may be leveraged to decrease the amount of radiotracer required, thereby permitting more frequent imaging or longer imaging periods during radiotracer decay. This is of particular value for imaging agents labeled with longer-lived radionuclides, such as ^{89}Zr, which have disadvantageous dosimetry properties and must therefore be administered in much smaller amounts than, for example, ^{18}F-labeled radiotracers. The combination of full field of view and enhanced temporal resolution in total-body PET imaging also allows for improved dynamic quantification of radiotracer uptake over time.

POTENTIAL FOR TOTAL-BODY PET IMAGING IN INFECTIOUS DISEASES

High-sensitivity total-body PET has potential to dramatically improve molecular imaging and systems biology approaches in such fields as oncology, bone metabolism, inflammation, and cardiovascular medicine,[19,28–31] as discussed elsewhere in this issue. However, applications to infectious disease research and clinical care are just now emerging, but may address several limitations of traditional PET imaging as follows:

1. *Direct visualization of low-level specific pathogen or host pathogen interactions.* The direct visualization, anatomic localization, and quantitation of viral and bacterial diseases are extremely challenging. For example, chronic viral infections that are able to maintain some state of latency under either natural immune control (eg, various human herpes viruses, such as cytomegalovirus and Epstein-Barr virus) or under the cover of antiviral therapy (eg, HIV) express low levels of viral proteins (ie, low infectious burden), and can persist in locations that are difficult, if not impossible, to sample directly.[7] For example, HIV may infect a small number of mononuclear cells in the setting of ART (eg, <1 infected CD4 T cell per million cells in the circulation), and much of the viral genetic material is quiescently integrated into the human genome.[15,16] HIV also largely resides in organized lymphoid or other tissues outside of the peripheral circulation, such as gut-associated lymphoid tissue or lymph nodes, and many anatomic regions are inaccessible to routine sampling. Chronic bacterial disease, such as latent *Mycobacterium tuberculosis*, may also persist in low burdens in immune-privileged anatomic sites, including tissue outside the pulmonary system.[1,2,32] In addition to low pathogen burden or protein production, there is potential for variability in gene sequences between and within individuals and suboptimal engagement of tracer molecule to targets. As a result, there is a need for whole-body molecular imaging platforms with high sensitivity and improved signal/noise ratios over standard PET imaging platforms to visualize the limited disease reservoirs. In addition to the previous examples, increased sensitivity from total-body immunoPET (eg, radiolabeled pathogen-specific monoclonal antibodies [mAb]) may also be particularly relevant in acute viral infections that manifest in highly morbid disease, such as COVID-19. Whereas individuals with SARS-CoV-2 infection may shed viral RNA in the respiratory tract weeks after onset of symptoms,[33] replication seems to be predominately restricted to respiratory mucosa. However, given the extent of multiple organ dysfunction and inflammatory cascade observed in COVID-19,[34] there may be more widespread tissue viral cytopathic effects that are far more subtle than that observed in the respiratory tract. These sites also present challenges to direct investigation through invasive means, necessitating PET imaging strategies that are highly sensitive and able to detect low-level signal from background noise.Highly sensitive, total-body PET also has the potential to enhance molecular imaging of cellular targets of viral infection required for efficient replication. For example, current immunoPET strategies are being used to image CD4 expression in the setting of HIV/SIV,[10,14] and there is intense interest in visualizing angiotensin-converting enzyme-2 expression in the setting of COVID-19. Whereas traditional PET may have sensitivity to visualize expression of such target in organized lymph node or pulmonary tissues, increased sensitivity and signal/noise ratios will likely be needed to identify and quantify expression in other tissues, which may play a role in whole-body pathogenesis and organ involvement. Such sensitive noninvasive, total-body surveys may also allow predictions of disease severity and clinical outcomes.

2. *Biokinetic imaging of immunologic response to infection.* Persistent cellular immune responses following viral infection may be subtle and require longitudinal imaging to understand pathogen-specific responses and to inform on systems-based immunology approaches. Specific examples of CD4 and CD8 T-cell imaging are discussed later, but will likely require high-sensitivity total-body imaging and longitudinal imaging requiring multiple doses of tracer with reduced radiation risk to individuals.

3. *Inflammatory consequences of infection and other pathogen-related comorbidities.* Inflammatory responses to various infections are profound and long lasting.[34] For example, SARS-CoV-2 can lead to dramatic increase in soluble markers of inflammation and coagulopathy that persist for weeks to months following cessation of viral shedding and resolution of viral replication.[34] Whether or not low-level, persistent immune activation is associated with individuals that experience chronic COVID-19 symptoms ("long haulers") is not known, but even in the setting of normalized circulating inflammatory markers, there may be more subtle and persistent tissue foci of cardiopulmonary,

lymph node, and other tissue inflammation or fibrosis that would require high-sensitivity imaging. A large body of FDG-PET imaging studies of SARS-CoV-2 has recently emerged reporting pulmonary hypermetabolism consistent with an active inflammatory process along with increased associated lymph node tracer uptake.[17] More recent published data suggest that these findings are not isolated to the lungs, and may involve other organs, such as the salivary glands,[18] bone marrow, spleen, and nasopharynx.[18] HIV also leads to chronic immune activation and inflammation leading to increased cardiac, immunologic, and neurologic morbidity, even in the setting of long-term antiretroviral use. FDG PET has been implemented in both of these viral infections[15,16] but limited by sensitivity in treated chronic HIV or convalescent COVID-19 and by the radiation dose limitations inherent in longitudinal imaging studies.

4. *Tissue distribution and kinetics of anti-infective agents.* PK/PD studies used in traditional early phase clinical development of antimicrobial and antiviral agents rely on frequent peripheral blood sampling to establish drug kinetics and elimination in the circulation. These data are also used to evaluate drug efficacy or biologic effects in vivo. However, there is a paucity of data regarding drug dynamics in tissues, which are the primary sites of antimicrobial and antiviral activity.[35,36] Drugs may distribute rapidly throughout tissues preventing whole-body PK evaluations. Examples of dichotomies between tissue and circulating blood drug levels are common. For example, cerebrospinal fluid drug levels may be different from levels within the brain parenchymal itself. As a result there has been interest in using PET imaging of radiolabeled drugs to look at the tissue-wide biodistribution and kinetics of various anti-infective agents.[37] The potential for PET imaging to inform on PK/PD was demonstrated by a recent animal and human study of [^{11}C] rifampin in the setting of tuberculous meningitis.[38] This study demonstrated that rifampin penetration into tuberculosis-infected brain lesions was limited, heterogeneous in distribution, and decayed rapidly over time.[38] PET data were used to establish PK models to predict a higher dose of drug to be used to achieve therapeutic parenchymal concentrations.[38] Our group is currently conducting clinical PET studies to determine the early tissue distribution and kinetics of raltegravir in people with HIV on ART. Raltegravir is a strand-transfer HIV integrase inhibitor, a commonly used class of antiretroviral in combination ART. Certain

immune-privileged environments are important foci of HIV persistence in the setting of ART and many of these loci may have achieved suboptimal ART drug levels, leading to ongoing low-level viral production and persistent immune activation.[39] These drugs are rapidly and efficiently absorbed and distribute rapidly throughout tissues. However, little information is known about tissue-penetration of drug where active HIV infection may persist. **Fig. 1** shows representative PET imaging of [^{18}F]Raltegravir using traditional imaging methods hours after intravenous drug administration. PET imaging of [^{18}F]Raltegravir provides a unique opportunity to image total-body drug PK. However, current PET methods using serial imaging time points to determine biokinetics of drug requires multiple bed positions and certain areas have revealed low to no detection of drug, such as the brain, which may represent radioactive drug concentrations that are lower than the sensitivity threshold. As a result, there is an urgent need for total-body PET platforms that have increased sensitivity and signal/noise ratios. In addition, these total-body scanners also allow imaging-derived arterial blood time course of a radiotracer providing an arterial input function to the body's tissue uptake. This information significantly simplifies the process of quantification of the tracer's binding in tissues, and the results may be presented as whole-body quantitative, functional parametric images.[24] The improved sensitivity also allows tracers to be followed over longer periods of time as the radionuclides decay.

5. *Tracking responses to biologic and immunotherapies for viral infections.* Similar to cancer research, there has been intense interest in using cell-based therapies for various chronic viral infectious diseases. These approaches range from exogenous infusions of allodonor viral-specific T cells to chimeric antigen receptor (CAR) T cells designed to target proteins, such as the HIV envelope.[40] Many of these therapies require expansion of pathogen-specific cells on engagement with target antigen, but it is challenging to determine the longitudinal kinetics of donor cells across tissues and time without invasive sampling.[40] These cells may have limited access to various anatomic compartments, such as lymph node follicles, which contain most of the HIV reservoir,[41] and the central nervous system, another important, but understudied area of viral persistence.[42] PET imaging of CAR-T cell therapies has been implemented in cancer,[43] and there is intense interest in having the ability to follow various

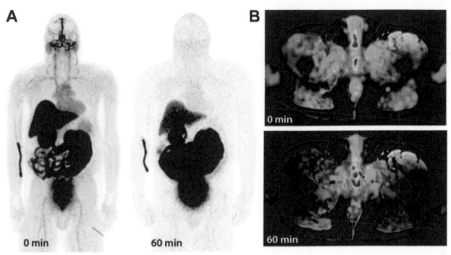

Fig. 1. [^{18}F]Raltegravir PET imaging in a participant with HIV on suppressive ART. (*A*) Maximum intensity projections acquired immediately and 60 minutes following intravenous injection demonstrate rapid elimination of tracer from tissues that may harbor persistent HIV. (*B*) Axial PET/MR imaging overlays of inguinal lymph nodes. Low tracer uptake was identified in inguinal lymph nodes highlighting the need for high-sensitivity total-body PET imaging that allows for dynamic temporal imaging of antiretroviral tissue distribution and kinetics.

cellular therapies in the setting of infection that can track cell distribution, turnover, and persistence over time. However, noninvasive PET imaging modalities will need high sensitivity and to allow for longitudinal imaging with several time points and multiple radiotracer administrations while keeping radiation doses to acceptable levels. Total-body PET is ideal for this undertaking.

EXAMPLE OF MOLECULAR IMAGING OF IMMUNE RESPONSES TO INFECTIOUS DISEASES HIGHLIGHTING THE NEED FOR TOTAL-BODY PET IMAGING
ImmunoPET Imaging of CD4 T-Cell Dynamics in Simian Immunodeficiency Virus/Human Immunodeficiency Virus Infection

CD4$^+$ T cells are the main target of HIV infection. Active disease leads to subsequent and profound reduction in CD4$^+$ lymphocytes throughout the blood and tissues. Although counts may improve in many individuals on ART, lasting perturbations to tissues, such as the lymph nodes and gut-associated lymphoid tissues, are common.[15,16] As a result, there has been interest in CD4$^+$ T cell–specific PET-based imaging techniques to follow CD4$^+$ T-cell dynamics and recovery during natural infection and following various immune-based interventions. For example, a recent investigation of the use of an α4β7 mAb in acute SIV infection in macaques demonstrated sustained virologic control in mAb-treated monkeys.[44] Although this major finding has yet to be confirmed

in subsequent studies using a different and more replication-competent SIV strain, the study involved PET/computed tomography imaging using a ^{64}Cu-labeled F(ab')2 antibody against CD4 to demonstrate repopulation of CD4 T cells in several tissues, including gut (**Fig. 2**).[14] The reconstitution of gut CD4 T cells was unexpected based on the original study hypothesis that the α4β7 mAb would interfere with CD4$^+$ T-cell trafficking to these areas.[44] As a result, this study is proof of concept of how imaging various cell-specific markers may provide critical information regarding whole-body immune responses over time. However, similar studies are challenging in the setting of HIV infection given the need for longitudinal study design incorporating multiple radiolabeled antibody infusions and the subsequent need to reduce radionuclide dose. Human studies would also benefit from the use of radiolabeled mAbs with longer half-lives (eg, incorporating ^{89}Zr). Whereas ^{89}Zr has a 78-hour $t_{1/2}$ and can be imaged up to a week or so following administration using traditional PET, high-sensitivity total-body imaging may allow serial imaging over 2 to 3 weeks following a single administration of tracer allowing for imaging dynamics of CD4 T-cell populations in near real-time.

Importance of CD8 T-Cell Immune Responses in Viral Infections

CD8 T cells play a major role in antiviral and antifungal immunity and are capable of secreting proimmune molecules, such as interferon-γ, tumor

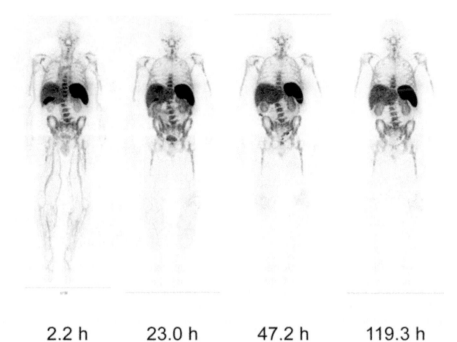

2.2 h   23.0 h   47.2 h   119.3 h

Fig. 2. Biodistribution. Whole-body images of a participant at various times after injection of ^{89}Zr-IAB22M2C (CD8 T cell–specific minibody; 1.5-mg dose). All images show most intense activity within spleen, followed by marrow, liver, and kidneys. (*From* Pandit-Taskar N, Postow MA, Hellmann MD, et al. First-in-Humans Imaging with (89)Zr-Df-IAB22M2C Anti-CD8 Minibody in Patients with Solid Malignancies: Preliminary Pharmacokinetics, Biodistribution, and Lesion Targeting. J Nucl Med. 2020;61(4):512-519; with permission.)

necrosis factor-α, and interleukin-2, and can release cytotoxic granules containing granyzme-B and perforin that help kill infected cells. Pathogen-specific immunity usually develops over a course of weeks following infection. The frequency of these cells in the circulation degrades with time, although they can mount an amnestic response following antigen exposure leading to rapid proliferation and increased effector T-cell phenotypes.[45] As a result, they are key players in controlling acute infection and protect from future viral challenge.

Memory T-cell responses likely play an important role in SARS-CoV-2 immunity and are likely an essential component of the coordinated immune response following vaccination.[46] Despite lymphopenia in SARS-CoV-1 and SARS-CoV-3, increased frequency of cells responding to various antigens, such as Spike, Nucleocapsid, membrane, and accessory (functional) protein (eg, ORF 1ab) peptide sequences, develops within the weeks following infection.[45,46] In addition, mucosal immune responses (eg, tissue resident memory T cells) may also play a crucial role in this response because this is the initial and major site of SARS-CoV-2 infection and replication. Cytotoxic CD8 T cells also play a critical role in controlling acute and chronic untreated HIV

infection and are important in maintaining viral latency during ART.[47,48] However, these cytolytic CD8 T cells may be excluded from various immune-privileged sites, such as B-cell follicles containing follicular CD4 T cells, a major component of the HIV reservoir. As a result, there is urgent need for direct PET imaging strategies to characterize the whole-body T-cell response in the setting of various infections. Noninvasive modalities have the potential to significantly increase the understanding of immune responses in vivo.

Direct ImmunoPET Imaging of CD8 T-Cell Immune Responses

^{89}Zr-Df-IAB22M2C[49] is a CD8 T cell–specific radiolabeled minibody that allows imaging, tracking and quantification of CD8-expressing T cells in vivo by PET imaging as shown in **Fig. 2**. Early phase human studies have demonstrated successful targeting of tumor tissue enriched in CD8 T cells. Therefore, there is clear rationale to pursue direct imaging of CD8 T-cell responses using ^{89}Zr-Df-IAB22M2C in the setting of infection. Total-body PET imaging has the potential to allow following radiolabeled CD8 T-cell turnover at sites of active infection and as they traffic from lymph node stores for several weeks following injection of tracer.[49] Repeat administration of tracer may also be performed if cumulative radiation dose can kept low to examine the temporal and anatomic dynamics and replenishment of CD8 T cells from acute through convalescent infection. There are several distinct advantages of total-body PET for studies of T-cell biology in response to viral and other infection. These include the ability to image with high temporal resolution the distribution throughout the entire body allowing for whole-body, quantitative, functional parametric images,[30,31] and to capitalize on its geometric efficiency to image with the highest sensitivity to allow the reconstruction of images with high statistical quality[50] with the potential for delineating, for the first time, T-cell activity within the lymphatic system. As a result, there is urgent need for further clinical implementation of CD8 T cell–specific immunoPET strategies in viral diseases, such as COVID-19 and HIV, among many others.

PET Imaging T-Cell Activation

Recent advances in molecular imaging have enabled PET imaging of T cell–specific immune activation and proliferation. More specifically, the radiofluorinated imaging agent, [^{18}F]F-AraG, was synthesized with a goal of development for human use. F-AraG is a fluorinated purine derivative with selective T-cell uptake.[51,52] [^{18}F]F-AraG is a high affinity substrate for deoxyguanosine kinase (dGK) and a low affinity substrate for deoxycytidine kinase (dCK). Both dGK and dCK are overexpressed in activated T cells. Blocking the expression of either dGK or dCK causes reduction in [^{18}F]F-AraG uptake, whereas overexpression of either dGK or dCK leads to increased accumulation of [^{18}F]F-AraG. [^{18}F]F-AraG PET has been used to investigate immune activation in murine models of various inflammatory disorders, malignancies, and allogeneic stem cell transplantation.[51–53] Data from these in vivo studies demonstrate that this approach yields highly sensitive imaging of activated T cells. Importantly, [^{18}F]F-AraG was more specific for activated CD8 and CD4 T cells than for monocytes/macrophages. As a result, this novel tracer has a role in imaging CD8 T-cell immune responses to infection and our group has several human studies enrolling or in development to study cellular responses to HIV and SARS-CoV-2 infection. However, high-sensitivity total-body PET imaging has the potential to greatly enhance the utility of such a tracer.

SUMMARY AND FUTURE DEVELOPMENT

The development of specific imaging biomarkers of infectious pathogens and immune responses is challenging. Several obstacles of this development, however, may be overcome with high-sensitivity total-body PET imaging technologies that allow for improved resolution and dynamic quantification of radiotracer uptake over time. The combination of full field of view and enhanced temporal resolution in total-body PET imaging allows for improved dynamic quantification of radiotracer uptake over time and may enable whole-body, noninvasive systems immunology approaches to infectious disease research.

ACKNOWLEDGMENTS

Dr Ian Wilson of ImaginAb, Inc is acknowledged for sharing his insight into T-cell activity in COVID patients and future developments of T-cell imaging biomarker.

CONFLICT STATEMENT

T.J. Henrich receives grant support from Gilead Sciences, Merck, and Bristol Myers Squibb. UC Davis has a revenue sharing agreement with United Imaging Healthcare.

REFERENCES

1. Jain SK. The promise of molecular imaging in the study and treatment of infectious diseases. Mol Imaging Biol 2017;19(3):341–7.
2. Ordonez AA, Sellmyer MA, Gowrishankar G, et al. Molecular imaging of bacterial infections: overcoming the barriers to clinical translation. Sci Transl Med 2019;11(508).
3. Rudd JH, Narula J, Strauss HW, et al. Imaging atherosclerotic plaque inflammation by fluorodeoxyglucose with positron emission tomography: ready for prime time? J Am Coll Cardiol 2010;55(23):2527–35.
4. Tawakol A, Migrino RQ, Bashian GG, et al. In vivo 18F-fluorodeoxyglucose positron emission tomography imaging provides a noninvasive measure of carotid plaque inflammation in patients. J Am Coll Cardiol 2006;48(9):1818–24.
5. Sathekge M, Maes A, Kgomo M, et al. FDG uptake in lymph-nodes of HIV+ and tuberculosis patients: implications for cancer staging. Q J Nucl Med Mol Imaging 2010;54(6):698–703.
6. Sathekge M, Maes A, Van de Wiele C. FDG-PET imaging in HIV infection and tuberculosis. Semin Nucl Med 2013;43(5):349–66.
7. Henrich TJ, Hsue PY, VanBrocklin H. Seeing is believing: nuclear imaging of HIV persistence. Front Immunol 2019;10:2077.
8. Polvoy I, Flavell RR, Ohliger M, Rosenberg O, Wilson DM. Nuclear imaging of bacterial infection- state of the art and future directions. J Nucl Med. Aug 6: jnumed.120.244939. doi:10.2967/jnumed.120.244939.

9. Ances BM, Hammoud DA. Neuroimaging of HIV-associated neurocognitive disorders (HAND). Curr Opin HIV AIDS 2014;9(6):545–51.

10. Santangelo PJ, Rogers KA, Zurla C, et al. Whole-body immunoPET reveals active SIV dynamics in viremic and antiretroviral therapy-treated macaques. Nat Methods 2015;12(5):427–32.

11. Weinstein EA, Ordonez AA, DeMarco VP, et al. Imaging Enterobacteriaceae infection in vivo with 18F-fluorodeoxysorbitol positron emission tomography. Sci Transl Med 2014;6(259):259ra146.

12. Li J, Zheng H, Fodah R, et al. Validation of 2-(18)F-fluorodeoxysorbitol as a potential radiopharmaceutical for imaging bacterial infection in the lung. J Nucl Med 2018;59(1):134–9.

13. Yao S, Xing H, Zhu W, et al. Infection imaging with (18)F-FDS and first-in-human evaluation. Nucl Med Biol 2016;43(3):206–14.

14. Santangelo PJ, Cicala C, Byrareddy SN, et al. Early treatment of SIV+ macaques with an alpha4beta7 mAb alters virus distribution and preserves CD4(+) T cells in later stages of infection. Mucosal Immunol 2018;11(3):932–46.

15. Deeks SG, Lewin SR, Ross AL, et al. International AIDS Society global scientific strategy: towards an HIV cure 2016. Nat Med 2016;22(8):839–50.

16. Estes JD, Kityo C, Ssali F, et al. Defining total-body AIDS-virus burden with implications for curative strategies. Nat Med 2017;23(11):1271–6.

17. Awulachew E, Diriba K, Anja A, et al. Computed tomography (CT) imaging features of patients with COVID-19: systematic review and meta-analysis. Radiol Res Pract 2020;2020:1023506.

18. Halsey R, Priftakis D, Mackenzie S, et al. COVID-19 in the act: incidental 18F-FDG PET/CT findings in asymptomatic patients and those with symptoms not primarily correlated with COVID-19 during the United Kingdom coronavirus lockdown. Eur J Nucl Med Mol Imaging 2020;1–13. https://doi.org/10.1007/s00259-020-04972-y.

19. Zhang YQ, Hu PC, Wu RZ, et al. The image quality, lesion detectability, and acquisition time of (18)F-FDG total-body PET/CT in oncological patients. Eur J Nucl Med Mol Imaging 2020;47(11):2507–15.

20. Badawi RD, Shi H, Hu P, et al. First human imaging studies with the EXPLORER total-body PET scanner. J Nucl Med 2019;60(3):299–303.

21. Pantel AR, Viswanath V, Daube-Witherspoon ME, et al. PennPET explorer: human imaging on a whole-body imager. J Nucl Med 2020;61(1):144–51.

22. Tan H, Gu Y, Yu H, et al. Total-body PET/CT: current applications and future perspectives. AJR Am J Roentgenol 2020;215(2):325–37.

23. Lv Y, Lv X, Liu W, et al. Mini EXPLORER II: a prototype high-sensitivity PET/CT scanner for companion animal whole body and human brain scanning. Phys Med Biol 2019;64(7):075004.

24. Cherry SR, Badawi RD, Karp JS, et al. Total-body imaging: transforming the role of positron emission tomography. Sci Transl Med 2017;9(381):eaaf6169.

25. Berg E, Zhang X, Bec J, et al. Development and evaluation of mini-EXPLORER: a long axial field-of-view PET scanner for nonhuman primate imaging. J Nucl Med 2018;59(6):993–8.

26. Karp JS, Viswanath V, Geagan MJ, et al. PennPET explorer: design and preliminary performance of a whole-body imager. J Nucl Med 2020;61(1):136–43.

27. Zeglis BM, Lewis JS. The bioconjugation and radiosynthesis of 89Zr-DFO-labeled antibodies. J Vis Exp 2015;(96):52521.

28. Saboury B, Morris MA, Nikpanah M, et al. Reinventing molecular imaging with total-body PET, Part II: clinical applications. PET Clin 2020;15(4):463–75.

29. Saboury B, Morris MA, Farhadi F, et al. Reinventing molecular imaging with total-body PET, Part I: technical revolution in evolution. PET Clin 2020;15(4):427–38.

30. Zhang X, Xie Z, Berg E, et al. Total-body dynamic reconstruction and parametric imaging on the uEXPLORER. J Nucl Med 2020;61(2):285–91.

31. Eftekhari F. Imaging assessment of osteosarcoma in childhood and adolescence: diagnosis, staging, and evaluating response to chemotherapy. Cancer Treat Res 2009;152:33–62.

32. Weinstein EA, Liu L, Ordonez AA, et al. Noninvasive determination of 2-[18F]-fluoroisonicotinic acid hydrazide pharmacokinetics by positron emission tomography in Mycobacterium tuberculosis-infected mice. Antimicrob Agents Chemother 2012;56(12):6284–90.

33. Lee S, Kim T, Lee E, et al. Clinical course and molecular viral shedding among asymptomatic and symptomatic patients with SARS-CoV-2 infection in a community treatment center in the Republic of Korea. JAMA Intern Med 2020;e203862. [Epub ahead of print].

34. Blanco-Melo D, Nilsson-Payant BE, Liu WC, et al. Imbalanced host response to SARS-CoV-2 drives development of COVID-19. Cell 2020;181(5):1036–45.e9.

35. Martinez-Picado J, Deeks SG. Persistent HIV-1 replication during antiretroviral therapy. Curr Opin HIV AIDS 2016;11(4):417–23.

36. Asmuth DM, Thompson CG, Chun TW, et al. Tissue pharmacologic and virologic determinants of duodenal and rectal gastrointestinal-associated lymphoid tissue immune reconstitution in HIV-infected patients initiating antiretroviral therapy. J Infect Dis 2017;216(7):813–8.

37. Huang SC. Role of kinetic modeling in biomedical imaging. J Med Sci 2008;28(2):57–63.

38. Tucker EW, Guglieri-Lopez B, Ordonez AA, et al. Noninvasive (11)C-rifampin positron emission tomography reveals drug biodistribution in tuberculous meningitis. Sci Transl Med 2018; 10(470).

39. Nettles RE, Kieffer TL, Kwon P, et al. Intermittent HIV-1 viremia (Blips) and drug resistance in patients receiving HAART. JAMA 2005;293(7):817–29.

40. Peterson CW, Kiem HP. Cell and gene therapy for HIV cure. Curr Top Microbiol Immunol 2018;417: 211–48.

41. Bronnimann MP, Skinner PJ, Connick E. The B-cell follicle in HIV infection: barrier to a cure. Front Immunol 2018;9:20.

42. Winston A, Antinori A, Cinque P, et al. Defining cerebrospinal fluid HIV RNA escape: editorial review AIDS. AIDS 2019;33(Suppl 2):S107–11.

43. Lee SH, Soh H, Chung JH, et al. Feasibility of real-time in vivo 89Zr-DFO-labeled CAR T-cell trafficking using PET imaging. PLoS One 2020;15(1):e0223814.

44. Byrareddy SN, Arthos J, Cicala C, et al. Sustained virologic control in SIV+ macaques after antiretroviral and alpha4beta7 antibody therapy. Science 2016;354(6309):197–202.

45. Swadling L, Maini MK. T cells in COVID-19: united in diversity. Nat Immunol 2020. [Epub ahead of print].

46. Jeyanathan M, Afkhami S, Smaill F, et al. Immunological considerations for COVID-19 vaccine strategies. Nat Rev Immunol 2020;20(10):615–32.

47. O'Connell KA, Bailey JR, Blankson JN. Elucidating the elite: mechanisms of control in HIV-1 infection. Trends Pharmacol Sci 2009;30(12):631–7.

48. McBrien JB, Mavigner M, Franchitti L, et al. Robust and persistent reactivation of SIV and HIV by N-803 and depletion of CD8(+) cells. Nature 2020; 578(7793):154–9.

49. Pandit-Taskar N, Postow MA, Hellmann MD, et al. First-in-humans imaging with (89)Zr-Df-IAB22M2C anti-CD8 minibody in patients with solid malignancies: preliminary pharmacokinetics, biodistribution, and lesion targeting. J Nucl Med 2020; 61(4):512–9.

50. Efthimiou N. New challenges for PET image reconstruction for total-body imaging. PET Clin 2020; 15(4):453–61.

51. Franc BL, Goth S, MacKenzie J, et al. In vivo PET imaging of the activated immune environment in a small animal model of inflammatory arthritis. Mol Imaging 2017;16. 1536012117712638.

52. Ronald JA, Kim BS, Gowrishankar G, et al. A PET imaging strategy to visualize activated T cells in acute graft-versus-host disease elicited by allogenic hematopoietic cell transplant. Cancer Res 2017; 77(11):2893–902.

53. Levi J, Lam T, Goth SR, et al. Imaging of activated T cells as an early predictor of immune response to anti-PD-1 therapy. Cancer Res 2019;79(13): 3455–65.

Total-Body PET Imaging of Musculoskeletal Disorders

Abhijit J. Chaudhari, PhD[a],[*],[1], William Y. Raynor, BS[b],[c],[1], Ali Gholamrezanezhad, MD[d], Thomas J. Werner, MSE[b], Chamith S. Rajapakse, PhD[b], Abass Alavi, MD[b]

KEYWORDS

- Arthritis • Fever of unknown origin • Osteoporosis • Sarcopenia • Cancer • Osteosarcoma
- PET/CT • PET/MR imaging

KEY POINTS

- A number of musculoskeletal disorders are systemic in nature or have systemic sequalae. Bio-markers that provide global assessment of disease activity across the entire body are urgently needed.
- Total-body PET/computed tomography (CT) can provide anato-molecular imaging-based measures across the entire human body at reduced dose, lower scan time, and higher spatial resolution.
- Total-body PET/CT measures can contribute toward an improved understanding of the underlying pathogenesis of musculoskeletal disorders and may provide new insights for the evaluation of and monitoring of interventions and therapy.
- Because total-body PET/CT includes images of the brain in the field of view, this approach may provide a means to detect and quantify the degree of pain that is associated with musculoskeletal disorders, potentially allowing further insight into the impact of opioids.

INTRODUCTION

Musculoskeletal disorders (MSDs) are broadly defined as diseases or injuries of the joints, bones, muscles, nerves, tendons, ligaments, supporting soft tissues, cartilage, and spinal discs, and comprise over 150 diagnoses.[1] Commonly encountered examples are arthritis (such as rheumatoid arthritis, systemic lupus erythematous, or osteoarthritis), osteoporosis/osteopenia, sarcopenia, infection, neoplasms, and neck and lower back pain. MSDs are a major cause of disability worldwide, second only to mental and substance use disorders,[2] and have a significant negative impact on global population health. They are prevalent across the lifespan and have an astronomical societal cost that comes in the form of limited mobility, dexterity and functional ability, persistent pain, inability to work, early retirement from work, inability to participate in societal roles, depression, and increased risk of developing other chronic disease conditions.[3]

Clinical evaluation of MSDs mostly relies on a combination of physical examination, serum biomarkers and pain- and health-assessment questionnaires. Outside of radiography, other imaging modalities have had a limited role in MSD evaluation. Anatomic imaging data from radiography, computed tomography (CT), and MR imaging have been shown to be only weakly correlated with clinical signs and disease pathogenesis or treatment response.[4] Therefore, precise image-based parameters that could allow assessment of the molecular and pathophysiologic processes that underlie the disease state and its progression over time could play a crucial role in the evaluation

[a] Department of Radiology, University of California Davis, 4860 Y Street, Sacramento, CA 95825, USA; [b] Department of Radiology, University of Pennsylvania, 3400 Spruce Street, Philadelphia, PA 19104, USA; [c] Drexel University College of Medicine, 2900 West Queen Lane, Philadelphia, PA 19129, USA; [d] Keck School of Medicine, University of Southern California, 1520 San Pablo Street, Los Angeles, CA 90033, USA
[1] These authors contributed equally to this work.
* Corresponding author.
E-mail address: ajchaudhari@ucdavis.edu

PET Clin 16 (2021) 99–117
https://doi.org/10.1016/j.cpet.2020.09.012

of MSDs. Molecular imaging with PET/CT and PET/MR imaging has been used for MSD evaluation, but only in a limited number of studies.[5] This has been a direct consequence of the associated high cumulative radiation dose, especially in the context of evaluating chronic MSDs, patient discomfort from the relatively long image acquisition time, and the inability to examine multiple body structures or systems that that are known to be affected by MSD. Furthermore, the limited spatial resolution of standard PET scanners is suboptimal for visualizing and quantifying disease activity in small joints or tissues, which appear to be a bellwether of pathology in several MSDs.

In this article we provide our perspective about the potential role of total-body PET/CT (TB PET/CT) in the management of patients with MSDs, with emphasis on autoimmune and degenerative arthritis, musculoskeletal infection, osseous disorders, sarcopenia, and musculoskeletal malignancies. Throughout this scientific communication, we elaborate on 3 major physical characteristics of TB PET/CT systems that are deemed crucial for successful evaluation of MSDs. : (1) the long axial field-of-view, which enables imaging multiple organs and systems simultaneously during the same phases of radiotracer distribution and uptake; (2) high geometric sensitivity, which allows the reduction of the administered radiotracer dose significantly and the shortening of the image acquisition time; and (3) higher spatial resolution compared with standard PET systems, which is essential for detecting and quantifying disease process in the small musculoskeletal structures such as small joints, tendons, and soft tissue structures.

RHEUMATOID AND PSORIATIC ARTHRITIS

Rheumatoid arthritis (RA) and psoriatic arthritis (PsA) are 2 common autoimmune disorders that are systemic in nature and cause an inflammatory reaction, particularly in the joints. They are a major cause of disability and loss of function in the adult population worldwide. The underlying causes of these disorders are unknown, and the majority of patients have no family history of these serious musculoskeletal disabilities. Although the prevalence of both conditions increases by age, juvenile idiopathic arthritis, formerly known as juvenile RA, is now recognized as an independent clinical entity in the broad class of autoimmune arthritis.

Joint inflammation is considered the hallmark of autoimmune arthritis, and tenosynovitis (inflammation of the synovium and the tendons) is commonly presented in both RA and PsA. The entity named enthesitis (inflammation of the entheses), which is unique to PsA, is considered the hallmark for early tissue damage. The existing treatment modalities include a vast number of established approaches and new therapeutics, such as tumor necrosis factor inhibitors, that target joint inflammation[6,7] and broadly show successful modification of the disease course.[8–10] Clinical evaluation of RA and PsA (based on a physical examination performed by a rheumatologist and serum biomarkers) underestimates disease burden and has limited sensitivity and specificity in assessing response to therapeutic interventions.[11,12] Conventional radiographs, MR imaging, and ultrasound scanning, while useful for assessing structural consequences of these disorders, do not directly determine disease activity at the cellular level, which is essential for early detection and determining response to therapy.[13] By now it is well established that structural abnormalities are a late manifestation of the disease process. As such, discrepancy and discordance between structural imaging findings in the evaluation of inflammatory arthropathies are not uncommon.[14] Recent advancement in quantitative and semiquantitative standard anatomic imaging, such as contrast-enhanced ultrasound,[15,16] quantitative MR imaging,[17] and dual-energy CT iodine maps[18] have been somewhat successful in the evaluation and staging of inflammatory arthropathies and their response to treatment. However, further studies are necessary to confirm their accuracy and practicality in this setting. PET/CT imaging with radiotracers such as ^{18}F-fluorodeoxyglucose (FDG) and ^{18}F-sodium fluoride (NaF) has been shown to be highly sensitive and accurate in examining MSDs, particularly those with significant inflammation (**Fig. 1**).[13]

FDG-based PET/CT imaging has been frequently used for assessing RA and PsA at various stages of the disease and monitoring response to treatment.[13,19–28] In one research study by Raynor and colleagues,[29] global synovial FDG activity was measured in 19 patients with RA. These investigators used a thresholding algorithm (ROVER software; ABX GmbH, Radeberg, Germany) to delineate focal FDG uptake in the synovial joints in the hands, elbows, shoulders, knees, and feet. PET parameters reflecting volume and uptake values with and without partial volume correction were found to be significantly higher in patients with RA compared with healthy control subjects and correlated significantly with clinical features such as C-reactive protein, erythrocyte sedimentation rate, and swollen joint count. In addition to the joints assessed by Raynor and colleagues,[29] FDG-PET/CT has been proposed to assess involvement of the hip and

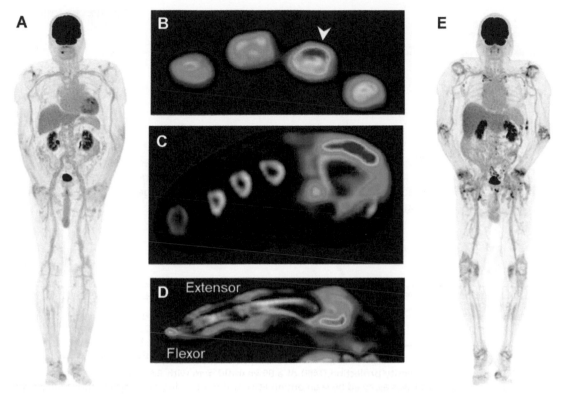

Fig. 1. TB PET in rheumatoid and psoriatic arthritis. Maximum intensity projection (MIP) from the TB PET scan of a 65-year-old man with established rheumatoid arthritis (*A*). Images of the subject in (*A*) showing classic ringlike patterns of radiotracer uptake consistent with synovitis in the joints of the hand (*B*), and foot (*C*). Extensor and flexor tenosynovitis and enthesitis in the right second digit of a 72-year-old man with established psoriatic arthritis (*D*), also shown in the MIP of the TB PET scan (*E*). These images were acquired on the uEXPLORER PET/CT scanner at the University of California Davis, with an injected dose of approximately 74 MBq. Images show static scans conducted over 20 minutes, starting at 40 minutes post-radiotracer injection. (*Courtesy of* Y. Abdelhafez, MD, University of California Davis.)

temporomandibular joint in patients with RA.[30,31] A study by Jonnakuti and colleagues[32] used PET imaging with NaF, a tracer that portrays osteoblastic activity, to assess knee involvement in RA. The investigators noted that increased NaF uptake was associated with increased knee degeneration determined by Kellgren-Lawrence grading; therefore, they concluded that NaF-PET/CT may have clinical utility in assessing bone changes in RA. These studies emphasize the utility of TB PET/CT in facilitating the assessment of joints throughout the body, which are frequently involved in systemic disorders such as RA and PsA and can be effectively evaluated with this technology (**Figs. 2 and 3**).

Several concerns have been raised about the role of PET/CT in the autoimmune arthritis population,[33] such as significant ionizing radiation exposure during the course of the disease and monitoring of treatment response, long scan times in a population that is functionally impaired, limited spatial resolution, which may be suboptimal for evaluating small joints such as those of the extremities that are affected early in the disease course, and examination of only a small anatomic segment of the body despite the clear need for systemic assessment. As noted above, the unique characteristics of TB PET/CT including the long axial field-of-view, high sensitivity, and excellent spatial resolution could overcome the challenges that are faced with conventional PET instruments. Particularly, TB PET/CT would enable (1) staging of RA or PsA disease activity in the entire body, as opposed to examining only a limited subset of joints, so that the appropriate therapy for each individual patient and disease state can be adopted and therefore improving the outcome[34,35]; (2) monitoring response to therapy in joint tissues to optimize the therapeutic window[36] and drug efficacy on a personalized basis,[37–39] switching promptly to another

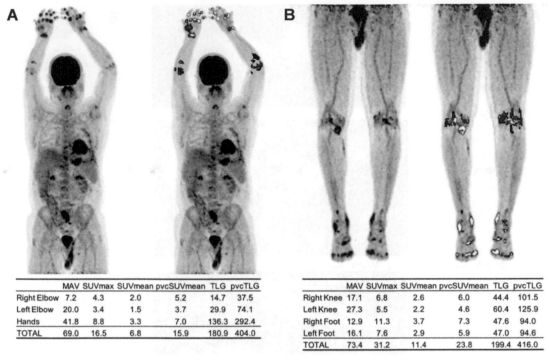

	MAV	SUVmax	SUVmean	pvcSUVmean	TLG	pvcTLG
Right Elbow	7.2	4.3	2.0	5.2	14.7	37.5
Left Elbow	20.0	3.4	1.5	3.7	29.9	74.1
Hands	41.8	8.8	3.3	7.0	136.3	292.4
TOTAL	69.0	16.5	6.8	15.9	180.9	404.0

	MAV	SUVmax	SUVmean	pvcSUVmean	TLG	pvcTLG
Right Knee	17.1	6.8	2.6	6.0	44.4	101.5
Left Knee	27.3	5.5	2.2	4.6	60.4	125.9
Right Foot	12.9	11.3	3.7	7.3	47.6	94.0
Left Foot	16.1	7.6	2.9	5.9	47.0	94.6
TOTAL	73.4	31.2	11.4	23.8	199.4	416.0

Fig. 2. FDG-PET maximum intensity projection (MIP) of a 69-year-old man with RA showing the upper body (*A*) and lower body (*B*). Synovitis was assessed by segmenting FDG-avid joints using an adaptive thresholding algorithm (ROVER software; ABX GmbH). Metabolically active volume (MAV), maximum standardized uptake value (SUV$_{max}$), mean SUV (SUV$_{mean}$), partial volume-corrected SUV$_{mean}$ (pvcSUV$_{mean}$), total lesion glycolysis (TLG = MAV × SUV$_{mean}$), and partial volume-corrected TLG (pvcTLG = MAV × pvcSUV$_{mean}$) were calculated and summed for each segmented region. The global pvcTLG for this patient was 820.0. These analyses could be enabled at a lower radiation dose and scan time, with more comprehensive body coverage in a single scan, using TB PET/CT. (*From* Saboury B, Morris MA, Nikpanah M, Werner TJ, Jones EC, Alavi A. Reinventing Molecular Imaging with Total-Body PET, Part II: Clinical Applications. *PET Clin.* 2020;15(4):463-475. https://doi.org/10.1016/j.cpet.2020.06.013; with permission.)

treatment in nonresponders[40,41]; and (3) assessing the influence of treatment on other crucial organ system, such as the cardiovascular system,[42] to reduce comorbidities and side-effects.[43–45] In the juvenile population, the potential of lowering radiation dose and shortening scan time will also be of great importance because the incidence of autoimmune arthritis is relatively high in this age group.

Based on published literature, most research studies in autoimmune arthritis have used FDG as the main PET tracer. Molecular and cellular events that underlie the inflammatory-proliferative cascade in autoimmune arthritis include activation and transmigration of leukocytes, aberrant pathways of T-cell activation, angiogenesis, hypoxia, and increased osteoclastic and impaired osteoblastic activity and appear to play an important role in the pathogenesis of these disorders.[46–48] There are significant gaps in the knowledge regarding the exact role of

these biological processes and their interactions during autoimmune arthritis pathogenesis. With the growing number of PET ligands,[49] these processes could be effectively examined by TB PET/CT to determine their role in these serious and yet treatable systemic inflammatory disorders. Such targeted research studies can also be of value in developing effective drugs in the future. Although most PET imaging studies are performed as a single static scan at a late time point (mostly at 1–2 hours after the administration of the tracer), performing dynamic imaging with TB PET/CT may lead to improved knowledge in these conditions.[50,51]

In summary, employing TB PET/CT imaging will lead to a significantly lower radiation dose, shorter scan time, and optimal quantification of the disease burden of autoimmune arthritides such as RA and PsA. This could address significant obstacles and longstanding challenges that have been faced in the fields of rheumatology

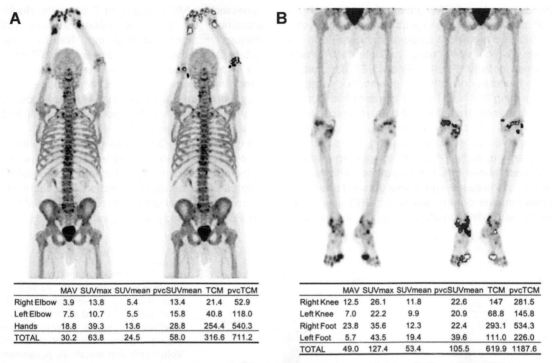

A

	MAV	SUVmax	SUVmean	pvcSUVmean	TCM	pvcTCM
Right Elbow	3.9	13.8	5.4	13.4	21.4	52.9
Left Elbow	7.5	10.7	5.5	15.8	40.8	118.0
Hands	18.8	39.3	13.6	28.8	254.4	540.3
TOTAL	30.2	63.8	24.5	58.0	316.6	711.2

B

	MAV	SUVmax	SUVmean	pvcSUVmean	TCM	pvcTCM
Right Knee	12.5	26.1	11.8	22.6	147	281.5
Left Knee	7.0	22.2	9.9	20.9	68.8	145.8
Right Foot	23.8	35.6	12.3	22.4	293.1	534.3
Left Foot	5.7	43.5	19.4	39.6	111.0	226.0
TOTAL	49.0	127.4	53.4	105.5	619.9	1187.6

Fig. 3. NaF-PET maximum intensity projection (MIP) of the same patient with RA as in **Fig. 2** showing the upper body (*A*) and lower body (*B*). ROVER software was used to segment focal areas of high bone formation in the joints. Metabolically active volume (MAV), maximum standardized uptake value (SUV_{max}), mean SUV (SUV_{mean}), partial volume-corrected SUV_{mean} ($pvcSUV_{mean}$), total calcium metabolism (TCM = MAV × SUV_{mean}), and partial volume-corrected TCM ($pvcTCM$ = MAV × $pvcSUV_{mean}$) were calculated and summed for each segmented region. The global pvcTCM for this patient was 1898.8. (*From* Saboury B, Morris MA, Nikpanah M, Werner TJ, Jones EC, Alavi A. Reinventing Molecular Imaging with Total-Body PET, Part II: Clinical Applications. *PET Clin.* 2020;15(4):463-475. https://doi.org/10.1016/j.cpet.2020.06.013.)

about staging disease activity, treatment options, long-term monitoring, and assessing treatment response.

OSTEOARTHRITIS AND DEGENERATIVE CONDITIONS

Osteoarthritis (OA) is a degenerative disease that is frequently associated with aging, obesity, and prior joint trauma or secondary to inflammatory arthropathies (such as RA and gout) or avascular necrosis.[52] This disorder represents one of the leading causes of impaired mobility in the elderly, and its prevalence is expected to increase as global life expectancy increases in the coming decades.[53] Although OA most commonly affects the spine, hip, knee, hands, and feet, it can potentially involve any synovial joint.[54] OA is characterized by systemic joint inflammation, exacerbated by proinflammatory changes that are related to aging as well as obesity,[55,56] and therefore this disease is an excellent candidate for imaging by PET/CT and PET/MR imaging.[57,58] In particular, FDG-

PET/CT, as a validated and effective method for detecting and quantifying synovitis due to OA, is ideally suited for assessing this very common joint disease.[57] Wandler and colleagues[59] found that uptake of FDG in the shoulder was associated with OA, bursitis, frozen shoulder, and rotator cuff injury. FDG uptake in the knee synovium of symptomatic OA patients has been found to be higher compared with that of control subjects.[60] In addition, FDG uptake in the knee has been associated with aging as well as clinical symptoms of OA unrelated to aging.[61,62]

In a recent study by Al-Zaghal et al.,[63] the role of FDG to assess degenerative changes in the knee was compared with that of NaF. CT segmentation was used to quantify uptake of FDG, as an inflammatory biomarker, and NaF, as a tracer that reflects subchondral bone formation and turnover. Soft tissue FDG uptake was correlated with aging, and uptake of both tracers was correlated with patient body mass index. In a study of 34 subjects, Khaw and colleagues[64] used NaF-PET/CT to evaluate bone turnover in the elbows, knees, hands, and feet. PET segmentation using ROVER software facilitated the quantification of the volumetric and metabolic parameters of NaF-avid regions, which were used to determine global disease activity (**Fig. 4**). Global PET parameters were found to correlate with subject body weight, suggesting that NaF-PET/CT is a sensitive method of determining the effects of biomechanical insufficiency on joint degeneration. To compare PET findings with those on MR imaging, Savic and colleagues[65] used NaF-PET/MR imaging to evaluate changes related to OA in 16 patients with varying levels of disease. The investigators found that bone turnover determined by NaF-PET was correlated with degenerative changes in cartilage assessed by MR imaging. In 2 separate studies examining the hip joint, Kobayashi and colleagues[66,67] demonstrated that NaF-PET can detect OA-related changes earlier than MR imaging and radiography and that NaF uptake correlated with pain severity. Other studies have suggested that NaF uptake in the knee can identify changes before manifestation of abnormal findings on MR imaging.[68,69]

In addition to OA involving the appendicular skeleton, degenerative processes affecting the spine such as disc degeneration and spondylosis also cause inflammatory reactions and increased bone turnover that are detected as abnormal sites on PET. In a study of 43 healthy subjects, FDG

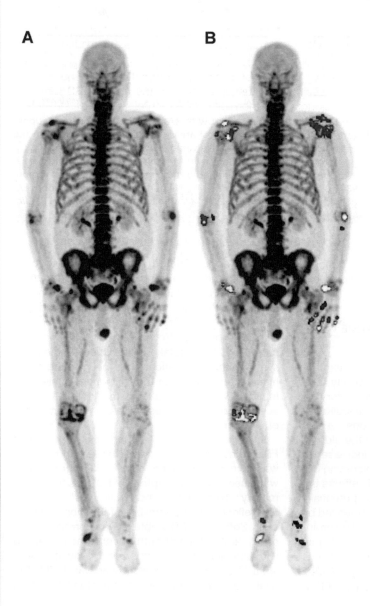

A   **B**

Fig. 4. NaF-PET maximum intensity projection (MIP) of a 72-year-old man showing tracer uptake in the joints before (*A*) and after (*B*) PET segmentation using an adaptive thresholding algorithm (ROVER software). Volumetric and metabolic parameters were automatically calculated and summed to determine total disease activity. The global partial volume-corrected total calcium metabolism for this patient was 338.6.

uptake in the thoracic and lumbar spine was found to correlate with body weight, likely representing early inflammatory changes related to degeneration.[70] A similar study demonstrated an association between body weight and increased NaF uptake in the cervical, thoracic, and lumbar spine.[71] Rosen and colleagues,[72] who analyzed FDG-PET/CT images from 150 subjects, found that degenerative disk and facet disease present on CT correlated with FDG uptake. PET imaging can also be used to diagnosis of other sources of back and neck pain that often cannot be visualized by other modalities and include radiculopathy, spondylitis, spondylodiscitis, and postsurgical complications and infections.[73-81] The findings from these studies suggest that PET has a potential role is assessing unknown causes of back pain in addition to detecting degenerative changes.

Because diseases affecting the skeleton can occur throughout the body, TB PET/CT is uniquely situated to diagnose and assess these common disorders. With the data available from TB PET/CT, future studies will be able to assess the total disease burden in the entire body rather than focusing on a subset of skeletal sites. FDG and NaF have been demonstrated to be feasible markers of degenerative processes, and global assessment of uptake of these tracers may have a future role in the determination of disease severity and response to therapy. PET tracers beyond FDG and NaF that target other pathologic processes involved in joint degeneration, such as angiogenesis or macrophage activity, potentially may reveal novel therapeutic targets.

FEVER OF UNKNOWN ORIGIN

The classic definition of fever of unknown origin (FUO) was first described in 1961 by Petersdorf and Beeson, who defined it as: "fever higher than 38.3°C (100.9°F) on several occasions, persisting without diagnosis for at least 3 weeks in spite of at least 1 week's investigation in hospital."[82,83] The definition of FUO was later revised and now includes cases in which 3 outpatient visits have not resulted in a diagnosis.[84] Causes of FUO include infection, inflammatory diseases, and malignancy, with more than 200 differential diagnoses being recognized.[84-86] Musculoskeletal infections are an important cause of FUO. Although conventional modalities, such as radiography, ultrasound, CT, and MR imaging are typically first-line options, by definition, in a majority of these cases no known musculoskeletal source of infection can be suspected and imaged specifically by these modalities. Therefore, a total-body imaging approach is of paramount importance and advantage in this setting. Moreover, equivocal findings on structural imaging modalities may warrant further evaluation with molecular modalities. In recent years, imaging with FDG-PET has become the study of choice in patients with FUO, which in the past was assessed by planar ^{67}Ga-citrate or ^{111}In-labeled white blood cell (^{111}In-WBC) scintigraphy.[84] In a prospective study that compared FDG-PET and ^{67}Ga-citrate imaging in 58 patients, FDG-PET successfully detected the source FUO in 35% of cases, whereas ^{67}Ga-citrate was helpful in 25% of the subjects examined.[87] Since all ^{67}Ga-citrate positive cases were also visualized by FDG-PET, the authors concluded that the latter could replace other techniques for this purpose. A prospective study of 23 patients found that FDG-PET had a sensitivity and specificity of 86% and 78% in determining the etiology of FUO, compared with 20% and 100% by ^{111}In-WBC scintigraphy.[88] A meta-analysis comparing the utility of FDG-PET/CT, FDG-PET, ^{67}Ga-citrate, and ^{111}In-WBC scintigraphy in evaluating FUO found that FDG-PET/CT had the highest sensitivity of 86% and the highest diagnostic yield of 58%.[89]

Among applications of FDG-PET/CT for the assessment of bone and soft tissue infections, that of diabetic foot has been studied the most over the past 2 decades.[90-96] The possibility of diabetic neuropathy resulting in neuropathic osteoarthropathy makes diagnosis of osteomyelitis in this setting difficult by traditional clinical and radiographic techniques.[93,97] In addition to its utility in assessing FUO with suspected osteomyelitis, FDG-PET/CT has also been shown to be able to differentiate osteomyelitis from neuropathic osteoarthropathy and soft tissue infections.[90-94,96] Besides FDG, other tracers such as NaF, ^{11}C-methionine, ^{68}Ga-citrate, ^{11}C-PK11195, and [124]I-FIAU have been used with PET imaging to detect and characterize osteomyelitis.[97,98] Alternatively, PET imaging with FDG-labeled autologous leukocytes has been reported to have a sensitivity of 83.3% and specificity of 100% in the diagnosis of osteomyelitis of the foot in patients with diabetes.[99,100] However, the role of the latter approach is very questionable and should not be considered for future clinical and research activities.

With increased validation for PET in the diagnosis of musculoskeletal infections and other differential causes of FUO, it becomes imperative that TB PET/CT be utilized in this domain. The nature of FUO often indicates that the underlying cause cannot be detected and localized by conventional means, and therefore only imaging of the entire body would be ideally suited to examine patients with this diagnosis. Although FDG will play a critical role in the setting of musculoskeletal infections, other PET tracers have shown some promise[49] and may also benefit from the unique capabilities of TB PET/CT.

OSTEOPENIA AND OSTEOPOROSIS

Osteoporosis, a disease characterized by increased osseous fragility and risk of fracture, has reached epidemic proportions. It affects 10 million Americans, resulting in 2 million fragility fractures per year.[101] Osteoporosis is known to be a systemic disease, and age-related bone fractures could happen in any part of the skeleton. Vertebral fractures are the most common fragility fractures. Of all the osteoporotic fractures, hip fractures have the most devastating consequences. The mortality rate in the year following a hip fracture is as high as 30%.[102,103] Fewer than half of patients who had a hip fracture regain their previous level of function.[103,104] Other skeletal sites for fragility fractures include the wrist, pelvis, humerus, ankle, and foot.

The current standard-of-care test for the assessment of metabolic bone diseases, including osteoporosis, involves the use of dual-energy X-ray absorptiometry (DXA).[105] DXA provides a measure of areal bone mineral density (BMD) at the hip or lumbar spine. Severity of the disease is typically quantified by the BMD T-score, which represents the standard deviations above or below the mean of a young healthy population. According to the World Health Organization (WHO) a T-score between −1.0 and −2.5 is defined as osteopenia and less than −2.5, osteoporosis.[106,107] DXA-derived BMD, a surrogate for bone quality, has many limitations, including the 2-dimensional nature and poor image quality. Also, the evaluation of BMD by DXA can be confounded by osteophytosis, resulting in erroneously high quantitative values.[108] As a consequence, over 50% of women who sustain a hip fracture have BMD T-scores greater than −2.5, that is, above the threshold for osteoporosis diagnosis and treatment.[109] Three-dimensional imaging modalities such as MR imaging[110,111] and CT[112–114] have been shown to have better performance in assessing metabolic bone diseases, particularly the bone strength, compared with DXA. However, the previously mentioned imaging modalities provide only structural information about bone. Because bone is a slow-changing organ at the macro and micro level, structural changes induced by age or disease or in response to therapy cannot be detected using conventional bone imaging modalities until several months to years have passed.

Limitations in current bone imaging modalities have resulted in the exploration of novel methodologies for better assessment of bone quality. In recent years, NaF-PET/CT has emerged as a modality that can quantify changes in bone health and integrity, including in benign conditions.[115–117] Affinity of NaF to bone involves the diffusion of the radiotracer through capillaries into the extracellular fluid of the bone and the exchange of the fluoride ion with a hydroxyl group in the hydroxyapatite mineral on bone surfaces during remodeling.[118] As a result, NaF uptake can be used as a measure of osteoblast activity and hence, bone turnover.

Quantification of both bone plasma clearance and bone uptake of NaF has been employed in the assessment of bone turnover. Both the Hawkins method and the Patlak Plot method are available to determine bone plasma clearance and require dynamic imaging. Alternatively, uptake is easily determined by a static scan and is often expressed as a standardized uptake value (SUV), which represents measured activity normalized to body weight and administered dose of tracer.[119] NaF uptake at the femoral neck was found to decrease with age and correlated with CT-derived BMD in a study that included 68 female subjects and 71 male subjects.[120] A study of 72 postmenopausal women classified as normal, osteopenic, or osteoporotic determined by DXA demonstrated decreased lumbar spine plasma clearance of NaF in osteoporotic subjects compared with both normal and osteopenic subjects.[121] Another study using NaF uptake showed similar findings of decreased bone turnover at the lumbar spine in patients diagnosed with osteoporosis compared with patients with a T-score above −2.5.[122] Besides osteoporosis, NaF-PET/CT has also shown utility in assessing metabolic bone diseases, including Paget disease of bone.[123,124]

Evaluating the effects of treatment for osteoporosis is a major potential application of NaF-PET/CT. Antiresorptive therapy with bisphosphonates such as alendronate and risedronate is known to rapidly decrease bone resorption, followed by a decrease in bone formation. Accordingly, treatment of 18 women with risedronate resulted in an 18% decrease in lumbar spine plasma clearance of NaF after 6 months.[125] Similarly, in a study of 24 postmenopausal women with glucocorticoid-induced osteoporosis treated with alendronate, NaF uptake decreased by 14% in the lumbar spine and by 24% in the femoral neck after 12 months.[122] Frost and colleagues[126] assessed changes after discontinuation of alendronate and risedronate on NaF uptake in the spine, hip, and femur of 20 postmenopausal women. The investigators found that although bone turnover in the spine remained suppressed, uptake in the hip and femur increased after 12 months in patients who had taken alendronate. Treatment with teriparatide results in an increase in both bone resorption and bone formation. In 18 postmenopausal women treated with teriparatide for 6 months, plasma clearance of NaF at the spine as well as uptake at the femoral shaft and pelvis were observed to increase significantly.[127]

In addition to the spine, pelvis, and femur, NaF-PET/CT has also been used to assess bone formation at the parietal bone, humerus, sternum, and tibia.[128,129] The calcaneus is a bone that presents with increased fracture risk due to osteoporosis. Although there have been several studies using MR imaging to assess calcaneal involvement in osteoporosis,[130,131] no studies have used NaF-PET/CT yet for this purpose. TB PET/CT would ensure that all areas of concern such as the calcaneus can be assessed for low bone turnover and therefore risk for fragility fracture. Using CT segmentation, metabolic activity in the whole skeleton can be quantified on PET (**Fig. 5**). Zirakchian Zadeh and colleagues[132] used this methodology to measure NaF uptake in the whole skeleton of patients with multiple myeloma to assess changes in bone turnover after therapy. A similar methodology could be applied to TB PET/CT images to determine systemic bone turnover in the entire skeleton in addition to the assessment of individual bones.

Due to scan time and radiation dose restrictions, conventional bone imaging modalities typically focus on one anatomic site for the assessment of metabolic bone diseases. Although osteoporosis and osteopenia are known to be systemic in nature bone quality at one skeletal site does not reflect the bone health at another site.[133] It is also known that bone metabolism is skeletal site dependent.[134] It is therefore useful to have the capability to assess the bone quality at all skeletal sites that are susceptible to osteoporotic fracture. TB PET/CT provides a unique opportunity to assess bone metabolism in the entire skeleton in one scan, and in the same phase of radiotracer distribution and uptake. In short, faster scan time, lower dose, and entire body coverage achievable by TB PET/CT could enable earlier detection of metabolic bone diseases before structural changes in bone could be detected by other imaging modalities.

SKELETAL MUSCLE

The human body consists of more than 500 skeletal muscles primarily responsible for contraction and relaxation and supporting other tissues of the skeletal system.[135] Skeletal muscles are distributed across the entire body, and play a crucial role in physical performance, glucose homeostasis and other metabolic functions.[136,137] Therefore, skeletal muscle loss or dysfunction can have severe health consequences, ranging from functional disability and institutionalization[138] to insulin resistance, metabolic syndrome, and obesity.[139] Sarcopenia, broadly defined as clinically significant loss of muscle mass and function, is now recognized as a hallmark of aging.[140] Besides aging, sarcopenia can also occur in other conditions such as autoimmune arthritis, heart failure, and cancer (commonly referred to as cachexia).[141] Sarcopenia presence increases both risk for hospitalization and cost of care during hospitalization,[142] with a two-fold or more increase in overall cost compared with those without the condition.[143] Sarcopenia is recognized as a muscle disease with an ICD-10-CM code that can be used to bill for care in some countries.[144]

To date, anatomic imaging methods, such as DXA, CT, MR imaging, and ultrasound have been used to assess surrogate measures of muscle mass and quality of relevance to sarcopenia.[140,145] Although muscle mass can be reliability estimated using these methods (via detailed image segmentation), there is no consensus on the metrics of muscle quality that best represent prognostic value.[146] For example, the degree of fat infiltration in muscle changes the latter's Hounsfield unit (HU) value in CT images and may provide an assessment of muscle quality; however, there is no standardization regarding CT thresholds to establish sarcopenia diagnosis across the different conditions.[146,147] Furthermore, these anatomic imaging modalities are unable to assess the molecular activity of skeletal muscle. On the other hand, PET has been shown to be sensitive to muscle blood flow, protein synthesis, and glucose metabolism, and has been used in the assessment of skeletal muscle with applications ranging from diabetes[148] and cancer-related dysfunction,[149,150] to exercise physiology.[151,152] Studies suggest that PET may provide information regarding skeletal muscle quality that is, unattainable from structural imaging modalities.[149,153] Commonly used PET radiotracers in the published literature to evaluate skeletal muscle are ^{15}O-water,[154-156] ^{11}C-methylmethionine[157] and FDG.[158-160] A number of other radiotracers targeting key pathologic processes

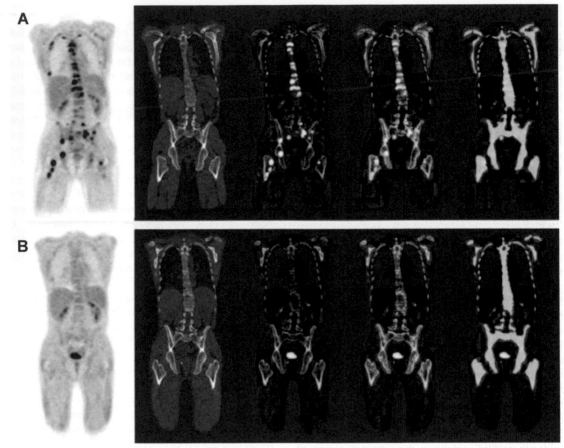

Fig. 5. Whole-body FDG-PET/CT images of a 60-year-old man with multiple myeloma. The cortical bone and bone marrow were segmented using a growing region algorithm based on Hounsfield units, followed by smoothing and closing algorithms (OsiriX software; Pixmeo SARL, Bernex, Switzerland). The global SUV$_{mean}$, which represents the whole bone marrow activity, before initiating treatment (*A*) was 2.02 and decreased to 1.10 after finishing the course of treatment (*B*). (*From* Raynor WY, Al-Zaghal A, Zadeh MZ, Seraj SM, Alavi A. Metastatic Seeding Attacks Bone Marrow, Not Bone: Rectifying Ongoing Misconceptions. *PET Clin.* 2019;14(1):135-144; with permission.)

underlying sarcopenia are under development or are being explored in early-stage human studies.[161-163]

Currently, PET/CT has a limited role in the clinical assessment of sarcopenia. However, TB PET/CT could overcome shortcomings of the existing methods. First, sarcopenia is not limited to just a few muscles,[164,165] meaning that no single muscle or muscle group is a robust representative of the systemic burden of sarcopenia.[166] TB PET/CT enables the assessment of the entire skeletal muscle in the body in the same phases of radiotracer distribution and uptake, and can therefore contribute toward a more comprehensive and global analysis of sarcopenia (**Fig. 6**). Second, TB PET/CT could play a critical role in the longitudinal monitoring of sarcopenia, as the cumulative doses will be significantly lower and

image acquisition is relatively fast. Third, the combination of higher spatial resolution and geometric sensitivity of TB PET/CT compared with current scanners will enable delineating activity of the different muscle groups to better understand sarcopenia pathogenesis,[167] and heterogeneity of radiotracer uptake,[152,168] which may provide insights for intervention. Lastly, TB PET/CT measures are quantitative and therefore provide reliable and reproducible data compared with those from physical examination and structural imaging.

In summary TB PET/CT measures may usher in several new biomarkers of sarcopenia that will be helpful both for understanding the underlying pathogenesis of the condition and for the evaluation of and monitoring of interventions and therapy.

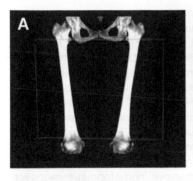
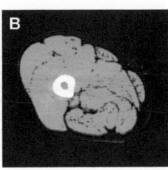

Fig. 6. Maximum intensity projection (MIP) of the CT image (*A*) showing a methodology used to segment muscle. Two lines (horizontal parallel green *lines*) corresponding to 5 cm above the intercondylar notch and 5 cm below the greater trochanter were manually delineated according to predetermined anatomic criteria. A growing region algorithm with lower and upper thresholds of 1 and 150 Hounsfield units, respectively, was used to segment the muscle (OsiriX software) (*B*). Applying this methodology to 71 subjects, thigh muscle volume was found to decrease with age, and uptake of FDG uptake was found to be significantly higher on the right side compared with the left. (*From* Kothekar E, Yellanki D, Borja AJ, et al. 18F-FDG-PET/CT in measuring volume and global metabolic activity of thigh muscles: a novel CT-based tissue segmentation methodology. *Nucl Med Commun.* 2020;41(2):162-168.; with permission.)

NEOPLASTIC MUSCULOSKELETAL DISEASES

Bone and soft tissue cancers of the musculoskeletal system are relatively uncommon but have significant impact on quality of life and are commonly associated with high morbidity and mortality in the affected population. These malignancies commonly metastasize to distant organs, which may not be successfully detected and monitored by conventional imaging techniques. Whole-body PET in this setting has the advantage of imaging both the primary lesion and the metastatic sites with a single image acquisition procedure.[169–171] Hybrid imaging with PET/MR imaging provides certain advantages over PET/CT, as PET/MR imaging allows higher reading confidence compared with PET/CT.

Most malignant tumors of the musculoskeletal system demonstrate increased FDG uptake due to their high glycolytic activity compared with the surrounding normal tissue structures. FDG-PET not only allows differentiation of soft tissue and osseous lesions that cannot be fully defined by structural imaging modalities alone, but is also a key component for staging/restaging of the disease and treatment planning (**Fig. 7**).[171–173] Erfanian and colleagues[172] reported a higher accuracy for PET/MR imaging compared with MR imaging alone in delineating soft tissue malignancies. In a recent study by Cleary and colleagues,[171] who examined patients with osteosarcoma, 81% were noted to have suspicious popliteal lymph nodes on the initial MR imaging. However, in contrast to MR imaging, only one node was presumed to be metastatic based on its increased metabolic activity on PET/CT, a finding that was further confirmed in the 12 months follow-up assessment.[171]

PET is commonly used for follow-up of aggressive bone and soft tissue tumors to evaluate therapy response and is often superior to structural imaging alone for this purpose. In fact, molecular imaging is the mainstay of personalized therapeutic approaches in musculoskeletal cancer treatment. A recent study reported by Lee and colleagues[174] described the impact of PET/CT in managing 73 patients with stage II osteosarcomas of the extremities who were treated with 2 cycles of neoadjuvant chemotherapy, surgical resection, and adjuvant chemotherapy. These patients underwent PET/CT before treatment (PET0), after 1 cycle of chemotherapy (PET1), and following the completion of neoadjuvant chemotherapy (PET2). They noted that evidence for response to treatment after the first cycle of preoperative chemotherapy was best predicted by PET.[174] This research demonstrated that PET was a powerful modality for early response monitoring by providing the opportunity of early modification of timing of local control. SUV_{max} on PET2, the delta (percentage change) of SUV_{max} between PET0 and PET1, and between PET0 and PET2 have been proposed by these researchers as the most accurate predictors of poor response and development of future metastatic events. Based on the data generated, patients with SUV of more than 5.9 on PET2 had a poor event-free survival compared with the others.[174] The features provided by PET have been further augmented by the incorporation of artificial intelligence, texture analysis, and machine learning into image interpretation.[175,176]

Despite all the advantages associated with this modality, some studies have warned about false-negative results with PET imaging. A retrospective study on 24 histopathologically confirmed cases of Ewing sarcoma who underwent MR imaging and

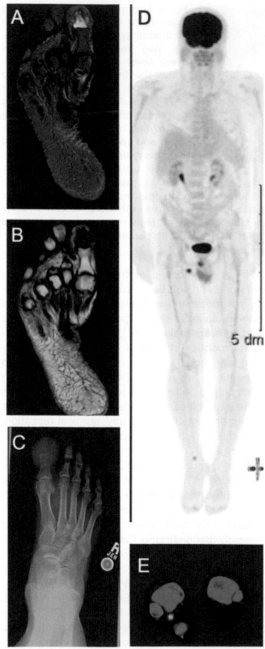

FDG-PET/CT within a 4-week interval demonstrated that some of the osseous metastases detected by MR imaging may not show increased metabolic activity on FDG-PET/CT, rendering them as false-negative results.[177] Therefore, it has been advised that caution should be exercised in interpreting FDG-PET/CT for the detection of skeletal metastases in Ewing sarcoma. Likely, the potential source of such false-negative results is due to the presence of low contrast resolution between bone metastases and the background hematopoietic marrow, hematopoietic reconversion due to recent chemotherapy, and/or due to the small size of the lesions that are not detectable by PET. In contrast, MR imaging may not be significantly affected by these factors.[177] We believe these findings emphasize the importance of integrated PET/MR imaging in these settings by combining the advantages of molecular imaging with those of MR imaging by providing structural details.[5,178,179] Also, it has been widely accepted that noncontrast chest CT is the modality of choice for the evaluation of pulmonary metastases of osteosarcoma and Ewing sarcoma due to suboptimal sensitivity of PET/CT in detecting lung nodules that are smaller than 2 cm and are located in the lower lobes (due to technical limitations of respiratory motion gating and misregistration of PET and CT scans).[180–182] However, TB PET/CT imaging may overcome some of these shortcomings by acquiring images over a shorter period of time and at later time points (at 3–4 hours).

DISCUSSION

As PET-based techniques become increasingly validated, their application in MSDs, such as arthritis, infection, osteoporosis, sarcopenia, and soft tissue and osseous neoplastic pathologies, will continue to grow. Many of these disorders are difficult to diagnose, stage, and evaluate over time with conventional imaging modalities. FDG and NaF among other tracers have the potential to reveal molecular processes before evidence of disease is present clinically or structurally on conventional imaging techniques. Although reported studies in the literature are based on examining individual joints, bones, and muscles, TB PET/CT will allow for a comprehensive and systematic evaluation of the MSDs that cannot easily be localized to one specific region. The introduction of TB PET/CT in this domain may allow for improved detection of many abnormalities throughout the body, accurate monitoring, and a better understanding of the effects of the current and future therapeutic intervention.

Fig. 7. A 58-year-old man with toe pain was evaluated with MR imaging of the foot. A marrow-replacing lesion of the first distal phalanx with T_2 hyper-signal (*A*) and T_1 hypo-signal intensity (*B*) was identified, the tissue sampling of which was consistent with osteosarcoma. After surgical resection and several courses of chemotherapy (*C*), the patient returned for restaging with whole-body FDG-PET/CT. A hypermetabolic right ankle (Kager fat pad, *D*, *E*) and inguinal lymph nodes (*D*) with respective SUV_{max} of 4.4 and 10.4 were identified, in keeping with metastatic lymphadenopathy.

However, before TB PET/CT can be widely adopted, certain aspects of this modality require further consideration and optimization. Regarding chronic conditions as well as pediatric applications, ionizing radiation dose may be a concern, and a cost-to-benefit analysis would be warranted to determine optimal scan frequency. Furthermore, depending on the kinetics of the radiotracer, the preferred scanning start time and duration may be disease-specific, causing difficulty in visualizing unrelated findings (such as evaluating cardiovascular disease in RA). Lastly, reconstruction parameters will also depend on the structure of interest. For example, imaging of small joints in RA would warrant parameters that produce high resolution, but high variance, while imaging of large muscles would warrant parameters that produce low variance, but lower resolution. Future research regarding the tradeoffs involved in each of these considerations would support the efficient use of TB PET/CT and facilitate wider applications of this new but very promising technology.

ACKNOWLEDGMENTS

The authors acknowledge support by the National Institutes of Health under award number R01AR076088.

DISCLOSURE

UC Davis has a revenue-sharing agreement with United Imaging Healthcare. The authors have no other matters to disclose.

CONFLICT OF INTEREST

The authors have declared no conflicts of interest.

REFERENCES

1. Briggs AM, Cross MJ, Hoy DG, et al. Musculoskeletal health conditions represent a global threat to healthy aging: a report for the 2015 World Health Organization World report on ageing and health. Gerontologist 2016;56(Suppl 2):S243–55.
2. Murray CJ, Barber RM, Foreman KJ, et al. Global, regional, and national disability-adjusted life years (DALYs) for 306 diseases and injuries and healthy life expectancy (HALE) for 188 countries, 1990–2013: quantifying the epidemiological transition. Lancet 2015;386(10009):2145–91.
3. March L, Smith EU, Hoy DG, et al. Burden of disability due to musculoskeletal (MSK) disorders. Best Pract Res Clin Rheumatol 2014;28(3):353–66.
4. Put S, Westhovens R, Lahoutte T, et al. Molecular imaging of rheumatoid arthritis: emerging markers, tools, and techniques. Arthritis Res Ther 2014; 16(2):208.
5. Gholamrezanezhad A, Guermazi A, Salavati A, et al. Evolving role of PET-computed tomography and PET-MR imaging in assessment of musculoskeletal disorders and its potential revolutionary impact on day-to-day practice of related disciplines. PET Clin 2018;13(4):xiii–xiv.
6. Cheung, T.T., McInnes, I.B. Future therapeutic targets in rheumatoid arthritis?. Semin Immunopathol 39, 487-500 (2017). https://doi.org/10.1007/s00281-017-0623-3
7. Tak PP. Analyzing synovial tissue samples. What can we learn about early rheumatoid arthritis, the heterogeneity of the disease, and the effects of treatment? J Rheumatol 2005;32(Suppl 72):25–6.
8. Singh JA, Hossain A, Tanjong Ghogomu E, et al. Biologics or tofacitinib for people with rheumatoid arthritis unsuccessfully treated with biologics: a systematic review and network meta-analysis. Cochrane Database Syst Rev 2017;3(3):CD012591.
9. Singh JA, Saag KG, Bridges SL Jr, et al. 2015 American College of Rheumatology guideline for the treatment of rheumatoid arthritis. Arthritis Rheumatol 2016;68(1):1–26.
10. Scott DL. Biologics-based therapy for the treatment of rheumatoid arthritis. Clin Pharmacol Ther 2012;91(1):30–43.
11. Forien M, Ottaviani S. Ultrasound and follow-up of rheumatoid arthritis. Joint Bone Spine 2017;84(5):531–6.
12. Kennish L, Labitigan M, Budoff S, et al. Utility of the new rheumatoid arthritis 2010 ACR/EULAR classification criteria in routine clinical care. BMJ Open 2012;2(5):e001117.
13. Mountz JM, Alavi A, Mountz JD. Emerging optical and nuclear medicine imaging methods in rheumatoid arthritis. Nat Rev Rheumatol 2012;8(12):719–28.
14. Serban O, Fodor D, Papp I, et al. Reasons for discordances between ultrasonography and magnetic resonance imaging in the evaluation of the ankle, hindfoot and heel of the patients with rheumatoid arthritis. Med Ultrason 2019;21(4):405–13.
15. Liu H, Huang C, Chen S, et al. Value of contrast-enhanced ultrasound for detection of synovial vascularity in experimental rheumatoid arthritis: an exploratory study. J Int Med Res 2019;47(11):5740–51.
16. Zhao C, Zhang R, Luo Y, et al. Multimodal VEGF-targeted contrast-enhanced ultrasound and photoacoustic imaging of rats with inflammatory arthritis: using dye-VEGF-antibody-loaded microbubbles. Ultrasound Med Biol 2020;46(9):2400–11.
17. Bennett JL, Wood A, Smith N, et al. Can quantitative MRI be used in the clinical setting to quantify the impact of intra-articular glucocorticoid injection

on synovial disease activity in juvenile idiopathic arthritis? Pediatr Rheumatol Online J 2019;17(1): 74.

18. Kayama R, Fukuda T, Ogiwara S, et al. Quantitative analysis of therapeutic response in psoriatic arthritis of digital joints with Dual-energy CT iodine maps. Sci Rep 2020;10(1):1225.

19. Fosse P, Kaiser MJ, Namur G, et al. (18)F- FDG PET/CT joint assessment of early therapeutic response in rheumatoid arthritis patients treated with rituximab. Eur J hybrid Imaging 2018;2(1):6.

20. Kubota K, Yamashita H, Mimori A. Clinical value of FDG-PET/CT for the evaluation of rheumatic diseases: rheumatoid arthritis, polymyalgia rheumatica, and relapsing polychondritis. Semin Nucl Med 2017;47(4):408–24.

21. Raynor W, Houshmand S, Gholami S, et al. Evolving role of molecular imaging with (18)F-sodium fluoride PET as a biomarker for calcium metabolism. Curr Osteoporos Rep 2016;14(4):115–25.

22. Chaudhari AJ, Ferrero A, Godinez F, et al. High-resolution 18F-FDG PET/CT for assessing disease activity in rheumatoid and psoriatic arthritis: findings of a prospective pilot study. Br J Radiol 2016; 89(1063):20160138.

23. Yamashita H, Kubota K, Mimori A. Clinical value of whole-body PET/CT in patients with active rheumatic diseases. Arthritis Res Ther 2014;16(5):423.

24. Kubota K, Ito K, Morooka M, et al. FDG PET for rheumatoid arthritis: basic considerations and whole-body PET/CT. Ann N Y Acad Sci 2011; 1228:29–38.

25. Chaudhari AJ, Bowen SL, Burkett GW, et al. High-resolution (18)F-FDG PET with MRI for monitoring response to treatment in rheumatoid arthritis. Eur J Nucl Med Mol Imaging 2010;37(5):1047.

26. Beckers C, Ribbens C, André B, et al. Assessment of disease activity in rheumatoid arthritis with 18F-FDG PET. J Nucl Med 2004;45(6):956–64.

27. Yun M, Kim W, Adam LE, et al. F-18 FDG uptake in a patient with psoriatic arthritis: imaging correlation with patient symptoms. Clin Nucl Med 2001;26(8): 692–3.

28. Polisson RP, Schoenberg OI, Fischman A, et al. Use of magnetic resonance imaging and positron emission tomography in the assessment of synovial volume and glucose metabolism in patients with rheumatoid arthritis. Arthritis Rheum 1995;38(6): 819–25.

29. Raynor WY, Jonnakuti VS, Zirakchian Zadeh M, et al. Comparison of methods of quantifying global synovial metabolic activity with FDG-PET/CT in rheumatoid arthritis. Int J Rheum Dis 2019;22(12): 2191–8.

30. Mupparapu M, Oak S, Chang YC, et al. Conventional and functional imaging in the evaluation of

temporomandibular joint rheumatoid arthritis: a systematic review. Quintessence Int 2019;50(9): 742–53.

31. Bhattarai A, Nakajima T, Sapkota S, et al. Diagnostic value of 18F-fluorodeoxyglucose uptake parameters to differentiate rheumatoid arthritis from other types of arthritis. Medicine (Baltimore) 2017; 96(25):e7130.

32. Jonnakuti VS, Raynor WY, Taratuta E, et al. A novel method to assess subchondral bone formation using [18F]NaF-PET in the evaluation of knee degeneration. Nucl Med Commun 2018;39(5):451–6.

33. Narayan N, Owen DR, Taylor PC. Advances in positron emission tomography for the imaging of rheumatoid arthritis. Rheumatology (Oxford) 2017; 56(11):1837–46.

34. Bastida C, Ruíz V, Pascal M, et al. Is there potential for therapeutic drug monitoring of biologic agents in rheumatoid arthritis? Br J Clin Pharmacol 2017; 83(5):962–75.

35. Woodrick RS, Ruderman EM. Safety of biologic therapy in rheumatoid arthritis. Nat Rev Rheumatol 2011;7(11):639–52.

36. Van Nies J, Krabben A, Schoones J, et al. What is the evidence for the presence of a therapeutic window of opportunity in rheumatoid arthritis? A systematic literature review. Ann Rheum Dis 2014; 73(5):861–70.

37. Zeman MN, Scott PJ. Current imaging strategies in rheumatoid arthritis. Am J Nucl Med Mol Imaging 2012;2(2):174–220.

38. Keen HI, Emery P. How should we manage early rheumatoid arthritis? From imaging to intervention. Curr Opin Rheumatol 2005;17(3):280–5.

39. Wunder A, Straub RH, Gay S, et al. Molecular imaging: novel tools in visualizing rheumatoid arthritis. Rheumatology (Oxford) 2005;44(11): 1341–9.

40. Favalli EG, Sinigaglia L, Becciolini A, et al. Two-year persistence of golimumab as second-line biologic agent in rheumatoid arthritis as compared to other subcutaneous tumor necrosis factor inhibitors: real-life data from the LORHEN registry. Int J Rheum Dis 2018;21(2):422–30.

41. Emery P, Gottenberg JE, Rubbert-Roth A, et al. Rituximab versus an alternative TNF inhibitor in patients with rheumatoid arthritis who failed to respond to a single previous TNF inhibitor: SWITCH-RA, a global, observational, comparative effectiveness study. Ann Rheum Dis 2015;74(6): 979–84.

42. Rose S, Sheth NH, Baker JF, et al. A comparison of vascular inflammation in psoriasis, rheumatoid arthritis, and healthy subjects by FDG-PET/CT: a pilot study. Am J Cardiovasc Dis 2013;3(4):273–8.

43. Humphreys J, Hyrich K, Symmons D. What is the impact of biologic therapies on common

co-morbidities in patients with rheumatoid arthritis? Arthritis Res Ther 2016;18(1):282.

44. Richards JS, Dowell SM, Quinones ME, et al. How to use biologic agents in patients with rheumatoid arthritis who have comorbid disease. BMJ 2015; 351:h3658.

45. Lahiri M, Dixon WG. Risk of infection with biologic antirheumatic therapies in patients with rheumatoid arthritis. Best Pract Res Clin Rheumatol 2015;29(2): 290–305.

46. Veale DJ, Fearon U. The pathogenesis of psoriatic arthritis. Lancet 2018;391(10136):2273–84.

47. Konisti S, Kiriakidis S, Paleolog EM. Hypoxia—a key regulator of angiogenesis and inflammation in rheumatoid arthritis. Nat Rev Rheumatol 2012; 8(3):153.

48. McInnes IB, Schett G. The pathogenesis of rheumatoid arthritis. N Engl J Med 2011;365(23): 2205–19.

49. Gholamrezanezhad A, Basques K, Batouli A, et al. Non-oncologic applications of PET/CT and PET/MR in musculoskeletal, orthopedic, and rheumatologic imaging: general considerations, techniques, and radiopharmaceuticals. J Nucl Med Technol 2017; 46(1). https://doi.org/10.2967/jnmt.117.198663.

50. Yaqub M, Verweij NJ, Pieplenbosch S, et al. Quantitative assessment of arthritis activity in rheumatoid arthritis patients using [11C] DPA-713 positron emission tomography. Int J Mol Sci 2020; 21(9):3137.

51. Kogan F, Broski SM, Yoon D, et al. Applications of PET-MRI in musculoskeletal disease. J Magn Reson Imaging 2018;48(1):27–47.

52. Fransen M, Simic M, Harmer AR. Determinants of MSK health and disability: lifestyle determinants of symptomatic osteoarthritis. Best Pract Res Clin Rheumatol 2014;28(3):435–60.

53. Nguyen US, Zhang Y, Zhu Y, et al. Increasing prevalence of knee pain and symptomatic knee osteoarthritis: survey and cohort data. Ann Intern Med 2011;155(11):725–32.

54. O'Neill TW, McCabe PS, McBeth J. Update on the epidemiology, risk factors and disease outcomes of osteoarthritis. Best Pract Res Clin Rheumatol 2018;32(2):312–26.

55. Greene MA, Loeser RF. Aging-related inflammation in osteoarthritis. Osteoarthritis Cartilage 2015; 23(11):1966–71.

56. Berenbaum F, Eymard F, Houard X. Osteoarthritis, inflammation and obesity. Curr Opin Rheumatol 2013;25(1):114–8.

57. Hayashi D, Roemer FW, Guermazi A. Imaging of osteoarthritis-recent research developments and future perspective. Br J Radiol 2018;91(1085): 20170349.

58. Al-Zaghal A, Raynor W, Khosravi M, et al. Applications of PET imaging in the evaluation of

59. Wandler E, Kramer EL, Sherman O, et al. Diffuse FDG shoulder uptake on PET is associated with clinical findings of osteoarthritis. AJR Am J Roentgenol 2005;185(3):797–803.

60. Parsons MA, Moghbel M, Saboury B, et al. Increased 18F-FDG uptake suggests synovial inflammatory reaction with osteoarthritis: preliminary in-vivo results in humans. Nucl Med Commun 2015;36(12):1215–9.

61. Saboury B, Parsons MA, Moghbel M, et al. Quantification of aging effects upon global knee inflammation by 18F-FDG-PET. Nucl Med Commun 2016;37(3):254–8.

62. Hong YH, Kong EJ. (18F)Fluoro-deoxy-D-glucose uptake of knee joints in the aspect of age-related osteoarthritis: a case-control study. BMC Musculoskelet Disord 2013;14:141.

63. Al-Zaghal A, Yellanki DP, Ayubcha C, et al. CT-based tissue segmentation to assess knee joint inflammation and reactive bone formation assessed by (18)F-FDG and (18)F-NaF PET/CT: effects of age and BMI. Hell J Nucl Med 2018; 21(2):102–7.

64. Khaw TH, Raynor WY, Borja AJ, et al. Assessing the effects of body weight on subchondral bone formation with quantitative (18)F-sodium fluoride PET. Ann Nucl Med 2020;34(8):559–64.

65. Savic D, Pedoia V, Seo Y, et al. Imaging bone-cartilage interactions in osteoarthritis using [(18) F]-NaF PET-MRI. Mol Imaging 2016;15:1–12.

66. Kobayashi N, Inaba Y, Tateishi U, et al. Comparison of 18F-fluoride positron emission tomography and magnetic resonance imaging in evaluating early-stage osteoarthritis of the hip. Nucl Med Commun 2015;36(1):84–9.

67. Kobayashi N, Inaba Y, Tateishi U, et al. New application of 18F-fluoride PET for the detection of bone remodeling in early-stage osteoarthritis of the hip. Clin Nucl Med 2013;38(10):e379–83.

68. Kogan F, Fan AP, McWalter EJ, et al. PET/MRI of metabolic activity in osteoarthritis: a feasibility study. J Magn Reson Imaging 2017;45(6):1736–45.

69. Draper CE, Quon A, Fredericson M, et al. Comparison of MRI and (1)(8)F-NaF PET/CT in patients with patellofemoral pain. J Magn Reson Imaging 2012; 36(4):928–32.

70. Ayubcha C, Zadeh MZ, Rajapakse CS, et al. Effects of age and weight on the metabolic activities of the cervical, thoracic and lumbar spines as measured by fluorine-18 fluorodeoxyglucose-positron emission tomography in healthy males. Hell J Nucl Med 2018;21(1):2–6.

71. Ayubcha C, Zirakchian Zadeh M, Stochkendahl MJ, et al. Quantitative evaluation of

normal spinal osseous metabolism with 18F-NaF PET/CT. Nucl Med Commun 2018;39(10):945–50.

72. Rosen RS, Fayad L, Wahl RL. Increased 18F-FDG uptake in degenerative disease of the spine: characterization with 18F-FDG PET/CT. J Nucl Med 2006;47(8):1274–80.

73. Peters M, Willems P, Weijers R, et al. Pseudarthrosis after lumbar spinal fusion: the role of (1)(8)F-fluoride PET/CT. Eur J Nucl Med Mol Imaging 2015;42(12):1891–8.

74. Seifen T, Rodrigues M, Rettenbacher L, et al. The value of (18)F-fluoride PET/CT in the assessment of screw loosening in patients after intervertebral fusion stabilization. Eur J Nucl Med Mol Imaging 2015;42(2):272–7.

75. Nakahara M, Ito M, Hattori N, et al. 18F-FDG-PET/CT better localizes active spinal infection than MRI for successful minimally invasive surgery. Acta Radiol 2015;56(7):829–36.

76. Inanami H, Oshima Y, Iwahori T, et al. Role of 18F-fluoro-D-deoxyglucose PET/CT in diagnosing surgical site infection after spine surgery with instrumentation. Spine (Phila Pa 1976) 2015;40(2):109–13.

77. Byrnes TJ, Xie W, Al-Mukhailed O, et al. Evaluation of neck pain with (18)F-NaF PET/CT. Nucl Med Commun 2014;35(3):298–302.

78. Quon A, Dodd R, Iagaru A, et al. Initial investigation of (1)(8)F-NaF PET/CT for identification of vertebral sites amenable to surgical revision after spinal fusion surgery. Eur J Nucl Med Mol Imaging 2012;39(11):1737–44.

79. Seifen T, Rettenbacher L, Thaler C, et al. Prolonged back pain attributed to suspected spondylodiscitis. The value of (1)(8)F-FDG PET/CT imaging in the diagnostic work-up of patients. Nuklearmedizin 2012;51(5):194–200.

80. Gamie S, El-Maghraby T. The role of PET/CT in evaluation of facet and disc abnormalities in patients with low back pain using (18)F-Fluoride. Nucl Med Rev Cent East Eur 2008;11(1):17–21.

81. Gratz S, Dorner J, Fischer U, et al. 18F-FDG hybrid PET in patients with suspected spondylitis. Eur J Nucl Med Mol Imaging 2002;29(4):516–24.

82. Petersdorf RG, Beeson PB. Fever of unexplained origin: report on 100 cases. Medicine (Baltimore) 1961;40:1–30.

83. Wright WF, Auwaerter PG. Fever and fever of unknown origin: review, recent advances, and lingering dogma. Open Forum Infect Dis 2020;7(5):ofaa132.

84. Hess S. FDG-PET/CT in fever of unknown origin, bacteremia, and febrile neutropenia. PET Clin 2020;15(2):175–85.

85. Al-Zaghal A, Raynor WY, Seraj SM, et al. FDG-PET imaging to detect and characterize underlying causes of fever of unknown origin: an unavoidable path for the foreseeable future. Eur J Nucl Med Mol Imaging 2019;46(1):2–7.

86. Mulders-Manders C, Simon A, Bleeker-Rovers C. Fever of unknown origin. Clin Med (Lond) 2015;15(3):280–4.

87. Blockmans D, Knockaert D, Maes A, et al. Clinical value of [(18)F]fluoro-deoxyglucose positron emission tomography for patients with fever of unknown origin. Clin Infect Dis 2001;32(2):191–6.

88. Seshadri N, Sonoda LI, Lever AM, et al. Superiority of 18F-FDG PET compared to 111In-labelled leucocyte scintigraphy in the evaluation of fever of unknown origin. J Infect 2012;65(1):71–9.

89. Takeuchi M, Dahabreh IJ, Nihashi T, et al. Nuclear imaging for classic fever of unknown origin: meta-analysis. J Nucl Med 2016;57(12):1913–9.

90. Kagna O, Srour S, Melamed E, et al. FDG PET/CT imaging in the diagnosis of osteomyelitis in the diabetic foot. Eur J Nucl Med Mol Imaging 2012;39(10):1545–50.

91. Nawaz A, Torigian DA, Siegelman ES, et al. Diagnostic performance of FDG-PET, MRI, and plain film radiography (PFR) for the diagnosis of osteomyelitis in the diabetic foot. Mol Imaging Biol 2010;12(3):335–42.

92. Schwegler B, Stumpe KD, Weishaupt D, et al. Unsuspected osteomyelitis is frequent in persistent diabetic foot ulcer and better diagnosed by MRI than by 18F-FDG PET or 99mTc-MOAB. J Intern Med 2008;263(1):99–106.

93. Basu S, Chryssikos T, Houseni M, et al. Potential role of FDG PET in the setting of diabetic neuro-osteoarthropathy: can it differentiate uncomplicated Charcot's neuroarthropathy from osteomyelitis and soft-tissue infection? Nucl Med Commun 2007;28(6):465–72.

94. Keidar Z, Militianu D, Melamed E, et al. The diabetic foot: initial experience with 18F-FDG PET/CT. J Nucl Med 2005;46(3):444–9.

95. Zhuang H, Duarte PS, Pourdehand M, et al. Exclusion of chronic osteomyelitis with F-18 fluorodeoxyglucose positron emission tomographic imaging. Clin Nucl Med 2000;25(4):281–4.

96. Kalicke T, Schmitz A, Risse JH, et al. Fluorine-18 fluorodeoxyglucose PET in infectious bone diseases: results of histologically confirmed cases. Eur J Nucl Med 2000;27(5):524–8.

97. Gholamrezanezhad A, Basques K, Batouli A, et al. Clinical nononcologic applications of PET/CT and PET/MRI in musculoskeletal, orthopedic, and rheumatologic imaging. AJR Am J Roentgenol 2018;210(6):W245–63.

98. Diaz LA Jr, Foss CA, Thornton K, et al. Imaging of musculoskeletal bacterial infections by [124I]FIAU-PET/CT. PLoS One 2007;2(10):e1007.

99. Dumarey N. Imaging with FDG labeled leukocytes: is it clinically useful? Q J Nucl Med Mol Imaging 2009;53(1):89–94.

100. Dumarey N, Egrise D, Blocklet D, et al. Imaging infection with 18F-FDG-labeled leukocyte PET/CT: initial experience in 21 patients. J Nucl Med 2006;47(4):625–32.

101. Burge R, Dawson-Hughes B, Solomon DH, et al. Incidence and economic burden of osteoporosis-related fractures in the United States, 2005-2025. J Bone Miner Res 2007;22(3):465–75.

102. Brauer CA, Coca-Perraillon M, Cutler DM, et al. Incidence and mortality of hip fractures in the United States. JAMA 2009;302(14):1573–9.

103. Leibson CL, Tosteson AN, Gabriel SE, et al. Mortality, disability, and nursing home use for persons with and without hip fracture: a population-based study. J Am Geriatr Soc 2002;50(10):1644–50.

104. Keene GS, Parker MJ, Pryor GA. Mortality and morbidity after hip fractures. BMJ 1993; 307(6914):1248–50.

105. de Bakker CMJ, Tseng WJ, Li Y, et al. Clinical evaluation of bone strength and fracture risk. Curr Osteoporos Rep 2017;15(1):32–42.

106. Messina C, Maffi G, Vitale JA, et al. Diagnostic imaging of osteoporosis and sarcopenia: a narrative review. Quant Imaging Med Surg 2018;8(1):86–99.

107. Assessment of fracture risk and its application to screening for postmenopausal osteoporosis. Report of a WHO Study Group. World Health Organ Tech Rep Ser 1994;843:1–129.

108. Kinoshita H, Tamaki T, Hashimoto T, et al. Factors influencing lumbar spine bone mineral density assessment by dual-energy X-ray absorptiometry: comparison with lumbar spinal radiogram. J Orthop Sci 1998;3(1):3–9.

109. Wainwright SA, Marshall LM, Ensrud KE, et al. Hip fracture in women without osteoporosis. J Clin Endocrinol Metab 2005;90(5):2787–93.

110. Rajapakse CS, Chang G. Micro-finite element analysis of the proximal femur on the basis of high-resolution magnetic resonance images. Curr Osteoporos Rep 2018;16(6):657–64.

111. Wehrli FW. Structural and functional assessment of trabecular and cortical bone by micro magnetic resonance imaging. J Magn Reson Imaging 2007; 25(2):390–409.

112. Keaveny TM, McClung MR, Genant HK, et al. Femoral and vertebral strength improvements in postmenopausal women with osteoporosis treated with denosumab. J Bone Miner Res 2014;29(1): 158–65.

113. Nishiyama KK, Ito M, Harada A, et al. Classification of women with and without hip fracture based on quantitative computed tomography and finite element analysis. Osteoporos Int 2014;25(2): 619–26.

114. Keyak JH, Sigurdsson S, Karlsdottir GS, et al. Effect of finite element model loading condition on fracture risk assessment in men and women: the AGES-Reykjavik study. Bone 2013;57(1):18–29.

115. Austin AG, Raynor WY, Reilly CC, et al. Evolving role of MR imaging and PET in assessing osteoporosis. PET Clin 2019;14(1):31–41.

116. Reilly CC, Raynor WY, Hong AL, et al. Diagnosis and monitoring of osteoporosis with (18)F-sodium fluoride PET: an unavoidable path for the foreseeable future. Semin Nucl Med 2018;48(6):535–40.

117. Jadvar H, Desai B, Conti PS. Sodium 18F-fluoride PET/CT of bone, joint, and other disorders. Semin Nucl Med 2015;45(1):58–65.

118. Costeas A, Woodard HQ, Laughlin JS. Depletion of 18F from blood flowing through bone. J Nucl Med 1970;11(1):43–5.

119. Blake GM, Siddique M, Frost ML, et al. Imaging of site specific bone turnover in osteoporosis using positron emission tomography. Curr Osteoporos Rep 2014;12(4):475–85.

120. Rhodes S, Batzdorf A, Sorci O, et al. Assessment of femoral neck bone metabolism using (18)F-sodium fluoride PET/CT imaging. Bone 2020;136: 115351.

121. Frost ML, Fogelman I, Blake GM, et al. Dissociation between global markers of bone formation and direct measurement of spinal bone formation in osteoporosis. J Bone Miner Res 2004;19(11): 1797–804.

122. Uchida K, Nakajima H, Miyazaki T, et al. Effects of alendronate on bone metabolism in glucocorticoid-induced osteoporosis measured by 18F-fluoride PET: a prospective study. J Nucl Med 2009; 50(11):1808–14.

123. Izadyar S, Gholamrezanezhad A. Bone scintigraphy elucidates different metabolic stages of melorheostosis. Pan Afr Med J 2012;11:21.

124. Installe J, Nzeusseu A, Bol A, et al. (18)F-fluoride PET for monitoring therapeutic response in Paget's disease of bone. J Nucl Med 2005;46(10):1650–8.

125. Frost ML, Cook GJ, Blake GM, et al. A prospective study of risedronate on regional bone metabolism and blood flow at the lumbar spine measured by 18F-fluoride positron emission tomography. J Bone Miner Res 2003;18(12):2215–22.

126. Frost ML, Siddique M, Blake GM, et al. Regional bone metabolism at the lumbar spine and hip following discontinuation of alendronate and risedronate treatment in postmenopausal women. Osteoporos Int 2012;23(8):2107–16.

127. Frost ML, Siddique M, Blake GM, et al. Differential effects of teriparatide on regional bone formation using (18)F-fluoride positron emission tomography. J Bone Miner Res 2011;26(5):1002–11.

128. Lundblad H, Karlsson-Thur C, Maguire GQ Jr, et al. Can spatiotemporal fluoride ((18)F(-)) uptake be

used to assess bone formation in the tibia? A longitudinal study using PET/CT. Clin Orthop Relat Res 2017;475(5):1486–98.

129. Win AZ, Aparici CM. Normal SUV values measured from NaF18- PET/CT bone scan studies. PLoS One 2014;9(9):e108429.

130. Rebuzzi M, Vinicola V, Taggi F, et al. Potential diagnostic role of the MRI-derived internal magnetic field gradient in calcaneus cancellous bone for evaluating postmenopausal osteoporosis at 3T. Bone 2013;57(1):155–63.

131. Link TM, Majumdar S, Augat P, et al. In vivo high resolution MRI of the calcaneus: differences in trabecular structure in osteoporosis patients. J Bone Miner Res 1998;13(7): 1175–82.

132. Zirakchian Zadeh M, Ostergaard B, Raynor WY, et al. Comparison of (18)F-sodium fluoride uptake in the whole bone, pelvis, and femoral neck of multiple myeloma patients before and after high-dose therapy and conventional-dose chemotherapy. Eur J Nucl Med Mol Imaging 2020. https://doi.org/10.1007/s00259-020-04768-0.

133. Rajapakse CS, Phillips EA, Sun W, et al. Vertebral deformities and fractures are associated with MRI and pQCT measures obtained at the distal tibia and radius of postmenopausal women. Osteoporos Int 2014;25(3):973–82.

134. Blake GM, Puri T, Siddique M, et al. Site specific measurements of bone formation using [(18)F] sodium fluoride PET/CT. Quant Imaging Med Surg 2018;8(1):47–59.

135. Jones HR Jr, Burns T, Aminoff MJ, et al. The netter collection of medical illustrations: nervous system, volume 7, part II-spinal cord and peripheral motor and sensory systems E-Book. 2nd Edition. Saunders, Philadelphia, PA, USA: Elsevier Health Sciences; 2013.

136. Tieland M, Trouwborst I, Clark BC. Skeletal muscle performance and ageing. J Cachexia Sarcopenia Muscle 2018;9(1):3–19.

137. Otto EB, Dworzecki T. The role of skeletal muscle in the regulation of glucose homeostasis. Endokrynol Diabetol Chor Przemiany Materii Wieku Rozw 2003; 9(2):93–7.

138. Reid KF, Fielding RA. Skeletal muscle power: a critical determinant of physical functioning in older adults. Exerc Sport Sci Rev 2012;40(1):4–12.

139. Stump CS, Henriksen EJ, Wei Y, et al. The metabolic syndrome: role of skeletal muscle metabolism. Ann Med 2006;38(6):389–402.

140. Boutin RD, Yao L, Canter RJ, et al. Sarcopenia: current concepts and imaging implications. AJR Am J Roentgenol 2015;205(3):W255–66.

141. Morley JE, Thomas DR, Wilson MM. Cachexia: pathophysiology and clinical relevance. Am J Clin Nutr 2006;83(4):735–43.

142. Cawthon PM, Lui LY, Taylor BC, et al. Clinical definitions of sarcopenia and risk of hospitalization in community-dwelling older men: the osteoporotic fractures in men study. J Gerontol A Biol Sci Med Sci 2017;72(10):1383–9.

143. Steffl M, Sima J, Shiells K, et al. The increase in health care costs associated with muscle weakness in older people without long-term illnesses in the Czech Republic: results from the Survey of Health, Ageing and Retirement in Europe (SHARE). Clin Interventions Aging 2017;12:2003.

144. Anker SD, Morley JE, von Haehling S. Welcome to the ICD-10 code for sarcopenia. J Cachexia Sarcopenia Muscle 2016;7(5):512–4.

145. Cruz-Jentoft AJ, Bahat G, Bauer J, et al. Sarcopenia: revised European consensus on definition and diagnosis. Age Ageing 2019;48(1):16–31.

146. Albano D, Messina C, Vitale J, et al. Imaging of sarcopenia: old evidence and new insights. Eur Radiol 2020;30(4):2199–208.

147. Lenchik L, Boutin RD. Sarcopenia: beyond muscle atrophy and into the new frontiers of opportunistic imaging, precision medicine, and machine learning. Paper presented at: Seminars in Musculoskeletal Radiology 2018; 22(03): 307 - 322. DOI: 10.1055/s-0038-1641573.

148. Raitakari M, Nuutila P, Ruotsalainen U, et al. Evidence for dissociation of insulin stimulation of blood flow and glucose uptake in human skeletal muscle: studies using [15O] H2O,[18F] fluoro-2-deoxy-D-glucose, and positron emission tomography. Diabetes 1996;45(11):1471–7.

149. Zhou C, Foster B, Hagge R, et al. Opportunistic body composition evaluation in patients with esophageal adenocarcinoma: association of survival with 18 F-FDG PET/CT muscle metrics. Ann Nucl Med 2020;34(3):174–81.

150. Kothekar E, Raynor WY, Al-Zaghal A, et al. Evolving role of PET/CT-MRI in assessing muscle disorders. PET Clin 2019;14(1):71–9.

151. Rudroff T, Kindred JH, Kalliokoski KK. [18F]-FDG positron emission tomography—an established clinical tool opening a new window into exercise physiology. J Appl Physiol 2015;118(10):1181–90.

152. Rudroff T, Weissman JA, Bucci M, et al. Positron emission tomography detects greater blood flow and less blood flow heterogeneity in the exercising skeletal muscles of old compared with young men during fatiguing contractions. J Physiol 2014; 592(2):337–49.

153. Foster B, Boutin RD, Lenchik L, et al. Skeletal muscle metrics on clinical (18)F-FDG PET/CT predict health outcomes in patients with sarcoma. J Nat Sci 2018;4(5):e502.

154. Ruotsalainen U, Raitakari M, Nuutila P, et al. Quantitative blood flow measurement of skeletal muscle

using oxygen-15-water and PET. J Nucl Med 1997; 38(2):314.

155. Nuutila P, Raitakari M, Laine H, et al. Role of blood flow in regulating insulin-stimulated glucose uptake in humans. Studies using bradykinin, [15O] water, and [18F] fluoro-deoxy-glucose and positron emission tomography. J Clin Invest 1996;97(7):1741–7.

156. Clyne CA, Jones T, Moss S, et al. The use of radioactive oxygen to study muscle function in peripheral vascular disease. Surg Gynecol Obstet 1979; 149(2):225–8.

157. Fischman AJ, Yu YM, Livni E, et al. Muscle protein synthesis by positron-emission tomography with L-[methyl-11C]methionine in adult humans. Proc Natl Acad Sci U S A 1998;95(22):12793–8.

158. Peltoniemi P, Lönnroth P, Laine H, et al. Lumped constant for [18F] fluorodeoxyglucose in skeletal muscles of obese and nonobese humans. Am J Physiology Endocrinol Metab 2000;279(5): E1122–30.

159. Nuutila P, Koivisto VA, Knuuti J, et al. Glucose-free fatty acid cycle operates in human heart and skeletal muscle in vivo. J Clin Invest 1992;89(6): 1767–74.

160. Mossberg KA, Rowe RW, Tewson TJ, et al. Rabbit hindlimb glucose uptake assessed with positron-emitting fluorodeoxyglucose. J Appl Physiol (1985) 1989;67(4):1569–77.

161. Chou TH, Stacy MR. Clinical applications for radiotracer imaging of lower extremity peripheral arterial disease and critical limb ischemia. Mol Imaging Biol 2020;22(2):245–55.

162. Barrington S, Blower P, Cook G. New horizons in multimodality molecular imaging and novel radiotracers. Clin Med (Lond) 2017;17(5):444–8.

163. Wu C, Yue X, Lang L, et al. Longitudinal PET imaging of muscular inflammation using 18F-DPA-714 and 18F-Alfatide II and differentiation with tumors. Theranostics 2014;4(5):546.

164. Lu Y, Karagounis LG, Ng TP, et al. Systemic and metabolic signature of sarcopenia in community-dwelling older adults. J Gerontol A Biol Sci Med Sci 2020;75(2):309–17.

165. Baracos VE. Psoas as a sentinel muscle for sarcopenia: a flawed premise. J Cachexia, Sarcopenia Muscle 2017;8(4):527–8.

166. Rutten IJ, Ubachs J, Kruitwagen RF, et al. Psoas muscle area is not representative of total skeletal muscle area in the assessment of sarcopenia in ovarian cancer. J Cachexia Sarcopenia Muscle 2017;8(4):630–8.

167. Ng JM, Bertoldo A, Minhas DS, et al. Dynamic PET imaging reveals heterogeneity of skeletal muscle insulin resistance. J Clin Endocrinol Metab 2014; 99(1):E102–6.

168. Kalliokoski KK, Kemppainen J, Larmola K, et al. Muscle blood flow and flow heterogeneity during exercise studied with positron emission tomography in humans. Eur J Appl Physiol 2000;83(4-5): 395–401.

169. Batouli A, Braun J, Singh K, et al. Diagnosis of non-osseous spinal metastatic disease: the role of PET/ CT and PET/MRI. J Neurooncol 2018;138(2): 221–30.

170. Behzadi AH, Raza SI, Carrino JA, et al. Applications of PET/CT and PET/MR imaging in primary bone malignancies. PET Clin 2018;13(4):623–34.

171. Cleary MX, Fayad LM, Ahlawat S. Popliteal lymph nodes in patients with osteosarcoma: are they metastatic? Skeletal Radiol 2020;49(11):1807–17.

172. Erfanian Y, Grueneisen J, Kirchner J, et al. Integrated 18F-FDG PET/MRI compared to MRI alone for identification of local recurrences of soft tissue sarcomas: a comparison trial. Eur J Nucl Med Mol Imaging 2017;44(11):1823–31.

173. Assadi M, Velez E, Najafi MH, et al. PET imaging of peripheral nerve tumors. PET Clin 2019;14(1):81–9.

174. Lee I, Byun BH, Lim I, et al. Early response monitoring of neoadjuvant chemotherapy using [(18)F] FDG PET can predict the clinical outcome of extremity osteosarcoma. EJNMMI Res 2020;10(1):1.

175. Sheen H, Kim W, Byun BH, et al. Metastasis risk prediction model in osteosarcoma using metabolic imaging phenotypes: a multivariable radiomics model. PLoS One 2019;14(11):e0225242.

176. Jeong SY, Kim W, Byun BH, et al. Prediction of chemotherapy response of osteosarcoma using baseline (18)F-FDG textural features machine learning approaches with PCA. Contrast Media Mol Imaging 2019;2019:3515080.

177. Bosma SE, Vriens D, Gelderblom H, et al. (18)F-FDG PET-CT versus MRI for detection of skeletal metastasis in Ewing sarcoma. Skeletal Radiol 2019;48(11):1735–46.

178. Gholamrezanezhad A, Guermazi A, Salavati A, et al. PET-computed tomography and PET-MR imaging and their applications in the twenty-first century. PET Clin 2019;14(1):xv–xvii.

179. Gholamrezanejhad A, Mirpour S, Mariani G. Future of nuclear medicine: SPECT versus PET. J Nucl Med 2009;50(7):16N–8N.

180. Batouli A, Gholamrezanezhad A, Petrov D, et al. Management of primary osseous spinal tumors with PET. PET Clin 2019;14(1):91–101.

181. Khalatbari H, Parisi MT, Kwatra N, et al. Pediatric musculoskeletal imaging: the indications for and applications of PET/computed tomography. PET Clin 2019;14(1):145–74.

182. Katal S, Gholamrezanezhad A, Kessler M, et al. PET in the diagnostic management of soft tissue sarcomas of musculoskeletal origin. PET Clin 2018;13(4):609–21.

Assessment of Total-Body Atherosclerosis by PET/Computed Tomography

Poul Flemming Høilund-Carlsen, MD, DMSc, Prof (Hon)[a,b,*], Reza Piri, MD[a,b], Oke Gerke, MSc, PhD[a,b], Lars Edenbrandt, MD, DMSc[c,d], Abass Alavi, MD, MD (Hon), PhD (Hon), DSc (Hon)[e]

KEYWORDS

- Atherosclerosis • Total body • FDG • NaF • Inflammation • Calcification • PET/CT

KEY POINTS

- It has recently been suggested that the atherosclerotic burden in various parts of the arterial system should be the focus of cardiovascular risk assessment using PET/computed tomography (CT) imaging rather than characterizing the individual vulnerable plaques.
- ^{18}F-fluorodeoxyglucose and ^{18}F-sodium fluoride, showing arterial wall inflammation and microcalcification, respectively, are presently the only PET tracers that have been studied extensively; their arterial uptakes rarely overlap in site and time.
- Arterial uptake of both tracers is modestly age dependent, albeit ^{18}F-sodium fluoride uptake is more consistently associated with risk factors than ^{18}F-fluorodeoxyglucose uptake and is more easily measured in the heart.
- Arterial ^{18}F-fluorodeoxyglucose uptake seems to come and go with time (months); recent preliminary data suggest that ^{18}F-sodium fluoride uptake may also be a more varying process than previously anticipated. These statements require confirmation in future prospective longitudinal studies.
- Total-body PET provides unique opportunities for studying atherosclerosis and its management more profoundly because of much higher sensitivity, ultrashort acquisition, and minimal radiation to the patient; this allows disease screening, delayed and repeat imaging with features such as global disease scoring, and parametric imaging to characterize the individual patients much better than was previously possible.

INTRODUCTION

The underlying premise of this forward-looking communication is the view put forth in recent years that the entire atherosclerotic process and disease burden should be the focus of cardiovascular risk assessment rather than characterizing the individual vulnerable plaques.[1–3] Until recently, there has been (and still is) an overwhelming interest in vulnerable or rupture-prone plaques, anticipating that, if such plaques can be identified and passivated, it would significantly improve the prognosis of patients with advanced atherosclerosis. A shift to assessing instead the

[a] Department of Nuclear Medicine, Odense University Hospital, Kløvervænget 47, 5000 Odense C, Denmark; [b] Department of Clinical Research, University of Southern Denmark, 5000 Odense C, Denmark; [c] Department of Clinical Physiology, Region Västra Götaland, Sahlgrenska University Hospital, Gothenburg, Sweden; [d] Department of Molecular and Clinical Medicine, Institute of Medicine, SU Sahlgrenska, 41345 Göteborg, Sweden; [e] Department of Radiology, Perelman School of Medicine, University of Pennsylvania, 3400 Spruce Street, PA 19104, USA
* Corresponding author. Department of Nuclear Medicine, Odense University Hospital, 5000 Odense C, Denmark.
E-mail address: pfhc@rsyd.dk

PET Clin 16 (2021) 119–128
https://doi.org/10.1016/j.cpet.2020.09.013

atherosclerotic burden in the heart, carotids, aorta, or other major arteries is a change of approach that places great demands on available imaging techniques, because atherosclerotic arterial wall changes are often scattered, diffuse, and mostly invisible by computed tomography (CT), meaning that they are difficult to segment properly (**Fig. 1**).

Apart from being able to show subtle arterial wall changes, an imaging test for measuring the atherosclerotic burden and prediction of cardiovascular risk based on the global atherosclerotic burden comprising the heart and major arteries must be easy and fast to perform and so specific, accurate, and reproducible that any clinician would be better off with that instead of conventional methods for assessment of diagnosis, prognosis, treatment triage, or therapeutic efficacy in individual patients.

This article elucidates and discusses potentials and challenges of a "transition from a focus on individual lesions to atherosclerotic disease burden in coronary and overall cardiovascular risk assessment," as Arbab-Zadeh and Fuster[2] put it, in light of novel total-body PET scanners and the rapid increase in artificial intelligence (AI) for interpretation of PET scans.

ATHEROSCLEROTIC DISEASE BURDEN OR VULNERABLE PLAQUE

Considerable effort has been put into modalities that can identify and characterize vulnerable plaques, which are considered as responsible for thrombosis and occlusion leading to acute myocardial infarction (MI) and stroke. They have a thin cap on the luminal side and a lipid-rich and often necrotic core that rarely gives rise to severe stenosis, properties that hamper their detection and have called for diagnostic criteria, primarily based on CT, ultrasonography, or magnetic resonance imaging,[4–12] none of which have reached general clinical application.

Therefore, arterial ^{18}F-sodium fluoride (NaF) PET imaging, initiated in 2010 by Derlin and colleagues,[13,14] who started studying the prevalence and topographic distribution of NaF uptake compared with CT calcification in major arteries, sparked an interest in studying NaF uptake in vulnerable coronary and carotid plaques[15–18] to achieve improved plaque characterization, because CT calcification could not precisely characterize individual patients.[19–21]

Postmortem studies of patients dying of cardiac arrest and acute MI have indicated that the

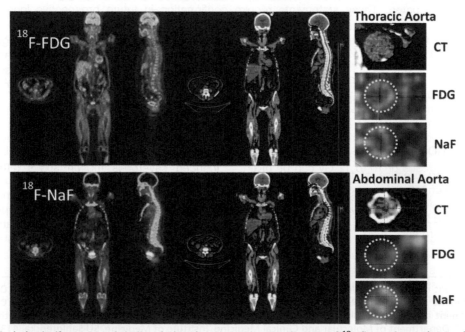

Fig. 1. Whole-body (from top of skull to below knee) uptake distribution of ^{18}F-fluorodeoxyglucose (FDG) and ^{18}F-sodium fluoride (NaF) in the axial, coronal, and sagittal planes shown on composite PET/CT and CT images in the left and right halves, respectively, of the panels). Note the intense uptake of NaF in the bones on PET images in the lower panel. The small images to the right show what is seen on axial slices of the thoracic aorta (upper 3 images) and the abdominal aorta (lower 3 images) by means of (from top to bottom) CT, FDG-PET/CT, and NaF-PET/CT and show some of the difficulties in delineating and segmenting the aortic wall correctly. The dotted circles circumscribe cross-sections of the aorta with its lumen in the middle.

percentage luminal area stenosis at sites of thrombus or at likely culprit lesions causing MI is high (≥75%) and that only 10% of culprit lesions had a diameter of less than 50% after thrombosis removal.[22–24] In the heart, it is a limitation that even advanced approaches examine plaques exclusively in the proximal parts of the coronary tree,[25,26] disregarding calcification in the distal and transmural branches supplying the subendocardial myocardial layers, where ischemia is more likely to trigger infarction and neuralgia. With global molecular imaging of the heart, this limitation does not apply and, thus, results of PET imaging may be a better indicator of cardiac atherosclerotic burden. Together with the observation that the atherosclerotic processes are more dynamic and changeable than previously thought,[27,28] this limitation has made leading cardiologists suggest that "our focus must remain on the entire atherosclerotic process and prevention of diffuse disease, and seeking individual plaques may not be the ultimate answer."[29]

Arbab-Zadeh and Fuster[2] conclude their review by stating that "there is no conclusive evidence that individual plaque assessment better predicts acute coronary event risk than established risk factors, such as the extent and severity of coronary artery disease." Because atherosclerotic plaque rupture occurs mostly without clinical symptoms, whereas the atherosclerotic disease burden is a consistent, strong predictor of adverse events, they suggest that, instead of focusing on individual coronary lesions, clinicians must strive for "comprehensive risk assessment that integrates specific information on the atherosclerotic plaque burden and systemic factors that increase the risk for disease activity and vascular thrombosis and is tailored to specific patient populations and individual patients."[2] Their point of view is reinforced by the fact that the literature on PET characterization of vulnerable plaques does not reveal such a close association between uptake of 18F-fluorodeoxyglucose (FDG) or NaF and alleged vulnerability that it is possible to predict with reasonable certainty the cardiovascular risks of individual patients.[18,30] Therefore, there may be a need for more elaborate schemes for risk assessment, taking into account, besides imaging results, also clinical, biochemical, and genetic data. This need calls for AI-based algorithms, as discussed later.

Assessment of total-body atherosclerosis is a new approach focusing on detection and grading of the extent and severity of disease, whether grading arterial wall inflammation (by FDG-PET) or microcalcification (by NaF-PET) as indicators of early-stage atherosclerosis or macrocalcification by CT as a representative of late-stage atherosclerosis.[31] With PET, this has been done by manual segmentation, summarizing uptake in multiple adjacent axial slices to get a single number representing the atherosclerotic burden in, for instance, the aorta. This task a cumbersome and time consuming; however, from experience in prostate cancer,[32,33] it seems that this can soon be done in atherosclerosis too in less than a minute or so by applying AI-based interpretation.[18,30] A major hope for this approach is to provide a means for monitoring effects of antiatherosclerotic intervention. Some of the challenges that must be dealt with before assessment of total-body atherosclerosis by molecular imaging can become a clinical reality are discussed here.

PET TRACERS FOR ATHEROSCLEROSIS IMAGING

Surprisingly few tracers have been found to be clinically useful in the study of atherosclerosis. Most tracers studied over the years never reached beyond the animal testing stage. This tendency goes for 18F-labeled resveratrol, offering some protection against atherosclerosis (including the inhibition of low-density lipoprotein),[34] 64Cu-DTPA-CLIO-VT680, a 64Cu-labeled triple reporter nanoparticle known to accumulate in macrophages located in inflamed lesions and carotid artery plaques after intravenous administration,[35] and 18F-4V, a tetrameric linear peptide targeting atherosclerotic plaques and myocardial ischemic lesions.[36] Other probes are 68Ga-NODAGA-AE105-NH2, a urokinase-type plasminogen activator receptor–targeting molecule[37]; 18F-AppCHFppA and 18F-SB209670, identifying the adenosine nucleotide receptor[38,39]; and 18F-ET-1, targeting the endothelin-1 receptor.[40] Common to these and many others are lack of specificity, because most of them target processes (eg, apoptosis) or elements (eg, metalloproteinases) of other types of disease, not least inflammation and cancer. When the Molecular Imaging and Contrast Agent Database (developed by the National Center for Biotechnology Information, at the National Institutes of Health) ceased in June 2013 to become updated, it contained only a single tracer that thus far had been used in humans for studies of atherosclerosis, namely FDG, whereas NaF was not mentioned for this purpose, or for imaging of bone metastases.[41]

18F-FLUORODEOXYGLUCOSE AND 18F-SODIUM FLUORIDE PET IMAGING IN ATHEROSCLEROSIS

Until now, only FDG and NaF have reached extensive human use, perhaps because of their early availability for other primary purposes (ie, studies of brain metabolism and bone mineral turnover, respectively).[42,43] FDG was first used by Yun and colleagues[44] almost 20 years ago, whereas NaF, as mentioned, was introduced about 10 years later by Derlin and colleagues.[13] Traditionally, in being a marker of glucose metabolism, FDG is known to show macrophage accumulation and thus inflammation, whereas NaF, in being adsorbed to micro-calcifications smaller than 50 μm, is a sensitive and specific marker of local tissue necrosis.[31] However, their interrelationship, temporal and topo-graphic relationships, and connection to CT-detectable arterial macrocalcification are still not known in detail. It was hoped that 1 or both tracers could be used to identify early-stage atheroscle-rosis and serve as precursors to the late-appearing macrocalcification and plaque develop-ment that cause organ damage. However, it seems that things are not that straightforward.

Recent reviews have pointed to NaF as perhaps the more valuable of the two, the reasons for which are 2-fold: (1) in animal studies, it shows some of the earliest changes observed in the atheroscle-rosis process[45]; (2) in human studies, it has, oppo-site to FDG, been consistently associated with cardiovascular risk in most parts of the arterial sys-tem.[17,18,46,47] Unlike FDG, NaF uptake is more easily detected and quantified in the heart, where it is assumed to represent early coronary artery atherosclerosis; NaF is not detectable in the myocardium of atherosclerotic pigs,[45] and pre-sumably not in the human myocardium either except in patients who have had an MI.[48]

There seems to be a missing link between arte-rial FDG uptake and existing or later-developed CT-detectable macrocalcification. Thus, multiple studies have shown a lack of overlap between FDG uptake and CT-detectable plaque,[12,14,48–51] although others could not show a significant corre-lation with cardiovascular risk factors.[51–54] In line with this, Meirelles and colleagues[55] showed that thoracic aorta FDG uptake in 100 consecutive pa-tients with cancer was a "waxing and waning pro-cess," as the investigators put it. FDG uptake was seen in 70% of the patients on the first scan and changed on the second in 55% of the patients af-ter a mean of 7 months (range, 21 days to 3 years). In 28 patients, vascular FDG uptake was less intense or had resolved on the second scan, whereas, in 27 patients, there was an increase at existing sites or appearance of new foci. There was a trend to unstable FDG uptake in older pa-tients and in women, no correlation between risk factors for cardiovascular disease and FDG vascular uptake, and FDG uptake and calcifica-tions were present at the same site in only 2

patients. Vascular calcifications were identified in 42 patients on the first or on the second PET/CT scan, were more commonly seen in older patients, and were generally stable from scan to scan. None of the patients progressed over time from FDG vascular uptake to calcifications at the same location.[55]

Recently, similar observations were made for NaF uptake in the abdominal aorta. Cecelja and colleagues[56] reported change in NaF uptake in the abdominal aorta of 21 postmenopausal women who underwent NaF-PET/CT for assess-ment of bone mineralization. They found no change in NaF target/background ratio after 3.8 years (standard deviation, 1.3 years) despite a significant 54% increase in abdominal aortic calcium volume.[56] Nakahara and colleagues,[57] who studied patients with prostate cancer with at least 3 NaF-PET/CT scans over at least 1.5 years, observed variable NaF uptake in the abdominal aorta from scan to scan, whereas cal-cium volumes remained constant or increased between scans.

Several studies showing significant correlations between NaF uptake and characteristics such as vulnerable or high-risk plaque used the term "pre-diction" for such associations,[51,56,58,59] as has been done multiple times in the past when a signif-icant correlation was observed between coronary calcification and risk of future cardiovascular events.[60–68] However, none of these associations was sufficiently close to allow such an accurate prediction in individual patients that it could be of use in the daily clinic. All showed that relationships were indicative rather than predictive, which leaves the question in limbo: despite increasing scientific activity, white spots remain on the map depicting the relationship between arterial wall FDG uptake, NaF uptake, and CT-detectable calcification. The unexplored areas call for longitu-dinal in-depth studies applying repeat FDG-PET and NaF-PET scans for comparison with CT calci-fication. The essence of what is known and not known about NaF uptake in atherosclerosis as of March 2020 (Høilund-Carlsen PF, Piri R, Constan-tinescu C, et al. Submitted for publication) can be summarized as follows:

By targeting arterial microcalcification, NaF up-take seems to be a marker of early-stage athero-sclerosis that is slightly age dependent, albeit with a large scatter, and consistently associated with cardiovascular risk. Increased arterial NaF uptake is uncommon in diabetics, as is NaF uptake in the renal arteries of hypertensive patients. Pro-gression of arterial wall NaF uptake has been stud-ied by retrospective analyses in the abdominal aorta only and indicates slow or variable progression over a period of some years despite constant or increasing calcium volumes. Therefore, it remains unknown whether NaF uptake is a reliable harbinger of CT-detectable calcification and whether intervention can modify NaF-associated microcalcification.

PET EQUIPMENT FOR PARTIAL-BODY OR TOTAL-BODY ASSESSMENT

With the advent of long-axial PET scanners with multiple detector rings that allow an elongated axial field of view of 70 or up to 200 cm, exemplified by the PennPET Explorer[69–71] and the United Imaging Explorer scanner,[72–76] respectively, clinicians will soon be able to collect information on illness in major parts or all over the body in a way and with a speed that has never been possible before. Thanks to the much higher sensitivity of these instruments (in theory, up to 40 times higher; in practice, presumably 8 to 10 times as high as with current PET/CT scanners), partial-body or total-body acquisitions can be made in seconds or in most cases probably a few minutes with the same fixed bed position. This kind of equipment places new major demands on logistics and investments, not to mention processing software, but offers benefits that health care will soon profit from. With regard to the physical characteristics and capabilities of these devices, reference is made to other literature[69–74]; here, the focus is on their possible importance for clinical PET/CT imaging of atherosclerosis.

A wide range of conditions and restrains that clinicians have not previously been able to take into account or deal with can now be addressed to optimize examination of individual patients. One is delayed imaging to reduce the amount of background activity, which is a problem with FDG in particular; another is improved motion correction because acquisition is so fast that it can be done in held inhalation or during a few breaths and with high resolution; a third is full-body recordings to elucidate disease activity in more than 1 or just a few locations in the body; and a fourth is dynamic recordings enabling parametric imaging to retrieve several essential disease parameters that have so far not been within practical reach. By means of dynamic imaging with high spatial and temporal resolution, total-body PET will allow kinetic analysis in patients that have hitherto only been able to be obtained in advanced experimental animal and human studies, many of which need real-life validation in patients.[73,76] In atherosclerosis, as in many other diseases, this would yield much more reliable estimates of metabolism, oxygen use, signal transduction, and pharmacodynamics

than have so far been able to be retrieved from static or conventional dynamic PET imaging within a limited field of view and insufficient time resolution.

Moreover, ultrashort acquisition times mean that patient placement on the scanner bed is more time consuming than the scan itself.[76] The much lower tracer doses needed result in effective doses to the patient that are much less than the natural background radiation, even in countries with low background levels. Such low effective patient doses mean that dual or triple tracer studies will become possible, whether performed in succession on the same day or on different days. Moreover, they will allow disease screening and repeat scans in longitudinal follow-up trials and studies monitoring therapy effect, which require a minimum of 3 scans (ie, baseline and 2 or more follow-up scans) to ensure reliable results.[77] The automation and advanced processing software needed with these devices will offset the greater uncertainty that comes with repeated imaging because all sources of error are in play every time a new scan is made.[78]

Thus, an entirely new series of possibilities open up with total-body PET imaging, for example:

- Mapping and quantification of atherosclerosis, its location, and relative activity throughout the body, something that may have both prognostic and therapeutic implications.
- Screening for incipient but threatening atherosclerotic processes in asymptomatic patients or patients with uncharacteristic symptoms, including cerebral atherosclerosis; carotid atherosclerosis as a forerunner of stroke; and accelerated cardiac, aortic, or peripheral arterial disease, all of which may be sensitive to early-onset therapy.
- Disease characterization with several different PET tracers in the same patient.
- Easy, fast, and risk-free monitoring of a variety of therapeutic interventions even in the same individual.
- Calculation of a single score, the global disease score, expressing the atherosclerotic burden in the body and its activity at diagnosis and as an easy, simple and reliable guidance for therapy.

ARTIFICIAL INTELLIGENCE–BASED INTERPRETATION

AI-based interpretation will become a necessity. Not only will it increase reproducibility and reduce differences caused by different scanners and scanner manufactures, it will significantly increase diagnostic accuracy, because it will never stop learning and optimizing, meaning that AI-based reporting will sooner or later become superior to that of a standard physician. In addition, the AI approach will take into account a wide range of paraclinical and clinical factors, all of which are not routinely considered or easy to interpret.[79–81]

In the long run, high-level AI will probably reach beyond the role of advanced medical decision aid by providing intelligent computer-generated suggestions for alternative diagnosis and treatment regimens. However, underlying paraclinical and clinical data must be permanently accessible to AI-based algorithms, and such data need to be updated continuously, a matter that, in times of increased data protection formalities, remains to be solved judiciously.

In practice, AI-based reporting will provide calculation in seconds of quantitative parameters that are practically impossible for individual physicians to obtain, primarily because manual segmentation is too uncertain and slow, in particular when it comes to discrimination between soft tissues (**Fig. 2**). With AI, such measures can be calculated for the entire body imaged by the UI Explorer scanner or for the torso, which is what the PennPET Explorer system with its 70-cm axial field of view can see in a single scan. The purpose is to provide clinicians with a tool, in this case a single number, that meets their 3 most important needs

when assessing individual patients: knowledge of whether (1) the disease is present and how widespread and active it is, (2) guidance for proper treatment triage, and (3) ability to judge whether the treatment is working or whether it is advisable to switch to another form of therapy. Total-body PET with AI-based interpretation may be the instrument that will make this vision come true.

With total-body PET, atherosclerosis development can be examined in known sites of predilection such as the heart and major arteries long before this is possible in the course of disease with other modalities. In addition, atherosclerosis can be studied in places where it is rarely done or where it is poorly practiced; for example, the brain, lungs, and arteries of smaller organs. However, to speculate further may be going too far while clinical total-body PET/CT is still in its infancy and needed sophisticated hardware and software are still works in progress. Nonetheless, the authors believe that total-body PET/CT has come to stay and that it will significantly change the perception, understanding, and treatment of many of the most important and debilitating diseases, including atherosclerosis.

COST-EFFECTIVENESS

The authors foresee that total-body PET will cause a complete change in the management of atherosclerosis, from diagnosis of late-onset

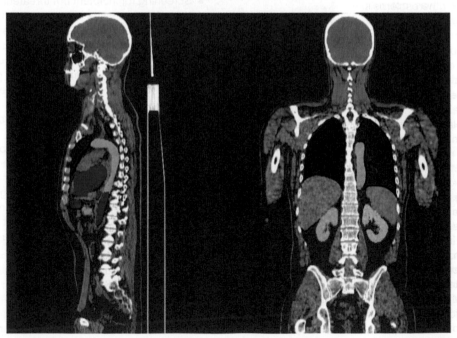

Fig. 2. AI-based segment of organs (color coded). Note the heart (*red*), thoracic aorta (*beige*), and abdominal aorta (*dark red*).

symptomatic lesions and their treatment, which is currently more repair than therapy, to detection in the early, symptom-free stages when there is a much greater chance of cure or inhibiting further development. The economic and patient-related benefits of such a strategy will be huge and difficult to estimate, although it will probably, as is customary with novel and advanced expensive equipment, be argued that this new technology is too complicated and costly to reach general clinical use. Only cost-effectiveness studies as well as or in prolongation to clinical studies will offer evidence to this end in the future. However, changing this is a matter of time. When these promising opportunities become apparent to colleagues, patients, and authorities, the production and clinical use of total-body PET will increase and reach a level where its advantages will more than counterbalance its gradually decreasing costs.

SUMMARY

Total-body PET imaging in atherosclerosis will, as in many other diseases, cause a change of perception of the illness, its development, and association with other disorders. In addition, it will allow prevention and/or earlier, more individualized, and more effective antiatherosclerotic intervention than is now common.

DISCLOSURE

This review was not funded. The authors have nothing to disclose.

REFERENCES

1. Narula J, Kovacic JC. Putting TCFA in clinical perspective. J Am Coll Cardiol 2014;64(7):681–3.
2. Arbab-Zadeh A, Fuster V. The myth of the "vulnerable plaque": transitioning from a focus on individual lesions to atherosclerotic disease burden for coronary artery disease risk assessment. J Am Coll Cardiol 2015;65(8):846–55.
3. Arbab-Zadeh A. Does "vulnerable" atherosclerotic plaque modify coronary blood flow?: how myths perpetuate. JACC Cardiovasc Imaging 2019. https://doi.org/10.1016/j.jcmg.2019.07.011 [pii: S1936-878X(19)30704-1].
4. Agatston AS, Janowitz WR, Hildner FJ, et al. Quantification of coronary artery calcium using ultrafast computed tomography. J Am Coll Cardiol 1990; 15(4):827–32.
5. Ehara S, Kobayashi Y, Yoshiyama M, et al. Spotty calcification typifies the culprit plaque in patients with acute myocardial infarction: an intravascular ultrasound study. Circulation 2004;110:3424–9.
6. Virmani R, Burke AP, Farb A, et al. Pathology of the vulnerable plaque. J Am Coll Cardiol 2006; 47(suppl):C13–8.
7. Motoyama S, Sarai M, Harigaya H, et al. Computed tomographic angiography characteristics of atherosclerotic plaques subsequently resulting in acute coronary syndrome. J Am Coll Cardiol 2009;54: 49–57.
8. Ricotta JJ, Aburahma A, Ascher E, et al. Updated Society for Vascular Surgery guidelines for management of extracranial carotid disease. J Vasc Surg 2011;54:e1–31.
9. Gauss S, Achenbach S, Pflederer T, et al. Assessment of coronary artery remodelling by dual-source CT: a head-to-head comparison with intravascular ultrasound. Heart 2011;97(12):991–7.
10. van Velzen JE, de Graaf FR, de Graaf MA, et al. Comprehensive assessment of spotty calcifications on computed tomography angiography: comparison to plaque characteristics on intravascular ultrasound with radiofrequency backscatter analysis. J Nucl Cardiol 2011;18(5):893–903.
11. Leipsic J, Abbara S, Achenbach S, et al. SCCT guidelines for the interpretation and reporting of coronary CT angiography: a report of the Society of Cardiovascular Computed Tomography Guidelines Committee. J Cardiovasc Comput Tomogr 2014; 8(5):342–58.
12. Marchesseau S, Seneviratna A, Sjöholm AT, et al. Hybrid PET/CT and PET/MRI imaging of vulnerable coronary plaque and myocardial scar tissue in acute myocardial infarction. J Nucl Cardiol 2018;25(6): 2001–11.
13. Derlin T, Richter U, Bannas P, et al. Feasibility of 18F-sodium fluoride PET/CT for imaging of atherosclerotic plaque. J Nucl Med 2010;51:862–5.
14. Derlin T, Wisotzki C, Richter U, et al. In vivo imaging of mineral deposition in carotid plaque using 18F-sodium fluoride PET/CT: correlation with atherogenic risk factors. J Nucl Med 2011;52:362–8.
15. Quirce R, Martínez-Rodríguez I, De Arcocha Torres M, et al. Contribution of 18F-sodium fluoride PET/CT to the study of the carotid atheroma calcification. Rev Esp Med Nucl Imagen Mol 2013;32:22–5.
16. Joshi NV, Vesey AT, Williams MC, et al. 18 F-fluoride positron emission tomography for identification of ruptured and high-risk coronary atherosclerotic plaques: a prospective clinical trial. Lancet 2014;383: 705–13.
17. Piri R, Gerke O, Høilund-Carlsen PF. Molecular imaging of carotid artery atherosclerosis with PET: a systematic review. Eur J Nucl Med Mol Imaging 2019. https://doi.org/10.1007/s00259-019-04622-y.
18. Høilund-Carlsen PF, Sturek M, Alavi A, et al. Atherosclerosis imaging with 18F-sodium fluoride PET: state-of-the-art review. Eur J Nucl Med Mol Imaging 2019. https://doi.org/10.1007/s00259-019-04603-1.

19. Ilangkovan N, Mogensen CB, Mickley H, et al. Prevalence of coronary artery calcification in a non-specific chest pain population in emergency and cardiology departments compared with the background population: a prospective cohort study in Southern Denmark with 12-month follow-up of cardiac endpoints. BMJ Open 2018;8(3):e018391.

20. Lindholt JS, Rasmussen LM, Søgaard R, et al. Baseline findings of the population-based, randomized, multifaceted Danish cardiovascular screening trial (DANCAVAS) of men aged 65-74 years. Br J Surg 2019;106(7):862–71.

21. Haase R, Schlattmann P, Gueret P, et al. Diagnosis of obstructive coronary artery disease using computed tomography angiography in patients with stable chest pain depending on clinical probability and in clinically important subgroups: meta-analysis of individual patient data. BMJ 2019;365: l1945.

22. Davies MJ, Thomas A. Thrombosis and acute coronary-artery lesions in sudden cardiac ischemic death. N Engl J Med 1984;310(18):1137–40.

23. Qiao JH, Fishbein MC. The severity of coronary atherosclerosis at sites of plaque rupture with occlusive thrombosis. J Am Coll Cardiol 1991;17: 1138–42.

24. Manohan G, Ntalianis A, Muller O, et al. Severity of coronary arterial stenoses responsible for acute coronary syndromes. Am J Cardiol 2009;103:1183–8.

25. Lassen ML, Kwiecinski J, Dey D, et al. Triple-gated motion and blood pool clearance corrections improve reproducibility of coronary 18F-NaF PET. Eur J Nucl Med Mol Imaging 2019;46(12):2610–20.

26. Kwiecinski J, Slomka PJ, Dweck MR, et al. Vulnerable plaque imaging using 18F-sodium fluoride positron emission tomography. Br J Radiol 2019; 20190797.

27. Tian J, Dauerman H, Toma C, et al. Prevalence and characteristics of TCFA and degree of coronary artery stenosis: an OCT, IVUS, and angiographic study. J Am Coll Cardiol 2014;64(7):672–80.

28. Kubo T, Maehara A, Mintz GS, et al. The dynamic nature of coronary artery lesion morphology assessed by serial virtual histology intravascular ultrasound tissue characterization. J Am Coll Cardiol 2010;55(15):1590–7.

29. Narula J, Nakano M, Virmani R, et al. Histopathologic characteristics of atherosclerotic coronary disease and implications of the findings for the invasive and noninvasive detection of vulnerable plaques. J Am Coll Cardiol 2013;61(10):1041–51.

30. Høilund-Carlsen PF, Edenbrandt L, Alavi A. Global disease score (GDS) is the name of the game! Eur J Nucl Med Mol Imaging 2019;46:1768–72.

31. Høilund-Carlsen PF, Moghbel M, Gerke O, et al. Evolving role of PET in detecting and characterizing atherosclerosis. PET Clin 2019;14:197–209.

32. Belal L, Sadik M, Kaboteh R, et al. Deep learning for segmentation of 49 segmented bones in CT scans: first step in automated PET/CT-based 3D quantification of skeletal metastases. Eur J Radiol 2019;113: 89–95.

33. Polymeri E, Sadik M, Kaboteh R, et al. Deep learning-based quantification of PET/CT prostate gland uptake: association with overall survival. Clin Physiol Funct Imaging 2019. https://doi.org/10. 1111/cpf.12611.

34. Norata GD, Marchesi P, Passamonti S, et al. Anti-inflammatory and anti-atherogenic effects of cathechin, caffeic acid and trans-resveratrol in apolipoprotein E deficient mice. Atherosclerosis 2007;191(2):265–71.

35. Coleman R, Hayek T, Keidar S, et al. A mouse model for human atherosclerosis: long-term histopathological study of lesion development in the aortic arch of apolipoprotein E-deficient (E0) mice. Acta Histochem 2006;108(6):415–24.

36. Nahrendorf M, Keliher E, Panizzi P, et al. 18F-4V for PET-CT imaging of VCAM-1 expression in atherosclerosis. JACC Cardiovasc Imaging 2009;2(10): 1213–22.

37. Liu J, Sukhova GK, Sun JS, et al. Lysosomal cysteine proteases in atherosclerosis. Arterioscler Thromb Vasc Biol 2004;24(8):1359–66.

38. Elmaleh DR, Fischman AJ, Tawakol A, et al. Detection of inflamed atherosclerotic lesions with diadenosine-5',5'''-P1,P4-tetraphosphate (Ap4A) and positron-emission tomography. Proc Natl Acad Sci U S A 2006;103(43):15992–6.

39. Johnstrom P, Fryer TD, Richards HK, et al. In vivo imaging of cardiovascular endothelin receptors using the novel radiolabelled antagonist [18F]-SB209670 and positron emission tomography (microPET). J Cardiovasc Pharmacol 2004;44:S34–8.

40. Johnstrom P, Harris NG, Fryer TD, et al. 18F-Endothelin-1, a positron emission tomography (PET) radioligand for the endothelin receptor system: radiosynthesis and in vivo imaging using microPET. Clin Sci (Lond) 2002;103(Suppl 48):4S–8S.

41. Molecular imaging and Contrast agent Database (MICAD). Bethesda (MD): National Center for Biotechnology information (US); 2004-2013. Available at: https://www.ncbi.nlm.nih.gov/books/ NBK5330/. Accessed February 3, 2020.

42. Alavi A, Reivich M. The conception of FDG-PET imaging. Semin Nucl Med 2002;32:2–5.

43. Bastawrous S, Bhargava P, Behnia F, et al. Newer PET application with an old tracer: role of 18F-NaF skeletal PET/CT in oncologic practice. Radiographics 2014;34:1295–316.

44. Yun M, Yeh D, Araujo LI, et al. F-18 FDG uptake in the large arteries: a new observation. Clin Nucl Med 2001;26:314–9.

45. McKenney-Drake ML, Moghbel MC, Paydary K, et al. 18F-NaF and 18F-FDG as molecular probes in the evaluation of atherosclerosis. Eur J Nucl Med Mol Imaging 2018;45(12):2190–200.

46. Moghbel M, Al-Zaghal A, Werner TJ, et al. The role of PET in evaluating atherosclerosis: a Critical review. Semin Nucl Med 2018;48(6):488–97.

47. Høilund-Carlsen PF, Piri R, Constantinescu C, et al. Atherosclerosis Imaging with 18F-Sodium Fluoride PET. Diagnostics (Basel) 2020 Oct 20;10(10):E852. https://doi.org/10.3390/diagnostics10100852.

48. Tatsumi M, Cohade C, Nakamoto Y, et al. Fluoro-deoxyglucose uptake in the aortic wall at PET/CT: possible finding for active atherosclerosis 1. Radiology 2003;229:831–7.

49. Ben-Haim S, Kupzov E, Tamir A, et al. Evaluation of 18F-FDG uptake and arterial wall calcifications using 18F-FDG PET/CT. J Nucl Med 2004;45:1816–21.

50. Dunphy MP, Freiman A, Larson SM, et al. Association of vascular 18F-FDG uptake with vascular calcification. J Nucl Med 2005;46:1278–84.

51. Dweck MR, Chow MW, Joshi NV, et al. Coronary arterial 18F-sodium fluoride uptake: a novel marker of plaque biology. J Am Coll Cardiol 2012;59: 1539–48.

52. Morbelli S, Fiz F, Piccardo A, et al. Divergent determinants of 18F–NaF uptake and visible calcium deposition in large arteries: relationship with Framingham risk score. Int J Cardiovasc Imaging 2014;30:439–47.

53. Blomberg BA, de Jong PA, Thomassen A, et al. Thoracic aorta calcification but not inflammation is associated with increased cardiovascular disease risk: results of the CAMONA study. Eur J Nucl Med Mol Imaging 2017;44:249–58.

54. Arani LS, Gharavi MH, Zadeh MZ, et al. Association between age, uptake of 18F-fluorodeoxyglucose and of 18F-sodium fluoride, as cardiovascular risk factors in the abdominal aorta. Hell J Nucl Med 2019;22(1):14–9.

55. Meirelles GS, Gonen M, Strauss HW. 18F-FDG uptake and calcifications in thoracic aorta on positron emission tomography/computed tomography examinations: frequency and stability of serial scans. J Thorac Imaging 2011;26:54–62.

56. Cecelja M, Moore A, Fogelman I, et al. Evaluation of aortic 18F-NaF tracer uptake using PET/CT as a predictor of aortic calcification in postmenopausal women: a longitudinal study. JRSM Cardiovasc Dis 2019;8. 2048004019848870.

57. Nakahara T, Narula J, Fox JJ, et al. Temporal relationship between 18F-sodium fluoride uptake in the abdominal aorta and evolution of CT-verified vascular calcification. J Nucl Cardiol 2019. https://doi.org/10.1007/s12350-019-01934-2.

58. Kitagawa T, Yamamoto H, Nakamoto Y, et al. Predictive value of (18)F-sodium fluoride positron emission tomography in detecting high-risk coronary artery disease in combination with computed tomography. J Am Heart Assoc 2018;7(20):e010224.

59. Kwiecinski J, Dey D, Cadet S, et al. Predictors of 18F-sodium fluoride uptake in patients with stable coronary artery disease and adverse plaque features on computed tomography angiography. Eur Heart J Cardiovasc Imaging 2019. https://doi.org/10.1093/ehjci/jez152 [pii:jez152].

60. Vesey AT, Jenkins WS, Irkle A, et al. 18F-Fluoride and 18F-fluorodeoxyglucose positron emission tomography after transient ischemic attack or minor ischemic stroke: case-control study. Circ Cardiovasc Imaging 2017;10(3) [pii:e004976].

61. Oliveira-Santos M, Castelo-Branco M, Silva R, et al. Atherosclerotic plaque metabolism in high cardiovascular risk subjects - a subclinical atherosclerosis imaging study with 18F-NaF PET-CT. Atherosclerosis 2017;260:41–6.

62. Raggi P, Callister TQ, Shaw LJ. Progression of coronary artery calcium and risk of first myocardial infarction in patients receiving cholesterol-lowering therapy. Arterioscler Thromb Vasc Biol 2004;24: 1272–7.

63. Irkle A, Vesey AT, Lewis DY, et al. Identifying active vascular microcalcification by (18)F-sodium fluoride positron emission tomography. Nat Commun 2015; 6:7495.

64. Murray CJ, Lopez AD. Measuring the global burden of disease. N Engl J Med 2013;369:448–57.

65. Vliegenthart R, Oudkerk M, Hofman A, et al. Coronary calcification improves cardiovascular risk prediction in the elderly. Circulation 2005;112:572–7.

66. Martin SS, Blaha MJ, Blankstein R, et al. Dyslipidemia, coronary artery calcium, and incident atherosclerotic cardiovascular disease: implications for statin therapy from the multi-ethnic study of atherosclerosis. Circulation 2014;129:77–86.

67. Doherty TM, Asotra K, Fitzpatrick LA, et al. Calcification in atherosclerosis: bone biology and chronic inflammation at the arterial crossroads. Proc Natl Acad Sci U S A 2003;100:11201–6.

68. Cocker MS, Spence JD, Hammond R, et al. [18F]-NaF PET/CT identifies active calcification in carotid plaque. JACC Cardiovasc Imaging 2017;10:486–8.

69. Cherry SR, Badawi RD, Karp JS, et al. Total-body imaging: transforming the role of positron emission tomography. Sci Transl Med 2017;9(381) [pii: eaaf6169].

70. Karp JS, Viswanath V, Geagan MJ, et al. PennPET explorer: design and preliminary performance of a whole-body imager. J Nucl Med 2020;61(1):136–43.

71. Pantel AR, Viswanath V, Daube-Witherspoon ME, et al. PennPET explorer: human imaging on a whole-body imager. J Nucl Med 2020;61(1):144–51.

72. Cherry SR, Jones T, Karp JS, et al. Total-body PET: maximizing sensitivity to create new opportunities

for clinical research and patient care. J Nucl Med 2018;59(1):3–12.

73. Zhang X, Zhou J, Cherry SR, et al. Quantitative image reconstruction for total-body PET imaging using the 2-meter long EXPLORER scanner. Phys Med Biol 2017;62(6):2465–85.

74. Badawi RD, Shi H, Hu P, et al. First human imaging studies with the EXPLORER total-body PET scanner. J Nucl Med 2019;60(3):299–303.

75. Zhang X, Xie Z, Berg E, et al. Total-body dynamic reconstruction and parametric imaging on the uEXPLORER. J Nucl Med 2020;61(2):285–91.

76. Zhang X, Cherry SR, Xie Z, et al. Subsecond total-body imaging using ultrasensitive positron emission tomography. Proc Natl Acad Sci U S A 2020;117(5):2265–7.

77. Gerke O, Ehlers K, Motschall E, et al. PET/CT-based response evaluation in cancer – a systematic review

of design issues. Mol Imaging Biol 2019. https://doi.org/10.1007/s11307-019-01351-4.

78. Høilund-Carlsen PF, Lauritzen SL, Marving J, et al. The reliability of measuring left ventricular ejection fraction by radionuclide cardiography: evaluation by the method of variance components. Br Heart J 1988;59:653–62.

79. Nensa F, Demircioglu A, Rischpler C. Artificial intelligence in nuclear medicine. J Nucl Med 2019;60(Suppl 2):29S–37S.

80. d'Amico A, Borys D, Gorczewska I. Radiomics and artificial Intelligence for PET imaging analysis. Nucl Med Rev 2020;23:36–9.

81. Oh KT, Lee S2, Lee H, et al. Semantic segmentation of white matter in FDG-PET using generative adversarial network. J Digit Imaging 2020. https://doi.org/10.1007/s10278-020-00321-5.

Potential Cardiovascular Applications of Total-body PET Imaging

Jose A. Rodriguez, MD[a], Senthil Selvaraj, MD, MA[b], Paco E. Bravo, MD[a,b,c],*

KEYWORDS

- Cardiovascular • Systemic • Whole body PET/CT

KEY POINTS

- Long axial field of view whole-body PET/CT systems is a hallmark in instrumentation development.
- It has the potential of impacting tremendously the performance of busy clinical services, but also facilitate the investigation of tissue kinetics at multiple levels simultaneously.
- It will also improve our understanding of the systemic effects and interactions of multiple cardiovascular disorders that until now had only been examined with single-frame whole body imaging.

INTRODUCTION/HISTORY/DEFINITIONS/BACKGROUND

The PennPET Explorer is a multiring system designed with a long (up to 140-cm) axial field of view (AFOV) that can image the major body organs simultaneously with higher sensitivity than that of commercial devices. The initial PennPET Explorer prototype was designed as a 3-ring–segment, 64-cm AFOV system; however, after the recent addition of 2 new ring segments, the AFOV was extended to 112 cm, and, eventually, will reach a length of 140 cm once all 6 ring segments be installed. The motivation for a long AFOV PET system is to use its high sensitivity to enhance clinical performance and to enable research applications requiring simultaneous measurement of biomarker uptake in multiple organ systems.[1,2]

This novel scanner allows a substantial improvement in dynamic imaging of the whole body with high temporal resolution, and the whole-body coverage enables simultaneous assessment of multiple organs and large vascular structures, opening previously unfathomable windows of opportunity for imaging cardiovascular disorders. There are preliminary studies that have proved the fine temporal sampling and excellent image quality of the PennPET Explorer that allows the identification of vascular structures as signal appears within the vessels.[2] This review discusses the potential cardiovascular applications for the PennPET Explorer.

POTENTIAL CARDIOVASCULAR APPLICATIONS
Multisystem Cardiovascular Disorders

Total-body PET has an immense array of opportunities that can change the methodologic research approach of multisystemic cardiovascular disorders, including amyloidosis and sarcoidosis. This new PET modality allows cardiovascular researchers to establish in an unprecedented holistic manner multiorgan dynamic PET analyses.[3] Although static PET provides an idea of a biomarker's uptake, dynamic PET with tracer kinetic modeling gives time-sensitive images that portray real-time behavior of the tissues with regards to

[a] Division of Nuclear Medicine and Clinical Molecular Imaging, Department of Radiology, Perelman School of Medicine, University of Pennsylvania, Philadelphia, PA, USA; [b] Division of Cardiovascular Medicine, Department of Medicine, Perelman School of Medicine, University of Pennsylvania, Philadelphia, PA, USA; [c] Division of Cardiothoracic Imaging, Department of Radiology, Perelman School of Medicine, University of Pennsylvania, Philadelphia, PA, USA
* Corresponding author. Hospital of the University of Pennsylvania, 3400 Civic Center Boulevard, 11-154 South Pavilion, Philadelphia, PA 19104.
E-mail address: paco.bravo@pennmedicine.upenn.edu

PET Clin 16 (2021) 129–136
https://doi.org/10.1016/j.cpet.2020.09.004
1556-8598/21/© 2020 Elsevier Inc. All rights reserved.

the tracer.[4] Furthermore, this new PET scanner has an incredibly high sensitivity, with the ability to detect throughout the whole body the location and kinetic behavior of focal pathologies, including cancer, infection, and inflammatory cardiovascular disorders, at considerably lower levels of disease activity than currently is possible with traditional PET scanners.[5]

Sarcoidosis

Sarcoidosis is an inflammatory granulomatous systemic disorder that can affect any organ, including the heart. In patients with cardiac sarcoidosis (CS), PET studies with various radiotracers show characteristic heterogenous areas of inflammation or disease activity. The role of the PennPET Explorer for CS could be to elucidate the pharmacokinetics of inflammatory radiotracers on multiple organs simultaneously. Radiotracers, such as fluorine-18 (18F)-FDG, Gallium-68-DOTA-tracers,[6] ^{18}F-FLT,[7] and ^{18}F-FMISO,[8] have the potential for assessing disease activity in CS, and the PennPET Explorer could make better use of them by studying their dynamic properties systemically. There have been previous studies that have looked into the cardiac dynamic properties of PET tracers for sarcoidosis, but the limited AFOV of standard PET scanner devices do not permit kinetic evaluation in multiple distant organs at the same moment in time. In a study by Lebasnier and colleagues[9] on 28 biopsy-proved patients with CS who underwent cardiac dynamic ^{18}F-FDG PET/computed tomography (CT) , the investigators found that ^{18}F-FDG PET/CT was significantly heterogeneous in patients with CS with that the quantitative indexes of glucose metabolism heterogeneity were significantly increased in patients with CS compared to controls.

Similarly, Dweck and colleagues[3] investigated the utility of dynamic ^{18}F-FDG imaging in 25 patients with clinical suspicion of CS on a hybrid PET–magnetic resonance (MR) system. They observed that 8 patients had increased myocardial FDG uptake without corresponding late gadolinium enhancement (LGE) on MR imaging. Patients with matching LGE and focal FDG uptake tended to have relatively little variation in myocardial FDG activity between 10 minutes and 70 minutes, whereas patients with diffuse uptake and those with focal uptake limited to the lateral wall had a clear stepwise increment of myocardial FDG activity over time, starting at 10 minutes and extending possibly beyond 70 minutes, strongly suggesting that, in the absence of LGE, these latter patterns most likely represent physiologic (from incomplete suppression) rather than pathologic FDG uptake.

It would be interesting from a research point of view to extrapolate the methodology implemented by Lebasnier and colleagues and Dweck and colleagues to assess the time to uptake of inflammatory cardiovascular biomarkers in all the commonly affected tissues in sarcoidosis simultaneously (Fig. 1). In clinical terms, a whole-body PET with high sensitivity would be ideal for isolating potential biopsy sites for diagnosis.[10]

Amyloidosis

Amyloidosis is a systemic disorder secondary to amyloid plaque deposition in any organ or tissue. The heart is one of the most frequently involved organs, and cardiac amyloidosis, if left untreated, confers a significantly worse long-term prognosis.[11] Several PET tracers, including Carbon-11 (11C)-Pittsburgh compound-B, ^{18}F-florbetaben, and ^{18}F-florbetapir, have shown high affinity and specificity for amyloid β, including myocardial amyloidosis after PET imaging. Similar to what was described previously about sarcoidosis, a whole-body dynamic PET study can make an assessment of the standardized uptake value time–activity curves for all the organs affected in amyloidosis, and identify which tissues have more avid disease. This recently was shown by Ehman and colleagues[12] in a work that included 40 patients with light chain amyloidosis who were imaged with static whole-body ^{18}F-flobetapir PET/CT to investigate light chain amyloidosis deposition in multiple organs (Fig. 2A–G). It also will be important to investigate if ^{18}F-florbetapir might be able to potentially differentiate between amyloid subtypes and/or assess treatment response based on tracer kinetics (see Fig. 2H, I). A long AFOV PET scanner, such as the PennPET Explorer, will be able to investigate the veracity of such hypotheses.

Vasculitis

Vasculitis is a heterogeneous group of disorders characterized by the presence of inflammation of blood vessel walls. Frequently, these vascular inflammatory diseases affect multiple blood vessels simultaneously.[13] Acquisition of dynamic uptake images delineating the large and middle arteries of the whole body can be done with the PennPET Explorer, expanding on the ability to understand the mechanisms of pathology of various cardiovascular disorders like vasculitis (Fig. 3).[14] Several biomarkers of inflammation bind to specific inflammatory cells, utilization of these tracers with the PennPET Explorer for vasculitis would allow a more thorough comprehension of how each specific cell is involved in the pathogenesis of specific types of vasculitis

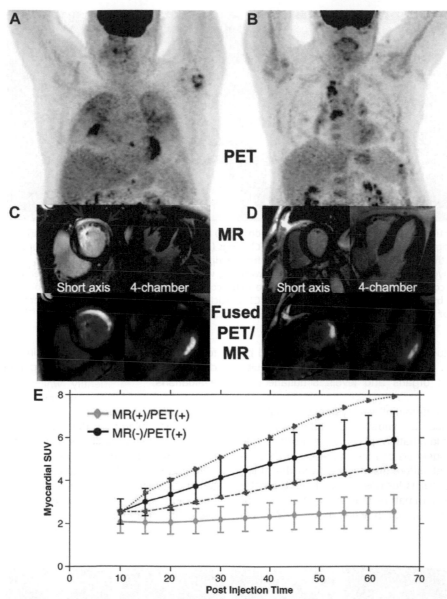

Fig. 1. Whole-body ^{18}F-FDG PET (*A-B*), cardiac MR(*C-D, upper rows*), and fused cardiac PET/MR images (*C-D, bottom rows*) of 2 individuals with sarcoidosis. Patient on the right (*A–C*) has LGE on MR (*arrows*) and FDG uptake on PET in the lateral wall (MR$^+$/PET$^+$), whereas, subject on the left (*B–C*) exhibits normal MR, but shows FDG uptake in the lateral wall on PET (MR−/PET$^+$). It was previously demonstrated that dynamic FDG kinetics (*E*) are different between MR$^+$/PET$^+$ and MR−/PET$^+$ individuals. ([*E*] *From* Dweck MR, Abgral R, Trivieri MG, et al. Hybrid Magnetic Resonance Imaging and Positron Emission Tomography With Fluorodeoxyglucose to Diagnose Active Cardiac Sarcoidosis. JACC Cardiovasc Imaging. 2018;11(1):94-107. https://doi.org/10.1016/j.jcmg.2017.02.021; with permission.)

and how these cells behave metabolically.[15] Moreover, the multiorgan changes regarding kinetic uptake of inflammatory radiotracers after appropriate treatment of vasculitis could be assessed with the PennPET Explorer, something that was not possible before the development of this total-body scanner.[16] Lamare and colleagues[17] proved with a limited AFOV PET scanner using dynamic tracing that inflammation is more prominent in symptomatic patients with vasculitis than those with clinical manifestations. In their study, the comparison of the time–activity curves of the aortic vessel wall showed that after the peak, the activity concentration in a symptomatic patients is 2-fold that in an asymptomatic patient.[17] With the PennPET

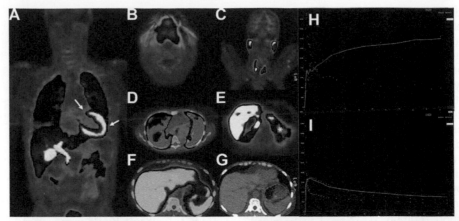

Fig. 2. Detection of multiorgan light chain amyloidosis (AL) by whole-body (*A*) ^{18}F-florbetapir PET/CT in the heart (*arrows*), tongue (*B*), parotid glands and thyroid (*C*), lungs (*D*), kidneys (*E*), and spleen (*F-G*). Florbetapir myocardial time activity curves (TAC) 0 to 60 minutes from 2 different patients. (*H*) Patient shows continuous and ascending myocardial activity over time without washout, whereas (*I*) subject exhibits no plateau of myocardial activity but constant washout. ([*A–G*] *From* Ehman and colleagues Early Detection of Multiorgan Light-Chain Amyloidosis by Whole-Body 18 F-Florbetapir PET/CT. J. Nucl. Med. 2019; 60:1234-1239; with permission; and [*H, I*] *Courtesy of* S. Dorbala, MD, Boston, MA.)

Explorer, studies, such as the that performed by Lamare and colleagues, could be done on multiple different organs and levels simultaneously (see **Fig. 3**).

The main differential with systemic vasculitis is the presence of widespread atherosclerosis, because inflammation plays an important role in the pathogenesis of atherosclerosis. PET usually excels at differentiating one from the other, because vasculitis lesions usually have a greater uptake of inflammatory biomarkers than atherosclerotic lesions, but a whole-body PET could

further characterize differences in these 2 cardiovascular entities using holistic dynamic PET evaluations.[18,19]

Myocardial infarction

Myocardial infarction (MI) is a cardiovascular emergency that constitutes one of the most common causes of morbidity and mortality worldwide. Although MI is not necessarily considered a systemic disorder, the local myocardial inflammation and injury seen after an acute MI do produce a systemic inflammatory response that has been

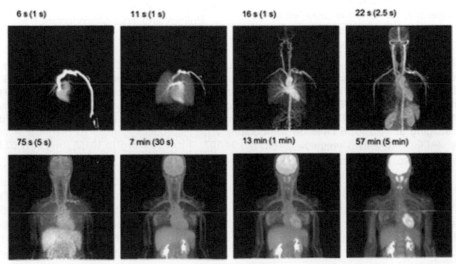

Fig. 3. ^{18}F-FDG whole-body dynamic images (frame rate in parenthesis) acquired on the PennPET Explorer with an AFOV of 64 cm. Notice the high definition of the large and medium-sized arteries in the thoracic and cerebral vasculature.

understudied until now. The PennPET Explorer allows a better assessment of this relationship and can provide further information in research of all the effects that an MI has in extracardiac tissues with dynamic PET studies. In a study on mice by Thackeray and colleagues[20] using PET imaging of the mitochondrial translocator protein (TSPO) as a marker of activated macrophages and microglia, abnormal uptake of TSPO signal in the brain correlated with cardiac signal over the full-time course of experiments. Thackeray and colleagues studied just 1 of the many organs that may be affected by the systemic effect of MI; the PennPET can provide kinetic simultaneous assessment of the impact on all organs during an MI.

Whole-body Perfusion and Blood Flow Quantification

Traditionally, PET perfusion imaging tracers have been used for detection of myocardial ischemia, but recently their pharmacodynamic properties have been studied in other vascular beds. Some of the most widely known biomarkers for perfusion include rubidium-82 (^{82}Rb), nitrogen-13 ammonia (^{13}NH$_3$), oxygen-15 water, and ^{11}C-acetate. PET imaging with perfusion radiotracers and their kinetic modeling enable noninvasive measurement of blood flow in patients with suspected or established ischemic disorders. Comparative quantification of regional blood flow can be established with the PennPET Explorer with dynamic studies in different organs at the same time, contrasting uptake differences between perfusion biomarkers in ischemic organs at distant locations. This new scanner also will allow a better pharmacokinetic comparison of perfusion radiotracers available to date, because it will be possible to assess their difference in uptake in different distant tissues.[21,22] It

will be particularly beneficial for assessment of radiotracers with short half-lives, like ^{82}Rb and ^{3}NH$_3$.[23] Individuals with coronary artery disease usually have widespread stenotic atherosclerotic plaques in other medium-to-large arteries, such as the ones located in the brain or kidneys.[24,25] The PennPET Explorer will provide cardiovascular researchers with the mean necessary to assess perfusion time–uptake defects in all vascular beds simultaneously. Moreover, this new imaging modality can help to better elucidate the physiologic fluctuations in perfusion that occur in organs, such as the heart, the brain, and the kidneys, at rest and during stress (**Fig. 4**).[26]

Additionally, there is a growing interest to investigate tumor perfusion and its relationship with prognosis and treatment response. In this sense, there are several reports on the feasibility of ^{82}Rb to assess tumor perfusion status in certain cases of multiple myeloma, lymphoma, lung, breast, and prostate cancer (**Fig. 5**).[27–29] At present, however, tumor perfusion imaging with ^{82}Rb is limited to single bed position because of the need to perform dynamic imaging for flow quantification and a very short half-life, which limit the possibility of assessing tumor flow status at distant lesions. Therefore, whole-body tumor perfusion imaging with simultaneous multisite quantification of tumor blood flow presents as an appealing future application of total-body PET imaging.

Myocardial and Peripheral Muscular Metabolism

Heart failure (HF) affects more than 6 million people in the United States and is associated with substantial morbidity and mortality in the contemporary era.[30] Although the pathophysiology remains complex, it has become increasingly clear

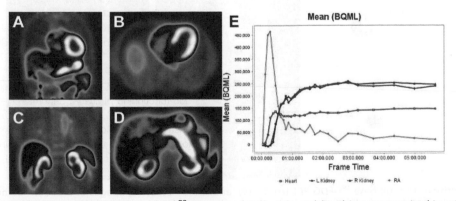

Fig. 4. Coronal (*A–C*) and axial (*B–D*) views of ^{82}Rb cardiac (*A, B*) and renal (*B–D*) images acquired in a PET/CT system with an AFOV of 26.3 cm. (*E*)^{82}Rb time activity curves (0–6 minutes) for heart and right (R) and left (L) kidneys. BQML, becquerel / milliliter; RA, right atrium.

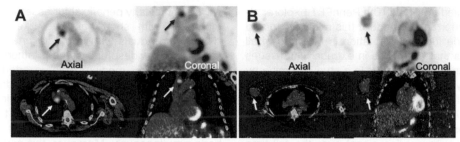

Fig. 5. ⁸²Rb PET (*top row*) and PET/CT (*bottom row*) images of 2 patients (*A, B*) exhibiting increased blood flow (*arrows*) within malignant masses. (*A*) Patient shows intense blood blow within a mediastinal mass due to poorly differentiated carcinoma. Similarly, (*B*) patient demonstrates moderately increased blood flow within a right-sided breast mass because of poorly differentiated invasive ductal carcinoma.

that metabolic derangements are relevant to the pathogenesis of HF.[31,32] The progression to clinical HF includes early impairments in myocardial fatty acid and glucose oxidation,[33] with an increasing reliance of ketone body utilization.[31,34,35] Yet, this provincial focus on the myocardium neglects the importance of the peripheral muscle in the constellation of HF symptoms,[36] because impairments in skeletal muscle fuel oxidation can impair exercise tolerance. Additionally, although sarcopenia is strongly prognostic in HF,[37] functional and metabolic assessment with radiotracers may further add to risk stratification efforts.

Because exercise limitation is the cardinal feature of patients with HF, whole-body dynamic imaging has the potential to yield substantial insights into central and peripheral muscular metabolism. Dynamic PET imaging after exercise is feasible,[38] and metabolic tracers, such as FDG or palmitate, can characterize carbohydrate and fat metabolism in different muscular beds. The PennPET Explorer scans a long AFOV of up to 140 cm (once completed), which will allow simultaneous assessment of the heart, and upper and lower extremity muscles with high sensitivity (**Fig. 6**), for example, enabling an assessment of metabolic kinetics at the peak of exercise and during recovery. Such information is useful for both understanding integrated disease pathophysiology and planning targeted therapy in HF. Ketone body–specific tracers, such as ¹¹C-acetoacetate, which are not widely available yet in the United States, will answer specific questions related to multiorgan uptake, particularly in states of ketone excess (ie, ketogenic diet or exogenous ketone

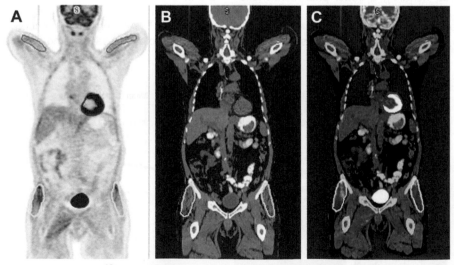

Fig. 6. Midthighs to skull base ¹⁸F-FDG PET (*A*), CT (*B*), and fused PET/CT (*C*) images of a patient demonstrating varying levels of FDG uptake in the biceps (blue contours), and quadriceps (yellow contours) muscles as well as intense FDG uptake in the heart (red contour). Dynamic quantification of multilevel muscle and heart uptake will be possible with AFOV PET/CT systems.

therapy).[31,39] Exploring such questions is not only important but timely. Sodium glucose cotransporter 2 (SGLT2) inhibitors are ketogenic and now standard of care in HF with reduced ejection fraction, given the dramatic reduction in HF hospitalizations and mortality observed with dapagliflozin.[40] Because SGLT2 inhibitors have pleiotropic effects on several different pathways and organ systems, dissecting the metabolic effects both centrally and peripherally will be important going forward.[31]

SUMMARY

In summary, the advent of long AFOV whole-body PET/CT systems is a hallmark in instrumentation development in radiology and has the potential not only of having a tremendous impact on the performance of busy clinical services but also of facilitating the investigation of tissue kinetics at multiple levels simultaneously. From a cardiovascular perspective, this unique methodology will improve significantly the understanding of the systemic effects and interactions of multiple cardiovascular disorders that until now had been examined only with single-frame, static, whole-body imaging.

DISCLOSURE

Dr S. Selvaraj receives research support from the Doris Duke Charitable Foundation (Physician Scientist Fellowship Award 2020061), the Measey Foundation, Institute for Translational Medicine and Therapeutics (Junior Investigator Preliminary/Feasibility Grant Program award), and the American Society of Nuclear Cardiology (Institute for the Advancement of Nuclear Cardiology award) for work related to ketone metabolism.

ACKNOWLEDGMENTS

The authors would like to thank Sharmila Dorbala, MD, from Brigham and Women's Hospital for facilitating some illustrations.

REFERENCES

1. Karp JS, Viswanath V, Geagan MJ, et al. Pennpet explorer: design and preliminary performance of a whole-body imager. J Nucl Med 2020;61:136–43.
2. Pantel AR, Viswanath V, Daube-Witherspoon ME, et al. Pennpet explorer: human imaging on a whole-body imager. J Nucl Med 2020;61(1):144–51.
3. Dweck MR, Abgral R, Trivieri MG, et al. Hybrid magnetic resonance imaging and positron emission tomography with fluorodeoxyglucose to diagnose active cardiac sarcoidosis. JACC Cardiovasc Imaging 2018;11(1):94–107.
4. Zhang X, Xie Z, Berg E, et al. Total-body dynamic reconstruction and parametric imaging on the uexplorer. J Nucl Med 2020;61(2):285–91.
5. Cherry SR, Jones T, Karp JS, et al. Total-body pet: maximizing sensitivity to create new opportunities for clinical research and patient care. J Nucl Med 2018;59:3–12.
6. Bravo PE, Bajaj N, Padera RF, et al. Feasibility of somatostatin receptor-targeted imaging for detection of myocardial inflammation: a pilot study. J Nucl Cardiol 2019. https://doi.org/10.1007/s12350-019-01782-0.
7. Martineau P, Pelletier-Galarneau M, Juneau D, et al. Imaging cardiac sarcoidosis with flt-pet compared with fdg/perfusion-pet: a prospective pilot study. JACC Cardiovasc Imaging 2019;12:2280–1.
8. Furuya S, Naya M, Manabe O, et al. (18)f-fmiso pet/ct detects hypoxic lesions of cardiac and extra-cardiac involvement in patients with sarcoidosis. J Nucl Cardiol 2019. https://doi.org/10.1007/s12350-019-01976-6.
9. Lebasnier A, Legallois D, Bienvenu B, et al. Diagnostic value of quantitative assessment of cardiac 18f-fluoro-2-deoxyglucose uptake in suspected cardiac sarcoidosis. Ann Nucl Med 2018;32:319–27.
10. Mañá J, Gámez C. Molecular imaging in sarcoidosis. Curr Opin Pulm Med 2011;17:325–31.
11. Baratto L, Park SY, Hatami N, et al. 18f-florbetaben whole-body PET/MRI for evaluation of systemic amyloid deposition. EJNMMI Res 2018;8:66.
12. Ehman EC, El-Sady MS, Kijewski MF, et al. Early detection of multiorgan light-chain amyloidosis by whole-body (18)f-florbetapir pet/ct. J Nucl Med 2019;60:1234–9.
13. Schnabel A, Hedrich CM. Childhood vasculitis. Front Pediatr 2019;6:421.
14. Drescher R, Freesmeyer M. Pet angiography: application of early dynamic pet/ct to the evaluation of arteries. AJR Am J Roentgenol 2013;201:908–11.
15. Goerres GW, Revesz T, Duncan J, et al. Imaging cerebral vasculitis in refractory epilepsy using [11c](r)-pk11195 positron emission tomography. AJR Am J Roentgenol 2001;176:1016–8.
16. Prieto-González S, Arguis P, Cid MC. Imaging in systemic vasculitis. Curr Opin Rheumatol 2015;27:53–62.
17. Lamare F, Hinz R, Gaemperli O, et al. Detection and quantification of large-vessel inflammation with 11c-(r)-pk11195 pet/ct. J Nucl Med 2011;52:33–9.
18. Bucerius J. Monitoring vasculitis with 18f-fdg pet. Q J Nucl Med 2016;60:219–35.
19. Belhocine T, Blockmans D, Hustinx R, et al. Imaging of large vessel vasculitis with 18fdg pet: Illusion or

reality? A critical review of the literature data. Eur J Nucl Med Mol Imaging 2003;30:1305–13.

20. Thackeray JT, Hupe HC, Wang Y, et al. Myocardial inflammation predicts remodeling and neuroinflammation after myocardial infarction. J Am Coll Cardiol 2018;71:263–75.

21. Khorsand A, Graf S, Pirich C, et al. Assessment of myocardial perfusion by dynamic n-13 ammonia pet imaging: comparison of 2 tracer kinetic models. J Nucl Cardiol 2005;12:410–7.

22. Maddahi J. Properties of an ideal pet perfusion tracer: new pet tracer cases and data. J Nucl Cardiol 2012;19:30–7.

23. Packard RRS, Huang S-C, Dahlbom M, et al. Absolute quantitation of myocardial blood flow in human subjects with or without myocardial ischemia using dynamic flurpiridaz f 18 pet. J Nucl Med 2014;55: 1438–44.

24. Kuller Lewis H, Lopez Oscar L, Gottdiener John S, et al. Subclinical atherosclerosis, cardiac and kidney function, heart failure, and dementia in the very elderly. J Am Heart Assoc 2017;6:e005353.

25. Tahari AK, Bravo PE, Rahmim A, et al. Initial human experience with rubidium-82 renal pet/ct imaging. J Med Imaging Radiat Oncol 2014;58:25–31.

26. Manabe O, Yoshinaga K, Katoh C, et al. Repeatability of rest and hyperemic myocardial blood flow measurements with 82rb dynamic pet. J Nucl Med 2009;50:68–71.

27. Mirpour S, Khandani AH. Extracardiac abnormalities on rubidium-82 cardiac positron emission tomography/computed tomography. Nucl Med Commun 2011;32:260–4.

28. Khandani AH, Commander CW, Desai H, et al. Visual and semiquantitative analysis of 82rb uptake in malignant tumors on pet/ct: first systematic analysis. Nucl Med Commun 2019;40:532–8.

29. Jochumsen MR, Tolbod LP, Pedersen BG, et al. Quantitative tumor perfusion imaging with (82)rb pet/ct in prostate cancer: analytic and clinical validation. J Nucl Med 2019;60:1059–65.

30. Benjamin EJ, Muntner P, Alonso A, et al, American Heart Association Council on Epidemiology and Prevention Statistics Committee and Stroke Statistics Subcommittee. Heart disease and stroke statistics-2019 update: a report from the American Heart Association. Circulation 2019;139:e56–528.

31. Selvaraj S, Kelly DP, Margulies KB. Implications of altered ketone metabolism and therapeutic ketosis in heart failure. Circulation 2020;141:1800–12.

32. Neubauer S. The failing heart–an engine out of fuel. N Engl J Med 2007;356:1140–51.

33. De Jong KA, Lopaschuk GD. Complex energy metabolic changes in heart failure with preserved ejection fraction and heart failure with reduced ejection fraction. Can J Cardiol 2017;33:860–71.

34. Horton JL, Davidson MT, Kurishima C, et al. The failing heart utilizes 3-hydroxybutyrate as a metabolic stress defense. JCI Insight 2019;4:e124079.

35. Nielsen R, Moller N, Gormsen LC, et al. Cardiovascular effects of treatment with the ketone body 3-hydroxybutyrate in chronic heart failure patients. Circulation 2019;139:2129–41.

36. Zamani P, Proto EA, Mazurek JA, et al. Peripheral determinants of oxygen utilization in heart failure with preserved ejection fraction: central role of adiposity. JACC Basic Transl Sci 2020;5:211–25.

37. Selvaraj S, Kim J, Ansari BA, et al. Body composition, natriuretic peptides, and adverse outcomes in heart failure with preserved and reduced ejection fraction. JACC Cardiovasc Imaging 2020. https://doi.org/10.1016/j.jcmg.2020.07.022.

38. Kemppainen J, Fujimoto T, Kalliokoski KK, et al. Myocardial and skeletal muscle glucose uptake during exercise in humans. J Physiol 2002;542:403–12.

39. Cuenoud B, Hartweg M, Godin JP, et al. Metabolism of exogenous d-beta-hydroxybutyrate, an energy substrate avidly consumed by the heart and kidney. Front Nutr 2020;7:13.

40. McMurray JJV, Solomon SD, Inzucchi SE, et al, DAPA-HF Trial Committees and Investigators. Dapagliflozin in patients with heart failure and reduced ejection fraction. N Engl J Med 2019;381(21): 1995–2008.

Frontiers in Neuroscience Imaging: Whole-Body PET

Ashesh A. Thaker, MD[a], Austin L. Chien, BA[b], Jacob G. Dubroff, MD, PhD[c],*

KEYWORDS

- Receptor • PET • Proteinopathy • Neurotransmitter • Pharmacokinetics • Pharmacodynamics
- Addiction • Dementia

KEY POINTS

- Neuroscience PET imaging has largely focused on the brain; however, the nervous system is present throughout the body with diverse receptors.
- Whole-body PET imaging will permit new insights into neuronal physiology. In turn, this could improve our understanding and treatment of neuropsychiatric disease, including addiction and depression.
- Understanding of abnormal protein accumulation, implicated in neurodegenerative diseases such as Alzheimer's and Parkinson's, continues to evolve and requires a whole-body approach.
- Direct visualization and measurement of drug distribution and metabolism using whole-body PET imaging will encourage nervous system-targeting drug development.

INTRODUCTION

The age of whole-body PET instrumentation will present unique opportunities across medicine and science. When Reivich and colleagues[1] published the first [^{18}F]fluorodeoxyglucose-PET image in 1979, no one could have predicted the magnitude of growth it would undergo, including instrumentation (ie, PennPET Explorer), radiochemistry, and clinical applications. In this article, the authors first provide an overview of whole-body nervous system organization because the field has principally focused on only the brain. They then examine different neuropsychiatric diseases and their respective interfaces with the nervous system from a more holistic view suited to match the broader lens of the Explorer instrument.

HUMAN NERVOUS SYSTEM OVERVIEW

The human nervous system can be organized into the central nervous system (CNS), comprising the brain and spinal cord, and the peripheral nervous system (PNS), comprising the somatic, autonomic, and enteric nervous system (ENS). The autonomic nervous system can be further subdivided into sympathetic and parasympathetic nervous systems.[2]

The brain serves as the primary hub of sensory reception and motor control. It includes the cerebral hemispheres, which harbor sensorimotor cortices and influence processes such as judgment, abstract reasoning, and emotion. Subcortically, the thalamus and hypothalamus relay sensory information to cortical regions and manage emotional responses, autonomic functions, and hormone synthesis. Basal ganglia occupy the gray matter space between the cortical surface and deep subcortical structures.[2–4] Within the posterior fossa, the cerebellum is involved in muscular control of balance and equilibrium. Purkinje cells within the cerebellum respond to excitatory glutamate neurotransmitters and deliver inhibitory signals using gamma-aminobutyric acid (GABA).[2–4]

[a] Department of Radiology, University of Colorado Anschutz Medical Campus, 12401 E 17th Ave, Aurora, CO 80045, USA; [b] Rutgers Robert Wood Johnson Medical School, 675 Hoes Lane West, Piscataway, NJ 08854, USA; [c] Division of Nuclear Medicine and Clinical Molecular Imaging, Perelman School of Medicine at the University of Pennsylvania, 3400 Spruce Street, 1 Silverstein, Philadelphia, PA 19104, USA
* Corresponding author.
E-mail address: jacob.dubroff@pennmedicine.upenn.edu

PET Clin 16 (2021) 137–146
https://doi.org/10.1016/j.cpet.2020.09.014
1556-8598/21/© 2020 Elsevier Inc. All rights reserved.

The brain stem comprises the midbrain, pons, and medulla, through which all descending and ascending tracts pass into the spinal cord or cerebral cortex, respectively. Most cranial nerve nuclei are located in the brain stem. The brain stem also conveys 3 monoaminergic pathways (serotonergic, noradrenergic, and dopaminergic).[2,3] The blood-brain barrier consists of capillary endothelial cells, which form tight junctions; adjoining astrocytes, which secrete chemicals to regulate endothelial permeability; and an underlying basement membrane. The blood-brain barrier thus forms a selectively permeable filter for substances to reach the CNS and is an important consideration for PET radiotracer development.[2,3]

The spinal cord is the source of 31 pairs of spinal nerves associated with individual vertebral levels. The conus medullaris terminates near the L1/L2 spinal level, with several nerves continuing inferiorly as the cauda equina. Spinal nerves begin in the gray matter of the spinal cord. The dorsal horn contains sensory cell bodies, the ventral horn has motor neuron cell bodies, and the intermediolateral horn has sympathetic nervous system cell bodies. Ventral and dorsal roots for a given vertebral level fuse to form a complete spinal nerve, which then subdivides into ventral and dorsal rami. White matter, made up of myelinated and unmyelinated nerve fibers, form columns and tracts that surround gray matter horns and relay information between the spine and other CNS components.[2,3,5]

The PNS has somatic and autonomic divisions. The somatic division provides signaling to and from body wall structures (skin, muscles, and mucous membranes). Spinal nerve ventral rami innervate muscles of the trunk and limbs and enable sensation from skin of the neck, ventrolateral torso, and limbs. Dorsal rami innervate vertebral facet joints and intrinsic back muscles and receive sensory information from skin of the back.[2,3] The autonomic nervous system includes sympathetic and parasympathetic divisions and controls many involuntary functions. Both divisions use preganglionic neurons and postganglionic neurons to transmit signals but differ in starting vertebral levels, and length of preganglionic signals.[2,3,5]

Sympathetic division nerves originate from lateral horns of vertebral levels T1-L2 (Fig. 1) and travel via ventral rami to reach trunk (paravertebral) ganglia where they synapse or pass through to reach collateral (prevertebral) ganglia, which can send postsynaptic signals to gut viscera as part of the ENS.[2–4] The first synapse of sympathetic signaling (at either trunk ganglia or collateral ganglia) always has a postsynaptic nicotinic receptor for acetylcholine neurotransmitters.

Terminal receptors of the sympathetic nervous system vary depending on the postsynaptic target. Most final sympathetic targets, including cardiac and smooth muscle, gland cells, and various nerve terminals, use adrenergic receptors, which respond to norepinephrine-binding. Other sympathetic targets include sweat glands, which have muscarinic receptors for acetylcholine; renal vasculature and smooth muscle, which have dopaminergic receptors for inhibitory dopamine signaling; and the adrenal medulla, which has nicotinic receptors for acetylcholine.[2,3,5]

The parasympathetic division of the autonomic nervous system begins in select cranial nerves from the brain (CN III, VII, IX, and X) and sacral levels S2-S4 (see Fig. 1). Preganglionic parasympathetic neurons synapse directly at terminal ganglia near target organs using nicotinic receptors for acetylcholine, while terminal parasympathetic neurons synapse at muscarinic tissue receptors for acetylcholine.[2,5]

The final division of the PNS is the ENS, which supplies muscles, glands, and sensory nerves of gastrointestinal organs. The ENS consists of millions of neurons that form ganglia interspersed throughout the gastrointestinal system. The interconnections of these ganglia form 2 plexuses: the myenteric plexus (or Auerbach plexus), which is located between the muscular layers of the gastrointestinal tract, and the submucosal plexus (or Meissner plexus) in the submucosa of the gastrointestinal tract. Both plexuses have sympathetic and parasympathetic components. The myenteric plexus's functions can be summarized as control of gastrointestinal muscular contraction and peristalsis, while the submucosal plexus controls fluid transport and secretion for the gastrointestinal system.[2,3]

Parasympathetic neurons synapse with enteric neurons using acetylcholine as a neurotransmitter for nicotinic and muscarinic receptors, which transmit excitatory signals. Conversely, sympathetic signals are received by adrenergic receptors for norepinephrine on enteric neurons. These sympathetic synapses occur at collateral ganglia, which include the celiac, superior mesenteric, and inferior mesenteric ganglia (see Fig. 1). Afferent signaling from the gastrointestinal system begins at sensory receptors and reaches the CNS via vagus and splanchnic nerves. Gastrointestinal afferent neuronal cell bodies are located in the inferior ganglion of the vagus nerve.[2,5]

There are different mechanisms of action for the numerous neuroreceptors throughout the nervous system. For example, nicotinic receptors respond to acetylcholine binding by triggering the opening of ligand-gated ion channels. Nicotinic

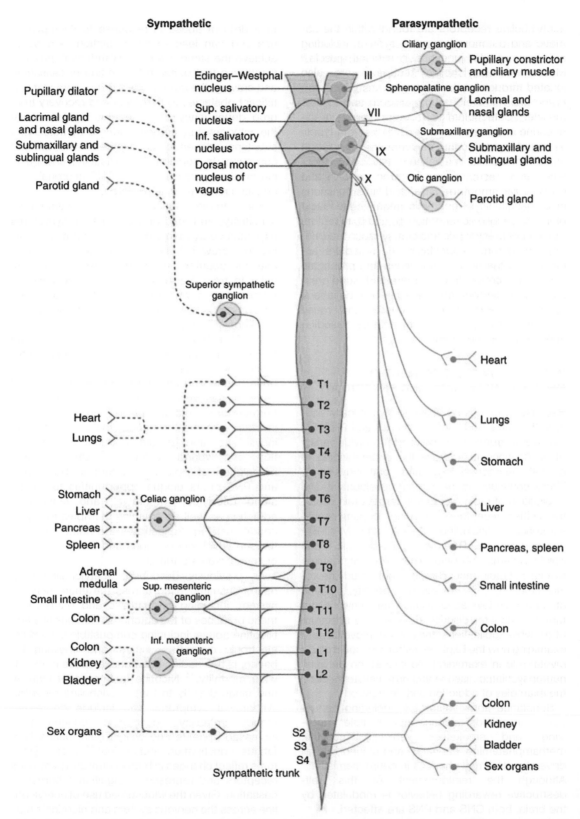

Fig. 1. The sympathetic nervous system and its sympathetic (thoracolumbar) and parasympathetic (craniosacral) divisions. Inf., inferior; Sup., superior. Waxman SG. The Autonomic Nervous System, *Clinical Neuroanatomy, 28e;* McGraw-Hill Education. 2017.

acetylcholine receptors are found within the somatic and autonomic nervous system, including at neuromuscular junctions in skeletal muscle.[6] Muscarinic acetylcholine receptors are also located throughout the nervous system, including in the brain as well as both smooth and cardiac muscle.[6] Catecholamine receptors bind norepinephrine and are categorized into α and β types. α_1 receptors are located on peripheral vasculature smooth muscle for mediation of vasoconstriction, whereas α_2 receptors are found in the CNS and on vascular smooth muscle, and have functions in preganglionic sympathetic negative-feedback, or in postganglionic reception. β_1 and β_2 receptors function as presynaptic and postsynaptic β-adrenergic receptors, respectively. β_1 receptors are located on the heart and kidneys and propagate signals to increase the heart rate and blood pressure. β_2 receptors are generally on peripheral vasculature and bronchial muscle and cause relaxation of target smooth muscle (ie, vasodilation and bronchodilation).[2,3]

WHOLE-BODY MEASUREMENT OF NEUROTRANSMISSION AND PHYSIOLOGY

Because of its unique ability to dynamically visualize the entire body, including CNS and PNS, the Explorer instrument can be used for a wide variety of applications to improve the understanding of normal neurophysiology and pathophysiology. There continues to be strong development and application of radiotracers that target brain neurotransmitter receptors, including dopaminergic,[7] serotonergic (including MAO-A and MAO-B),[8] cholinergic,[9–11] GABAergic,[12] glutamatergic,[13] and opioid systems.[14] Additional neurologically focused avenues of radiotracer development include neuroinflammation,[15–18] synaptic density,[19] and abnormal protein accumulation (ie, amyloid and tau),[20–23] as later discussed. Given the spectrum of possible applications, the authors move forward examining how the Explorer instrument could play a pivotal role in examining the interaction between neuropsychiatric disease and organ systems using the examples of addiction and depression.

Substance abuse disorders, including dependence on opioids, nicotine (combustible, vaporizing, and smokeless vehicles), cocaine, methamphetamine, cannabis, and alcohol, are all driven by abnormal changes in neurochemistry.[24] Although the reinforcement of this self-destructive rewarding behavior is modulated by the brain, both CNS and PNS are affected.

Tolerance, withdrawal, and craving are important behaviors associated with drug dependence and recovery. Tolerance is a diminished reaction to a drug of abuse in response to its repeated use and can lead to an escalation in dose to achieve the same reward.[25] Withdrawal, physical symptoms that occur in the setting of cessation, and craving, the urge to use a drug, represent significant obstacles to treatment and recovery from drug dependency.[26,27] The PNS can modulate the withdrawal symptoms endured by those with substance dependence disorders who attempt cessation. In addition, the plasticity, change in neuronal networking, of extra-CNS neuronal connections remains underexplored.

For example, nausea, diarrhea, sweating, pain sensitivity, and loss of libido are all symptoms experienced by opiate use disorder patients during withdrawal.[28] Loperamide is a common, over-the-counter μ-opioid receptor agonist used to treat diarrhea because of its ability to decrease parasympathetic tone of smooth muscle contractions in the intestines. μ-opioid receptor agonist abused drugs, such as heroin or oxycodone, have the same effect. As a substrate of P-glycoprotein, however, loperamide in pharmacologic doses does not cross the blood-brain barrier and interact with CNS receptors.[29] Thus, it has very limited potential for abuse. Furthermore, opioids act as neurotransmitters in other systems throughout the body affecting insulin secretion, steroid production, inflammation, and wound healing.[30–32] Understanding modulation of opioid receptors in both CNS and PNS offers unique opportunities to understand tolerance, withdrawal, and craving in addiction as well as optimize therapies for other conditions. **Fig. 2** illustrates the numerous systems in which endogenous and exogenous opioids can regulate function.[33]

As previously described, acetylcholine is a neurotransmitter used across the entire nervous system, including sympathetic and parasympathetic branches of the autonomic nervous system. Nicotine abuse, including combustible cigarettes, electronic cigarettes, cigars, and chewing tobacco, is the leading preventable cause of worldwide mortality.[34] Nicotine imitates acetylcholine and binds directly to the acetylcholine receptor. Withdrawal symptoms can include depressed mood, irritability, decreased concentration, increased appetite and weight gain, headaches, fatigue, constipation, and anxiety.[35] These symptoms reflect changes in both central and peripheral receptors and represent a significant barrier to cessation. Given the widespread use of acetylcholine across the nervous system and nicotine's high affinity for many of them (nicotinic vs muscarinic), one can see how nicotine abuse and cessation affect the entire body.

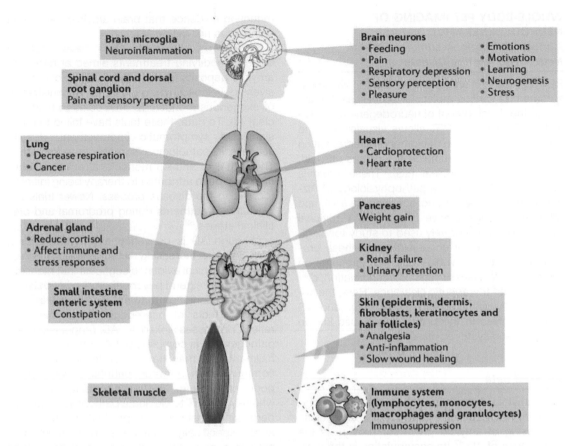

Fig. 2. The human body naturally synthetizes opioids, which are used as neurotransmitters to regulate many vital functions. Endogenous and exogenous opioids act through receptors found peripherally on nerve terminals innervating the adrenal glands, pancreas, and gastrointestinal tract and on immune, epidermal, and dermal cells, thus modulating steroid production, body weight via insulin secretion, opioid-induced constipation, inflammation, and wound healing. *From* Kibaly, C., Xu, C., Cahill, C.M. et al. Non-nociceptive roles of opioids in the CNS: opioids' effects on neurogenesis, learning, memory and affect. Nat Rev Neurosci 20, 5–18 (2019); with permission.

Depression remains a clinically significant problem.[36] When pharmacotherapy is required, serotonergic-specific reuptake inhibitors (SSRIs) are often used.[36] During the decades that these drugs have been successfully developed and implemented, the connections between CNS and gastrointestinal tract, lined with smooth muscle and largely governed by the parasympathetic nervous system, have been explored. Anatomists have long recognized the dorsal nucleus of the vagus nerve, which originates in the medulla and carries parasympathetic efferents to the gut. However, work pioneered by Gershon[37] has shown that serotonin, the same neurotransmitter targeted by pharmacotherapy for depression, is used by myenteric interneurons. More than 90% of serotonin in the body is produced in the gut.[38,39] There is an elevated prevalence of depression and anxiety in patients with inflammatory bowel disease (IBD), such as Crohn disease.[40,41]

More recently, the relationship between gut microbiota and brain has been better elucidated,[42,43] particularly in the setting of depression.[43,44] There is evidence that suggests gut microbiota regulate serotonin synthesis.[45] Furthermore, SSRIs can modulate gut microbiota.[46] Although PET has been used to characterize SSRI serotonergic neurotransmission and receptor effects in brain, PET has not yet been used to examine the whole body, including the enteric system. The Explorer instrument appears well poised to examine serotonergic signaling in the brain and gut, simultaneously, in studying the guts of patients with depression and the brains of patients with IBD (and vice versa).

WHOLE-BODY PET IMAGING OF NEURODEGENERATIVE DISEASE
Abnormal Protein Accumulation and Neurodegenerative Disease

PET represents a unique tool to allow in vivo measurement of various molecular processes that are key to the development of neurodegenerative disorders. Specifically, PET allows visualization and quantifiable evaluation of biomarkers representing abnormal protein accumulation, such as amyloid, tau, and alpha-synuclein (αS). These proteins play a critical role in the pathophysiology of Alzheimer disease (AD), Parkinson disease (PD), and other neurodegenerative diseases. Traditional PET has been extensively used to study topological and longitudinal accumulation of these proteins in the brain; whole-body PET presents an opportunity to assess systemic accumulation, distribution, and therapeutic clearance. Here, the authors briefly summarize amyloid, tau, and αS proteinopathies in the brain and discuss known and theoretic systemic dissemination.

Amyloid Beta

The amyloid hypothesis proposes that beta-amyloid (Aβ), a peptide produced by proteolytic processing of amyloid precursor protein, is the main cause of AD.[47] Its accumulation is the main component of senile plaques seen at brain autopsy and distributed widely throughout the neocortex in AD-affected individuals.[48] In the amyloid cascade hypothesis, increasing Aβ production and accumulation results in deposition of diffuse plaques within the brain, which in turn causes microglial and astrocytic activation, ultimately leading to progressive synaptic and neuronal dysfunction and injury. The most widely studied amyloid imaging agent is Pittsburgh compound-B (PIB), a C-11 radiotracer, which specifically binds extracellular and intravascular fibrillar Aβ. Neuropathologic studies have shown strong correlations between regional in vivo PET signal and in vitro measures of Aβ pathologic condition found at autopsy.[49] PIB distribution, binding, and kinetics have been extensively studied in the brain.[50,51] Newer F-18 tracers, such as florbetapir, have recently been approved by the Food and Drug Administration, have a longer half-life, and do not require on-site cyclotron production. Although found in high cortical concentration in AD patients, many studies have demonstrated imaging biomarker evidence of brain amyloid pathologic condition in cognitively normal patients and those with mild cognitive impairment.[49] Varying symptoms among these populations supports

mounting evidence that brain amyloid deposition alone does not define AD.

Several recent clinical trials have explored disease-modifying treatments aimed at removing amyloid deposits from the brain. The most extensively developed approach uses administration of exogenous monoclonal antibodies to bind and clear Aβ. To date, these trials have failed to show significant symptomatic improvement, despite success in pathologic clearance from the brain. The failure of anti-Aβ monoclonal antibody trials has often been attributed to therapy being initiated too late in the disease process. Newer trials are evaluating treatments during prodromal and preclinical stages.[52]

Although AD is conventionally regarded as a CNS disorder, increasing experimental, epidemiologic, and clinical evidence suggests that manifestations of AD extend beyond the brain.[53] Systemic pathologic condition may not simply reflect secondary effects of neurodegeneration but may reflect processes linked to AD progression. AD pathogenesis is complex, but Aβ remains a major hallmark and may have a systemic role, given communication between peripheral and central pools of Aβ (**Fig. 3**). An opportunity exists for whole-body PET to elucidate pathophysiologic underpinnings between Aβ production and clearance. Specifically, radiotracer biomarkers may provide a more thorough understanding of how peripheral systems may be involved in Aβ production and clearance, working synergistically to clear Aβ from the brain. Moreover, several systemic abnormalities have been found in AD, including disorders of immunity and inflammation, cardiovascular systems, hepatic and renal dysfunction, metabolic disorders, and gut microbiome disturbances.[53] A systemic view of AD is a novel perspective for understanding the role of Aβ in AD pathogenesis and offers opportunities for the development of new treatments and diagnostic biomarkers for AD.

Tau

Hyperphosphorylation and abnormal aggregation of tau, a microtubule-associated protein essential to neuronal stability and functioning, are implicated in various neurodegenerative diseases known as tauopathies, the most common of which is AD. In addition to formation and deposition of Aβ plaques, the aggregation of tau into paired helical filaments and subsequently neurofibrillary tangles (NFTs) is a hallmark and defining feature of AD.[48,54] Neuropathologic studies indicate a stereotyped topology of NFTs, defined according to successive "Braak stages" initially involving entorhinal and mesial temporal regions (I-II), before

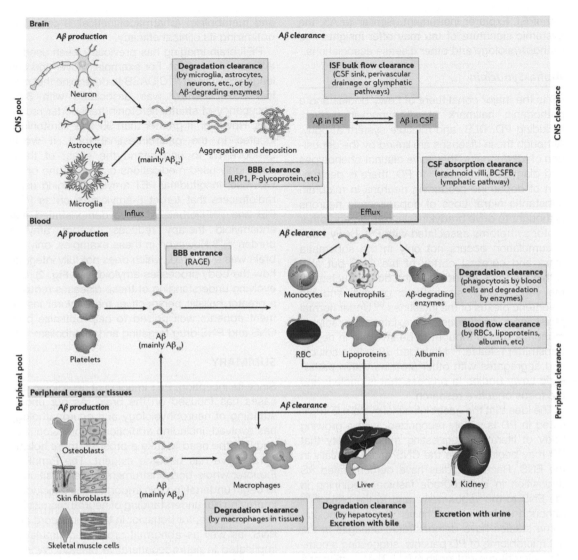

Fig. 3. Aβ is generated by neurons, microglia, and astrocytes in the brain, and by platelets, skin fibroblasts, osteoblasts, and skeletal muscle cells in the periphery. The CNS and peripheral pools of Aβ can interact; some Aβ peptides in the CNS are cleared via phagocytosis or proteolytic degradation, whereas others are released into the blood via the blood-brain barrier (BBB), interstitial fluid (ISF), bulk flow, or cerebrospinal fluid (CSF) egress pathways. Some Aβ peptides in blood are phagocytosed, including by monocytes or neutrophils; some are degraded by Aβ-degrading enzymes; and some are transported by carriers (such as erythrocytes, albumin, and lipoproteins) to peripheral organs or tissues, where they are degraded by macrophages or hepatocytes, or excreted via the liver or kidney. BCSFB, blood-CSF barrier; RAGE, receptor for advanced glycation end products; RBC, red blood cell. *From* Wang, J., Gu, B., Masters, C. et al. A systemic view of Alzheimer disease — insights from amyloid-β metabolism beyond the brain. Nat Rev Neurol 13, 612–623 (2017); with permission.

spreading to limbic (III-IV), and neocortical regions (V-VI).[55] Other types of tau deposits are present in various tauopathies, including progressive supranuclear palsy, corticobasal degeneration, and related conditions, such as Down syndrome, Parkinson disease (PD), and dementia with Lewy bodies (DLB).[56] Several tau radiotracers have recently been developed and are now in second generation, with increased specificity. Although

hyperphosphorylated tau resides predominantly intracellularly, studies have demonstrated clearance of extracellular tau via dural lymphatic or "glymphatic" paravascular channels.[57,58] Cerebrospinal fluid phosphorylated tau and total tau are routine biomarkers assessed in AD. Nonetheless, systemic clearance and distribution of extracellular tau beyond the CNS are largely unknown, offering an avenue of investigation for the

PennPET Explorer instrument. Similar to Aβ, the systemic signature of tau may offer insights into pathophysiology and other disease associations.

Alpha-Synuclein

αS is the major constituent of Lewy bodies and a pathogenic hallmark of all synucleinopathies, including PD, DLB, and multiple system atrophy. Although these diseases are linked by the deposition of αS deposits, they have distinct phenotypes and diagnostic criteria.[59] In PD, there is destruction of dopamine-producing neurons in midbrain substantia nigra. Loss of dopaminergic neurons is thought to drive bradykinesia, tremor, and other motor symptoms associated with PD. Lewy body accumulation occurs not only in the substantia nigra and cerebral cortex of the CNS but also within the PNS, including at the dorsal nucleus of the vagus nerve, sympathetic ganglia, and the myenteric plexus of the intestines.[60] Under normal physiologic conditions, αS exists as a soluble monomer and is thought to be involved in neurotransmitter release.[61] Misfolded αS is less soluble and aggregates with other proteins within pathologic Lewy bodies, a process that is unclear and the focus of active research.

The idea that the gastrointestinal system is implicated in PD is widely recognized, with a growing body of literature suggesting the possibility that PD may begin outside the CNS and potentially in the ENS. Recent studies have demonstrated αS deposition in a retrograde fashion, beginning in the ENS to the vagus nerve and to the brain.[60,62] Although underlying mechanisms remain unclear, some studies have demonstrated changes in the gut microbiome of PD patients, suggesting a complex microbiome-gut-brain axis.[60] The creation of a specific PET ligand for αS is an area of active research, highly suitable for whole-body PET imaging using the Explorer instrument.

EVALUATION OF PHARMACOTHERAPIES: PHARMACOKINETICS AND PHARMACODYNAMICS

CNS dysfunction has been implicated in the disorders touched upon in this review. Appropriately, their respective treatments have largely targeted the CNS. However, as our understanding of these diseases evolves, it is becoming more evident that whole-body pathophysiology remains underexplored. Furthermore, design and targeting of pharmacotherapy for these diseases such as consideration of blood-brain barrier kinetics also need to be addressed. When developing a therapeutic approach, understanding a drug's effect (pharmacodynamics) as well as its breakdown

and metabolism (pharmacokinetics) is critical to optimizing its clinical efficacy.

PET brain imaging has previously been used to evaluate drug effect. For example, Meyer and colleagues[63,64] used [11C]DASB to determine that clinical SSRI therapy was associated with 80% occupancy of striatal serotonin transporter receptors. However, if greater than 90% of serotonin is located in the gastrointestinal tract, it would behoove us to understand the effect of these commonly used medications outside of the brain. Likewise, longitudinal PET amyloid imaging using radiotracers that target β-amyloid, such as [11C]PiB and [18F]florbetapir, have demonstrated that antiamyloid therapy reduces cerebral amyloid burden.[65,66] However, in these examples, only the brain was evaluated, which does not fully integrate how the body processes amyloid (see **Fig. 2**). Our evolving understanding of these diseases requires a greater holistic perspective; the Explorer instrument appears well poised to help optimize both CNS and PNS drug targeting and metabolism.

SUMMARY

Since its inception, PET imaging of neurologic diseases has focused on the brain. As our understanding of neurophysiology and neuropathology has evolved, including addiction, depression, AD, and PD, the need to take a broader, more holistic perspective has become evident. The PennPET Explorer whole-body instrument is well positioned to begin undertaking this important task, including improving our understanding of neurotransmission and neuroreceptor behavior in the spinal cord and PNS, as well as abnormal protein accumulation implicated in neurodegenerative disease. Whole-body PET imaging will be critical for the design and development of new pharmacotherapies to understand their metabolism and efficacy. The PennPET Explorer's generous 1.4-m axial field of view permits simultaneous, high-resolution measurement of brain, spinal cord, and all organs in the chest, abdomen, and pelvis. This enables investigators to use a multitude of novel approaches, including examples outlined in this review. New radiotracers will be required; however, advancements in radiochemistry will spur additional avenues of research.

DISCLOSURE

The authors have nothing to disclose.

REFERENCES

1. Reivich M, Kuhl D, Wolf A. The [18F]fluorodeoxyglucose method for the measurement of local cerebral

glucose utilization in man. Circ Res 1979;44(1): 127–37.

2. Waxman S. Clinical Neuroanatomy. 29th edition. New York: McGraw-Hill; 2020.

3. Haines DE, Mihailoff GA, Cunningham WK, et al. Fundamental neuroscience for basic and clinical applications. 5th edition. Philadelphia, PA: Elsevier; 2018.

4. Purves D, Augustine GJ, Fitzpatrick D, et al, editors. Neuroscience. 6th edition. New York: Oxford University Press; 2017.

5. Kandel ER, Schwartz JH, Jessell TM, et al, editors. Principles of neural science. 5th edition. New York: McGraw-Hill; 2013.

6. Carlson AB, Kraus GO. Physiology, cholinergic receptors. In: StatPearls. Treasure Island, FL: StatPearls Publishing; 2018.

7. Doot RK, Dubroff JG, Labban KJ, et al. Selectivity of probes for PET imaging of dopamine D3 receptors. Neurosci Lett 2019;691:18–25.

8. Paterson LM, Kornum BR, Nutt DJ, et al. 5-HT radioligands for human brain imaging with PET and SPECT. Med Res Rev 2013;33(1):54–111.

9. Coughlin JM, Slania S, Du Y, et al. 18F-XTRA PET for enhanced imaging of the extrathalamic $\alpha4\beta2$ nicotinic acetylcholine receptor. J Nucl Med 2018; 59(10):1603–8.

10. Smits R, Fischer S, Hiller A, et al. Synthesis and biological evaluation of both enantiomers of [18F]flubatine, promising radiotracers with fast kinetics for the imaging of $\alpha4\beta2$-nicotinic acetylcholine receptors. Bioorg Med Chem 2014;22(2):804–12.

11. Horti AG. Development of [18F]ASEM, a specific radiotracer for quantification of the $\alpha7$-nAChR with positron-emission tomography. Biochem Pharmacol 2015;97(4):566–75.

12. Murrell E, Pham JM, Sowa AR, et al. Classics in neuroimaging: development of positron emission tomography tracers for imaging the GABAergic pathway. ACS Chem Neurosci 2020;11(14):2039–44.

13. Bhatt S, Hillmer AT, Girgenti MJ, et al. PTSD is associated with neuroimmune suppression: evidence from PET imaging and postmortem transcriptomic studies. Nat Commun 2020;11(1):1–11.

14. Li S, Zheng MQ, Naganawa M, et al. Development and in vivo evaluation of a k-opioid receptor agonist as a PET radiotracer with superior imaging characteristics. J Nucl Med 2019;60(7):1023–30.

15. Hou C, Hsieh CJ, Li S, et al. Development of a positron emission tomography radiotracer for imaging elevated levels of superoxide in neuroinflammation. ACS Chem Neurosci 2018;9(3):578–86.

16. Janssen B, Vugts DJ, Windhorst AD, et al. PET imaging of microglial activation - beyond targeting TSPO. Molecules 2018;23(3):607.

17. Shrestha S, Kim MJ, Eldridge M, et al. PET measurement of cyclooxygenase-2 using a novel radioligand: upregulation in primate neuroinflammation and first-in-human study. J Neuroinflammation 2020;17(1):140.

18. Jain P, Chaney AM, Carlson ML, et al. Neuroinflammation PET imaging: current opinion and future directions. J Nucl Med 2020;61(8):1107–12.

19. Finnema SJ, Nabulsi NB, Eid T, et al. Imaging synaptic density in the living human brain. Sci Transl Med. 2016 Jul 20;8(348):348ra96.

20. Ikonomovic MD, Buckley CJ, Heurling K, et al. Postmortem histopathology underlying β-amyloid PET imaging following flutemetamol F 18 injection. Acta Neuropathol Commun 2016;4(1):130.

21. Clark CM, Schneider JA, Bedell BJ, et al. Use of florbetapir-PET for imaging β-amyloid pathology. JAMA 2011;305(3):275–83.

22. Hammes J, Bischof G, Bohn K, et al. One stop shop: flortaucipir PET differentiates amyloid positive and negative forms of neurodegenerative diseases. jnumed. J Nucl Med 2020;120:244061. Published online.

23. Marquié M, Normandin MD, Vanderburg CR, et al. Validating novel tau positron emission tomography tracer [F-18]-AV-1451 (T807) on postmortem brain tissue. Ann Neurol 2015;78(5):787–800.

24. Volkow ND, Boyle M. Neuroscience of addiction: relevance to prevention and treatment. Am J Psychiatry 2018;175(8):729–40.

25. Harrison LM, Kastin AJ, Zadina JE. Opiate tolerance and dependence: receptors, G-proteins, and antiopiates. Peptides 1998;19(9):1603–30.

26. Koob GF. Drug addiction: the yin and yang of hedonic homeostasis. Neuron 1996;16(5):893–6.

27. Koob GF, Volkow ND. Neurobiology of addiction: a neurocircuitry analysis. Lancet Psychiatry 2016; 3(8):760–73.

28. Schuckit MA. Treatment of opioid-use disorders. N Engl J Med 2016;375(4):357–68.

29. Linnet K, Ejsing TB. A review on the impact of P-glycoprotein on the penetration of drugs into the brain. Focus on psychotropic drugs. Eur Neuropsychopharmacol 2008;18(3):157–69.

30. Wen T, Peng B, Pintar JE. The MOR-1 opioid receptor regulates glucose homeostasis by modulating insulin secretion. Mol Endocrinol 2009;23(5):671–8.

31. Stein C, Küchler S. Targeting inflammation and wound healing by opioids. Trends Pharmacol Sci 2013;34(6):303–12.

32. Kapas S, Purbrick A, Hinson JP. Action of opioid peptides on the rat adrenal cortex: stimulation of steroid secretion through a specific mu opioid receptor. J Endocrinol 1995;144:503–10.

33. Kibaly C, Xu C, Cahill CM, et al. Non-nociceptive roles of opioids in the CNS: opioids' effects on neurogenesis, learning, memory and affect. Nat Rev Neurosci 2019;20(1):5–18.

34. Gakidou E, Afshin A, Abajobir AA, et al. Global, regional, and national comparative risk assessment

of 84 behavioural, environmental and occupational, and metabolic risks or clusters of risks, 1990-2016: a systematic analysis for the Global Burden of Disease Study 2016. Lancet 2017;390(10100): 1345–422.

35. Mclaughlin I, Dani JA, De Biasi M. Nicotine withdrawal medial habenula. Curr Top Behav Neurosci 2015;99–123.

36. Park LT, Zarate CA. Jr.Depression in the Primary Care Setting. N Engl J Med 2019;380(6):559–68.

37. Gershon MD. Enteric serotonergic neurones... finally! J Physiol 2009;587(3):507.

38. Gershon MD, Tack J. The serotonin signaling system: from basic understanding to drug development for functional GI disorders. Gastroenterology 2007; 132(1):397–414.

39. Hata T, Asano Y, Yoshihara K, et al. Regulation of gut luminal serotonin by commensal microbiota in mice. PLoS One 2017;12(7):1–13.

40. Keefer L, Kane SV. Considering the bidirectional pathways between depression and IBD: recommendations for comprehensive IBD care. Gastroenterol Hepatol 2017;13(3):164–9.

41. Byrne G, Rosenfeld G, Leung Y, et al. Prevalence of anxiety and depression in patients with inflammatory bowel disease. Can J Gastroenterol Hepatol 2017; 2017:6496727.

42. Mayer EA, Tillisch K, Gupta A. Gut/brain axis and the microbiota. J Clin Invest 2015;125(3):926–38.

43. Foster JA, McVey Neufeld KA. Gut-brain axis: how the microbiome influences anxiety and depression. Trends Neurosci 2013;36(5):305–12.

44. Valles-Colomer M, Falony G, Darzi Y, et al. The neuroactive potential of the human gut microbiota in quality of life and depression. Nat Microbiol 2019;4(4):623–32.

45. Yano JM, Yu K, Donaldson GP, et al. Indigenous bacteria from the gut microbiota regulate host serotonin biosynthesis. Cell 2015;161(2):264–76.

46. Fung TC, Vuong HE, Luna CDG, et al. Intestinal serotonin and fluoxetine exposure modulate bacterial colonization in the gut. Nat Microbiol 2019;4(12):2064–73.

47. Hardy J, Selkoe DJ. The amyloid hypothesis of Alzheimer's disease: progress and problems on the road to therapeutics. Science 2002;297(5580):353–6.

48. Jack CR, Bennett DA, Blennow K, et al. NIA-AA research framework: toward a biological definition of Alzheimer's disease. Alzheimers Dement 2018; 14(4):535–62.

49. Rabinovici GD, Jagust WJ. Amyloid imaging in aging and dementia: testing the amyloid hypothesis in vivo. Behav Neurol 2009;21(1–2):117–28.

50. Price JC, Klunk WE, Lopresti BJ, et al. Kinetic modeling of amyloid binding in humans using PET imaging and Pittsburgh Compound-B. J Cereb Blood Flow Metab 2005;25(11):1528–47.

51. Lopresti BJ, Klunk WE, Mathis CA, et al. Simplified quantification of Pittsburgh compound B amyloid imaging PET studies: a comparative analysis. J Nucl Med 2005;46(12):1959–72.

52. van Dyck CH. Anti-amyloid-β monoclonal antibodies for Alzheimer's disease: pitfalls and promise. Biol Psychiatry 2018;83(4):311–9.

53. Wang J, Gu BJ, Masters CL, et al. A systemic view of Alzheimer disease - insights from amyloid-β metabolism beyond the brain. Nat Rev Neurol 2017; 13(10):612–23.

54. Bloom GS. Amyloid-β and tau. JAMA Neurol 2014; 71(4):505.

55. Braak H, Braak E. Neuropathological stageing of Alzheimer-related changes. Acta Neuropathol 1991;82(4):239–59.

56. Wang Y, Mandelkow E. Tau in physiology and pathology. Nat Rev Neurosci 2016;17(1):5–21.

57. Patel TK, Habimana-Griffin L, Gao X, et al. Dural lymphatics regulate clearance of extracellular tau from the CNS. Mol Neurodegener 2019; 14(1):1–9.

58. Iliff JJ, Chen MJ, Plog BA, et al. Impairment of glymphatic pathway function promotes tau pathology after traumatic brain injury. J Neurosci 2014;34(49): 16180–93.

59. Meade RM, Fairlie DP, Mason JM. Alpha-synuclein structure and Parkinson's disease - lessons and emerging principles. Mol Neurodegener 2019;14(1):1–14.

60. Fitzgerald E, Murphy S, Martinson HA. Alpha-synuclein pathology and the role of the microbiota in Parkinson's disease. Front Neurosci 2019;13(APR): 1–13.

61. Calo L, Wegrzynowicz M, Santivañez-Perez J, et al. Synaptic failure and α-synuclein. Mov Disord 2016; 31(2):169–77.

62. Holmqvist S, Chutna O, Bousset L, et al. Direct evidence of Parkinson pathology spread from the gastrointestinal tract to the brain in rats. Acta Neuropathol 2014;128(6):805–20.

63. Meyer JH, Wilson AA, Ginovart N, et al. Occupancy of serotonin transporters by paroxetine and citalopram during treatment of depression: a [11C] DASB PET imaging study. Am J Psychiatry 2001; 158(11):1843–9.

64. Meyer JH, Wilson AA, Sagrati S, et al. Serotonin transporter occupancy of five selective serotonin reuptake inhibitors at different doses: an [11C]DASB positron emission tomography study. Am J Psychiatry 2004;161(5):826–35.

65. Salloway S, Sperling R, Fox NC, et al. Two phase 3 trials of Bapineuzumab in mild-to-moderate Alzheimer's disease. N Engl J Med 2014;370(4):322–33.

66. Sevigny J, Chiao P, Bussière T, et al. The antibody aducanumab reduces Aβ plaques in Alzheimer's disease. Nature 2016;537(7618):50–6.

Moving?

Make sure your subscription moves with you!

To notify us of your new address, find your **Clinics Account Number** (located on your mailing label above your name), and contact customer service at:

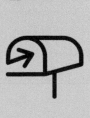

Email: journalscustomerservice-usa@elsevier.com

800-654-2452 (subscribers in the U.S. & Canada)
314-447-8871 (subscribers outside of the U.S. & Canada)

Fax number: 314-447-8029

Elsevier Health Sciences Division
Subscription Customer Service
3251 Riverport Lane
Maryland Heights, MO 63043

*To ensure uninterrupted delivery of your subscription, please notify us at least 4 weeks in advance of move.

Printed and bound by CPI Group (UK) Ltd, Croydon, CR0 4YY

03/10/2024

01040370-0017